OKANAGAN UNIV/COLLEGE LIBRARY

P9-DUJ-443

K

Autism and Asperger Syndrome

RC   88 H68 2004
          ricia.

Autism and related disorders affect almost every area of an individual's life. Yet little has been written about the long-term outcome, particularly for those adults who are of high ability but who continue to be handicapped by their social, communication and behavioural difficulties.

Autism and Asperger Syndrome reviews what is known about adults with autism in terms of their social functioning and educational and occupational status. Focusing mainly on the problems experienced by high-functioning people with autism – and those working with and caring for them – the book offers practical ways of dealing with their difficulties. Each chapter makes use of clinical case material to illustrate the kinds of problems faced and ways in which these may be overcome. First-hand accounts from people with autism are included and links with psychiatric illness in later life are explored.

This new edition of a book for professionals, families and people with autism has been completely updated to take account of the latest research in the field. It also includes an additional chapter on the differences between autism and Asperger syndrome.

Patricia Howlin is Consultant Clinical Psychologist and Professor of Clinical Psychology at St. George's Hospital Medical School, University of London.

OKANAGAN UNIVERSITY COLLEGE
LIBRARY
BRITISH COLUMBIA

Autism and Asperger Syndrome

Preparing for adulthood

Second edition

Patricia Howlin

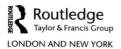 Routledge
Taylor & Francis Group

LONDON AND NEW YORK

First published 1997
by Routledge
11 New Fetter Lane, London EC4P 4EE

Simultaneously published in the USA and Canada
by Routledge
29 West 35th Street, New York, NY 10001

Reprinted 1998, 2000, 2003 (twice)

Second edition first published 2004

Routledge is an imprint of the Taylor & Francis Group

© 1997, 2004 Patricia Howlin

Typeset in 10/12pt Times NR by Graphicraft Limited, Hong Kong
Printed and bound in Great Britain by TJ International,
Padstow, Cornwall

All rights reserved. No part of this book may be reprinted or
reproduced or utilised in any form or by any electronic,
mechanical, or other means, now known or hereafter
invented, including photocopying and recording, or in any
information storage or retrieval system, without permission in
writing from the publishers.

British Library Cataloguing in Publication Data
A catalogue record for this book is available
from the British Library

Library of Congress Cataloging in Publication Data
A catalog record for this book has been requested

ISBN 0-415-30967-0 (hbk)
ISBN 0-415-30968-9 (pbk)

Dedication

This book is dedicated to the memory of Rosemary Hemsley, with whom this work first began, and to Ros Blackburn and all those like her whose stories fill this book.

Contents

Figures

Tables

Foreword

I deem it both a privilege and a pleasure to write the foreword to this book.

Professor Howlin has a remarkable knowledge of autism – not just autism the condition, but more importantly, autism the people – and her many years' experience in working with, supporting and informing people across the autism spectrum is clearly apparent in her writing.

What I like about this book is that the author clearly accepts and addresses the reality that children with autism do in fact grow into adults with autism, and this publication deals with the continuing and changing issues which this raises. A detailed series of follow-up studies helps to provide a better general picture of ASD across the age span and also highlights how specialist schemes such as supported employment can make a difference to people's lives.

The real value of this book, however, is that while it serves as an informative reference for parents, professionals and practitioners it is also a wonderful handbook and self-help guide for people with autism and Asperger syndrome themselves. Using real case scenarios the author examines a variety of issues which face a large cross section of people with autism-spectrum disorders and describes how the individuals have helped themselves or been helped to cope with many of these. Her approach is positive whilst remaining realistic.

Professor Howlin never promises perfection or miraculous results but instead suggests ways in which individuals can attain their maximum potential whatever that may be.

Ros Blackburn, adult with autism

Acknowledgements

First and foremost thanks must go to the many individuals on whose stories this book relies. All the anecdotal accounts are based on true scenarios, although occasionally circumstances have been be altered to preserve anonymity. I am particularly grateful to Ros Blackburn for her permission to quote directly from some of her own experiences. The clinical and research expertise of many other colleagues over the years has also been invaluable. There are too many to name individually but I have been especially grateful to the continuing support of Michael Rutter, Sue Goode, Pam Yates, and Lorna Wing to mention but a few.

Finally, special thanks must go to my secretary Jill Rolfe for her painstaking work in checking the document and the accuracy of references etc. and without whose help the book would never have seen the light of day.

Thanks to Pyramid Educational Consultants (UK) for the right to print PECS pictures

Introduction

The first edition of this book was written only six years ago, but in those few intervening years much has changed. At that time I noted that very little had been written about adults with autistic-spectrum disorders and that, other than a few impressive autobiographical accounts, most reports tended to focus on difficulties and challenging behaviours. However, the last six years have witnessed an explosion of books about adults, many written from personal experience. There have also appeared many accounts by or about individuals who are of normal or above normal intellectual ability, in other words those who are described as being 'high-functioning', 'more able' or as having Asperger syndrome (or, in the United States, Asperger disorder).

These present a much more positive picture of autism than had generally been the case throughout previous decades. It is now clear that many individuals with autism who do not have additional cognitive impairments are able to succeed well as adults. Many attain high academic levels and have successful careers. Many marry and many have children of their own: children who, because of the high level of heritability of autism, are also likely to share some of the characteristics associated with the condition. Unfortunately, those who do succeed tend to do so *despite* the lack of adequate provision rather than because of any special help or understanding, although it has become increasingly clear that outcome is significantly influenced – both positively and negatively – by the support structures available from childhood through adulthood.

Despite advances in our knowledge about the causes of autism, and about more effective approaches to intervention, autism remains a lifelong, pervasive and sometimes devastating disorder that can affect almost every aspect of an individual's functioning. Impairments in communication limit the ability to understand what is happening or why, and can result in major problems in relating to other people or in effectively controlling the daily environment. Difficulties with reciprocal social contacts may mean that even the simplest personal interactions are fraught with hazards. Problems in coping with change, and the need to adhere to fixed routines and patterns of behaviour can also have a major impact on day-to-day life.

Research into ways of ameliorating such difficulties has helped to identify general strategies that are likely to offer hope to people with autism and their families. Thus, it is now well established that in environments that are highly structured, predictable, and consistent, and where cues are largely visual rather than verbal, the limitations imposed by autism can be greatly reduced and potential skills significantly enhanced. It is clear, too, that if appropriate support and *practical* advice are offered to families in the early years following diagnosis many of the behavioural problems that can subsequently make life so difficult can be minimised or even avoided altogether. This has resulted in an intensive focus on early intervention programmes, with many resources, both clinical and educational, being devoted to the under-five age group. Whilst any increase in resources for those with autism and their families is to be welcomed, there is the danger that such a focus could actually limit opportunities for older individuals. It is true that the first five years are crucial ones in any child's life, and this may be particularly so for children with autism. However, most individuals are likely to live on for at least a further sixty years, and it is unrealistic to expect that the skills acquired in even the most successful pre-school programmes will be the same as those needed to cope successfully over the following six decades. Thus, while improved funding for toddler and pre-school programmes can only be applauded, it is crucial that the long–term and often very special needs of people with autism continued to be recognised and provided for as they move through childhood into adulthood and eventually into old age. Claims for the miraculous effects of particular therapies (see Chapter 3) remain, so far, unsupported by empirical evidence, but adult outcome studies (see Chapter 2) indicate that prognosis in autism is greatly influenced by access to adequate educational provision and, subsequently, to support structures that can enable individuals to progress through college and into appropriate employment. Adult outcome is also dependent on the degree of help available in finding appropriate accommodation, in coping with the demands of daily life, and in integrating as fully as possible into the wider social community.

There is a particular need, too, to explore how the needs of more intellectually able people with autism can be appropriately met. If a child with autism has little or no speech and additional cognitive impairments, there are now many services to which parents can turn. Interventions such as Early Bird, the Hanen Program or Portage are but a few of the schemes that may be readily available – although, of course, opportunities vary depending on local facilities. Early and often highly intensive pre-school programmes may be provided and, later, specialist schooling is almost certain to be offered. Provision for sheltered or supported employment and living is also likely to be available for adults with intellectual impairments and autism. In contrast, the parents of a child with autism who has good language and normal or above normal intellectual ability are likely to face a much harder battle, not only in obtaining a diagnosis in the first place (Howlin and Asgharian 1999) but in accessing adequate help thereafter. Home-based intensive interventions are only likely to be available to families with adequate financial resources. Placement in 'integrated' or 'inclusive' schooling often means no specialist support whatsoever, and once individuals move on to college or work autism-specific provision is almost unknown.

Society in general also tends to be less sympathetic towards individuals whose needs or disabilities are perceived as relatively mild. Thus, the demands made on someone who is clearly very disabled, has little or no speech and withdraws from social contact into a life of solitary routine are unlikely to be excessive. But for someone who appears 'nearly normal', who has had the benefit of a 'good' education, and who possesses considerable ability, at least in certain areas, expectations are often unrealistically high. When the adolescent or adult with autism is unable to meet these expectations he or she may well be faced with criticism and rejection, which in turn does little to improve confidence, self-esteem or social functioning. He or she may be unable to find a job, make friends or form close relationships. All too often he or she is well aware of being 'different', but without help there is little they can do to improve the situation. There is the additional frustration of knowing that although such individuals have skills – and sometimes very special gifts – they are unable to make full use of these. Yet apart from their families they often have no one to whom they can turn for comfort or guidance.

It is for this reason that this book focuses mainly, although not entirely, on the needs of those people with autism who, though in many ways very able, are likely to require as much, if not even more support if they are to fulfil their true and considerable potential. Ros Blackburn, a woman with autism who is well known for her lecturing skills, often claims, 'My biggest disability is my ability.' By this she means that throughout her adult life, attempts to obtain the help she needs to live truly independently (instead of having always to turn to her parents when problems arise) have always been thwarted, because social and other services view her as quite competent to cope alone.

She has a job and her own flat, and is able to lecture about autism to an audience of several hundred people without a qualm. The fact that almost every minute of every day is fraught with anxiety, and that the slightest change to routine can result in intense distress, is something services simply do not consider to be of relevance, even though access to support when needed could have a major impact on her life and that of her parents.

Most of the chapters in this revised edition are new or substantially rewritten. To begin with, there is a discussion of the controversy concerning the relationship between autism and Asperger syndrome; whether they should be viewed as different conditions; the evidence (or lack of it) for the distinction, and whether terminology should affect access to intervention. Studies of outcome in adults with autism are also reviewed, as information about prognosis generally is vital if we are to be able to judge the long-term effectiveness of specific treatments. These, too, are discussed, as is the evidence for their success. Later chapters focus on issues such as college life, employment and close relationships. This last-named topic was barely discussed in the earlier edition, but thanks largely to personal accounts by people with autism or those living with them we now have far more insight not only into the problems that close personal relationships may entail but also – more importantly – into ways of circumventing or dealing with these more effectively. The chapters that have changed least are those covering the specific difficulties associated with autism: communication, social interactions and ritualistic and stereotyped behaviours. These remain central to the condition and, on the whole, approaches to modifying these difficulties have not changed substantially over recent years. The final chapter, on increasing independence, also – unfortunately – remains little changed. Thus, while there have been important and positive incentives designed to improve access to further education and later employment the situation regarding support for independent living remains far from adequate. In many cases there are still few options between the two extremes of highly restrictive and expensive residential care and no systematic support at all. This is an area that, over the next few years, must be the focus of far more research and funding.

Note

The examples used throughout the book are all taken from real life, although individual characteristics and circumstances have been changed to preserve anonymity.

1 Is there a distinction between autism and Asperger syndrome?

Historical Background

At much the same time that Kanner was writing about children with autism in the United States (Kanner 1943) Asperger, in Austria, was describing the group of children who eventually came to be named after him (Asperger 1944). With an ocean and a world war between them, collaboration was hardly to be expected. However, gradually clinicians and researchers began to recognise the striking similarities between these two conditions. Both authors described difficulties with reciprocal social interaction, communication, and ritualistic and stereo-typed routines, usually beginning within the first two years of life. Both stressed the contrast between the children's profound social deficits and their 'purposeful, and intelligent relation to objects' (Kanner 1946). Behavioural problems such as aggression, destructiveness and outbursts of temper were also noted, as were various developmental problems. Interestingly, too, both accounts contained descriptions of other family members who exhibited 'autistic' traits. It is true that Asperger's accounts tend to focus on more able individuals, whilst many of Kanner's children were seen to have intellectual impairments. Never-theless, Asperger also referred to individuals 'with considerable intellec-tual retardation' and noted that 'The fate of (these) cases is often very sad'. Likewise, Kanner described some individuals who had achieved highly, both in terms of education and employment, in adult life.

Linguistic and political considerations meant that Asperger's work received little publicity: papers published in German gained little favour in much of Europe or America in the years shortly after the Second World War. In contrast, Kanner's accounts were rapidly published in reputable journals. It was not until 1981, when Lorna Wing first brought Asperger's original writings to the attention of clinicians, that the con-dition began to be more widely recognised. It was first included within the major classification systems, under the broader category of Pervasive Developmental Disorders (PDD), in the early 1990s (DSM-IV 1994, ICD-10 1993). Wing's main purpose for highlighting Asperger's work was to draw attention to the fact that typically autistic features could be found in individuals with well-developed language and cognitive skills as well as in those of low IQ. But as many clinicians failed to recognise their problems as falling within the autistic spectrum, access to correct diagnosis and treatment was often denied. Wing considered the term Asperger syndrome to be a useful 'shorthand' label, indicating that autism could affect people with a high IQ and extensive vocabulary as well as those who had no language and significant learning difficulties. In other words, Asperger syndrome represented the more cognitively able end of the 'autistic continuum'.

There can be no doubt that her work resulted in many high-functioning individuals finally obtaining an appropriate diagnosis. Nevertheless, two decades later Wing has expressed doubts about the wisdom of introducing the term into clinical practice (Wing 2000). The 'Pandora's box' she opened has, she believes, resulted in a 'belief that Asperger syndrome and autism are different conditions – quite the opposite of my intention'. Her original purpose – to emphasise the fact that there was no evidence for a distinction between Asperger syndrome and autism – has frequently been overlooked. Instead, the question of whether the two are different conditions (albeit part of the same spectrum of disorders) has been a source of continuing debate over recent years, as recent volumes by Klin *et al.* (2000) and Schopler *et al.* (1998) testify.

Formal diagnostic criteria for Asperger syndrome note that the social deficits and ritualistic and stereotyped behaviours have the same features as in autism (World Health Organization 1992, American Psychiatric Association 1994). The two main distinguishing features are the presence of relatively normal cognitive skills and the lack of early language delays in the Asperger group (see Table 1.1). Although Volkmar and Klin (2000) state that these diagnostic criteria should be considered as 'tentative and in need of empirical validation', both systems are explicit that Asperger syndrome and autism are mutually exclusive categories. DSM-IV guidelines also specify that if criteria for autism are met then this diagnosis takes precedence over Asperger syndrome, However, as a number of authors have pointed out, if strict DSM/ICD criteria are applied, a diagnosis of Asperger syndrome becomes unlikely or even impossible (Eisenmajer *et al.* 1996, Ghaziuddin *et al.* 1992a, Manjiviona and Prior 1995, Mayes *et al.* 2001, Miller and Ozonoff 1997, Szatmari *et al.* 1994).

Table 1.1 ICD-10 research criteria for Asperger syndrome

ICD-10 research criteria for Asperger syndrome
A No clinically significant general delay in language or cognitive development. Single words present by 2 years; phrases by 3 years. Self-help/adaptive behaviours/curiosity about environment in first 3 years normal. Motor development may be delayed, with clumsiness evident later.
B Qualitative abnormalities in reciprocal social interaction. **Criteria as for autism.**
C Intense, circumscribed interests or restricted, repetitive and stereotyped patterns of behaviour, interests and activities. **Criteria as for autism** although less usual for motor mannerisms/preoccupations with parts of objects etc. to occur.

Research into the association between autism and Asperger syndrome

In a review of recent studies comparing individuals with Asperger syndrome and high-functioning autism (HFA), it was apparent that inadequate group matchings, small samples, and above all a lack of agreement on diagnostic criteria made it almost impossible to reach a definite conclusion about the similarities and/or differences between the two conditions (Howlin 2003). The review included only those studies in which a *direct* comparison between individuals with high-functioning autism (IQ 70+) and Asperger syndrome had been conducted and in which diagnostic criteria and measures of IQ were adequately specified. However, as can be seen from Tables 1.2 and 1.3, in many cases strict DSM-IV criteria for Asperger disorder were *not* used, principally because, as noted above, if these guidelines are followed only a minority of individuals meet the necessary criteria. Instead, researchers tended to use the term for individuals who, though often meeting criteria for autism, had not shown early language delays. Many studies also failed to match participants with Asperger syndrome and those with high-functioning autism on the basis of IQ. Thus, any reported differences between the groups could be due to cognitive disparities rather than a true diagnostic differentiation.

Table 1.2 Summary of studies comparing individuals with Asperger syndrome and high-functioning autism (Asperger syndrome groups higher IQ)

Principal area of study, author (and criteria for AS)	Age Mean/range	N HFA:AS	Conclusions
General clinical characteristics			
1 Szatmari *et al.* 1995 (modified ICD-10 criteria)	5 years	47:21	HFA > social and adaptive problems, rituals and early language delays. No differences in current non-verbal/communication/motor skills
2 Eisenmajer *et al.* 1996 (clinical diagnosis)	10 years	48:69	Few differences on any variables, delayed language only significant difference in HFA group
3 Kurita 1997 (ICD-10)	5–6 years	16:26	Few significant differences but HFA > on some CARS items
4 Gilchrist *et al.* 2001 (ICD-10)	HFA 21 years; AS 14 years	13:20	HFA > ADI problems age 4–5 years. No difference in current functioning on ADI or ADOS
Obstetric/early history and motor skills			
5 Ghaziuddin *et al.* 1994 (ICD-10)	12–13 years	9:11	No significant differences in motor skills
6 Ghaziuddin *et al.* 1995b (ICD-10)	13–14 years	9:11	No significant differences in neonatal optimality scores
7 Ghaziuddin and Butler 1998 (DSM-IV/ICD-10)	10–11 years	12:12	No significant differences in motor skills when IQ controlled for
8 Manjiviona and Prior 1999 (modified ICD-10)	11 years	9:12	AS > PIQ but no differences in motor skills

Neuropsychological and language profiles

9	Ghaziuddin and Gerstein 1996 (ICD-10)	15–16 years	13:17	AS > pedantic speech
10	Ehlers *et al.* 1997 (Gillberg criteria)	10 years	40:40	Differences in cognitive profiles; AS higher scores on most subtests
11	Pomeroy, 1998 ('non-language impaired' PDD)	7–8 years	13:15	AS > VIQ; also > language comprehension and expression
12	Manjiviona and Prior, 1999 (Modified/strict DSM-IV)	10–11 years	21:35	AS > VIQ no differences on neuropsychological profiles
13	Miller and Ozonoff, 2000 (DSM-IV)	10 years	26:14	No significant differences in motor skills, executive function or TOM when IQ co-varied

Behavioural and psychiatric problems

14	Ghaziuddin *et al.* 1995a (ICD-10)	12 years	8:12	AS > disorganised thought; few other significant differences
15	Tonge *et al.* 1999 (DSM-IV)	AS 9.9; HFA 7.4 years	75:52	AS > psychopathology
16	Kim *et al.* 2000 (modified DSM-IV)	12 years	40:19	No differences in depression/anxiety/mood

Table 1.3 Summary of studies comparing individuals with Asperger syndrome and high-functioning autism matched for full-scale IQ

Principal area of study, author (and criteria for AS)	Age Mean/range	N HFA:AS	Conclusions
General clinical characteristics			
1 Szatmari et al. 1990 (Wing's criteria)	HFA 23, AS14 years	17:26	HFA > social impairments, language problems, stereotypes and preoccupations
2 Mayes et al. 2001 (Modified DSM-IV)	6.0 years	23:24	No difference on any of 71 variables (IQ, language, symptomatology, motor co-ordination, emotion or behaviour)
3 Ozonoff and McMahon Griffith 2000 (DSM-IV)	13.5 years	23:12	HFA > ADI scores at 4; few differences in current scores. No differences in social functioning. AS > special interests HFA > insistence on sameness
Obstetric/early history and motor abnormalities			
4 Szatmari et al. 1989a (Wing's criteria)	HFA 23 AS 14	25:28	HFA > early abnormalities in social, language and behaviour
5 Gillberg and Gillberg 1989 (Gillberg criteria)	10 years	23:23	AS > clumsy

Neuropsychological and language profiles

6	Szatmari et al. 1990 (DSM-III)	HFA 23, AS14		17:26	Few differences in IQ profiles, motor or other test scores
7	Ozonoff et al. 1991 (modified ICD-10)		11–12 years	13:10	AS > VIQ and > VIQ-PIQ difference. AS > verbal memory, executive function and TOM scores. HFA > CARS scores
8	Fine et al. 1994 (Wing's criteria)	HFA 23; AS 14		18:23	Cohesive discourse > in AS group
9	Klin et al. 1995 (modified ICD-10)		15–16 years	19:21	HFA > PIQ and better motor skills; AS >VIQ and higher verbal ability
10	Iwanaga et al. 2000 (DSM-IV)		5–6 years	15:10	No significant differences on gross or fine motor tasks, and most non-verbal tests. AS > HFA on some verbal tasks
11	Klin, 2000 (DSM-IV)		19–20 years	20:20	No differences on social attribution task
12	Rinehart et al. 2001 (DSM-IV)		10 years	12:12	HFA > problems in shifting attention
13	Ozonoff et al. 2002 (DSM-IV)		13.5 years	23:12	Few differences but AS > VIQ-PIQ different; HFA > expressive problems. No differences on executive function/TOM tasks

Behavioural and psychiatric disturbance

14	Szatmari 1989b (Wing's criteria)	HFA 25 AS 14		25:28	HFA > bizarre preoccupations; AS? > psychiatric problems

Nevertheless, even when the Asperger groups were of higher overall IQ than the HFA groups, the differences were often small and inconsistent. Among the reports with a focus on early history, general clinical severity or motor problems, most reported few differences. Ghaziuddin and Butler (1998) identified more motor difficulties in their HFA group, but the difference disappeared when IQ was controlled for and both groups were relatively impaired compared to population norms. Szatmari *et al.* (1994) found that early group differences in language abilities diminished over time, and Gilchrist *et al.* (2001) also noted that initial differences in symptom severity tended to decline with age. Thus, although there were differences on ADI scores in early childhood (with the HFA group showing more difficulties) there were no significant differences in adolescence and early adulthood. Of five reports on neuropsychological and linguistic functioning the Asperger groups generally showed superior verbal skills; but, again, these differences tended to disappear when IQ was controlled for. Evidence for differences in behavioural or psychiatric disturbance was also inconsistent, with Ghaziuddin *et al.* (1995) and Tonge *et al.* (1999) reporting increased pathology in the Asperger groups, although this was not found in the study of Kim and colleagues (2000).

The findings were variable even when the groups were matched for IQ. Of five reports on early history and general clinical characteristics, three suggested higher rates of problems in the HFA groups, but Ozonoff and colleagues (Ozonoff *et al.* 2002) found that these differences were not necessarily maintained as children grew older. Stereotyped and ritualistic behaviours occurred in both groups, but in the Ozonoff study there was greater evidence of special interests in the Asperger group whilst insistence on sameness was more common in the autism group. Although many clinical accounts of individuals with Asperger syndrome have reported problems of motor coordination, the only study to find evidence of increased clumsiness was that of Gillberg and Gillberg (1989).

Amongst those studies examining neuropsychological or linguistic functioning, several studies reported higher verbal skills in the Asperger groups, even though the groups had been matched for overall IQ. There were few differences in scores on tasks of social understanding, theory of mind or executive function, and although individuals with Asperger syndrome showed some superiority in these areas in Ozonoff's study, this difference may have been related to their higher verbal skills. Rates of psychiatric disturbance did not differ markedly, although Szatmari and colleagues found that individuals with HFA tended to show more bizarre preoccupations.

Most of the comparative studies of autism and Asperger syndrome have involved children or adolescents, but there were indications from several (Gilchrist *et al.* 2001, Ozonoff *et al.* 2002, and Szatmari *et al.* 1994) that even if differences could be identified in childhood, these tended to disappear with age. To investigate this possibility further, Howlin (2003) compared past history and current functioning in adults with a diagnosis of HFA or Asperger syndrome. Diagnosis of an autistic disorder was confirmed on the basis of the Autism Diagnostic Interview – Revised (ADI-R; Lord *et al.* 1994) and all participants had a non-verbal IQ of 70 or above. The sample comprised thirty-four individuals who had been delayed in their language development (the HFA group) and forty-two who had shown no early language delays (the Asperger group). The average age in both groups was around twenty-six to twenty-seven years.

The findings indicated that parents did report certain differences between the groups when they were younger. Parents of children with autism were initially more concerned about language delays. Children with Asperger syndrome tended to be older when parents first noted abnormalities in their development (average age twenty-one months as compared to an average of fifteen months in the autism group), and their parents' first concerns were split fairly evenly between general behaviour problems, ritualistic and stereotyped behaviours/interests, and motor delays/difficulties. However, on the Autism Diagnostic Interview (ADI-R) parental ratings of their children's development suggested that these early differences decreased over time. Thus, by the age of four to five years, no significant group differences were found in social or communication skills. As adults, average IQ scores in both groups were almost identical (100 in the HFA group and 101 in the Asperger group) and age-equivalent scores on tests of language use and comprehension were also similar, at around fifteen to sixteen years. On the ADI-R, ratings of social functioning, communication and ritualistic/stereotyped behaviours were remarkably close, and outcome in terms of friendships, employment and independent living did not differ. Only two individuals in the Asperger group and three in the autism group were reported to have developed close friendships, although rather more (ten with autism, fifteen with Asperger syndrome) had acquaintances whom they met outside home or work. Three men (two autistic, one Asperger) were married or living with a partner, and one of the married men in the autism group had children. One woman in the Asperger group was divorced. The majority in both groups (nineteen with autism, twenty-six with Asperger syndrome) still lived with their parents, and of those who did live independently most (seven out of eleven in the autism group; nine out of fifteen in the Asperger group) continued to require support either from their families or social services. Three people with autism and one with Asperger syndrome were in specialist residential provision, and one man with autism was in a long-stay psychiatric hospital. In terms of employment, fifteen individuals in each group had never had a job, and only two in each group had relatively well-paid, permanent employment. Three individuals in each group were in sheltered placements or worked with the family firm; the remainder was in short-term, low-paid or voluntary posts that did not provide them with sufficient money to live independently.

Even ratings of motor clumsiness, a variable that has frequently been claimed to characterize individuals with Asperger syndrome (see Volkmar and Klin 2000), failed to differentiate between the groups. The number of individuals with an additional psychiatric diagnosis was also similar in both groups, with depressive disorders appearing to be the most common. Use and understanding of language was somewhat better among the Asperger adults, although the differences were small and insignificant. The only area in which a significant group difference emerged was in academic attainment, with more individuals among the Asperger group obtaining graduate or postgraduate qualifications. However, this advantage in terms of academic attainment did not seem to have resulted in higher levels of achievement in later life.

The finding that early differences between individuals with a diagnosis of Asperger syndrome or high-functioning autism may reduce with age is supported by a number of other recent studies. Gilchrist *et al.* (2001), for example, found that scores on the Autism Diagnostic Interview, which had differed significantly between individuals with autism and Asperger syndrome at the age of four to five years, had disappeared by adolescence or early adulthood. Szatmari (2000) has suggested that any differences identified in the early years may not represent a true diagnostic 'splitting' between the groups but instead are probably related to the severity of early language delays, which can lead to children following somewhat different trajectories over time. Both he and Wing (2000) have reported that young children with apparently typical autism may 'shift' to follow an 'Asperger-type' pathway subsequently, especially if they develop good language. If, on the other hand, language development is markedly delayed, children are likely to remain at a disadvantage in their ability to 'catch up' linguistically and this in turn will affect many other aspects of their cognitive and social functioning.

A further recent review of research in this area by Macintosh and Dissanayake (2004) also suggests that there is no empirical basis for classifying Asperger syndrome as a condition distinct from high-functioning autism. However, comparisons between these two groups will only produce meaningful conclusions if participants are appropriately matched for intellectual level. The age at which data are collected will also influence the findings, as differences between the two groups seem to become less evident as they grow older. The superiority of individuals with Asperger syndrome with respect to some aspects of their language is not enough to indicate a distinction between the two conditions. Instead, the fact that individuals with a diagnosis of autism are, by definition, so much further behind in their early language development may be the prime reason for the relative severity of their communication difficulties in later life.

It is important to be aware that the distinction made between the two conditions in DSM-IV and ICD-10 criteria does not rest on sound empirical data but is based largely on clinical descriptions. Clearly, there are major differences between individuals with autism who are of normal IQ and language ability and those of very low IQ with little or no language. These differences also have important implications for service provision. However, within the higher-functioning range, experimental studies have failed to identify distinct subgroups. Moreover, diagnostic instruments designed for more able individuals, such as the Asperger Syndrome Diagnostic Interview (Gillberg *et al.* 2001), the Autism-Spectrum Quotient (Baron-Cohen *et al.* 2001) or the Childhood Asperger Syndrome Test (Scott *et al.* 2002) have failed to delineate any specific characteristics that differentiate between Asperger syndrome and autistic individuals of normal intelligence. Furthermore, the finding that the language abilities of high-functioning individuals, whether or not they had marked delays in their early language development, are frequently well below chronological age in adulthood, raises further problems in terms of the validity of the DSM-IV/ICD-10 distinction. (Howlin 2003). Thus, although Asperger syndrome is, by definition, not associated with impairments in spoken language, more detailed assessments indicate that, in many cases, this criterion is not met as comprehension, vocabulary and social use of language remain well below chronological age levels.

The results of comparative studies are also of clinical importance since they not only highlight the *lack* of any substantial difference between the two diagnostic groups in adulthood but also illustrate the poor prognosis, even for high-functioning individuals within the autistic spectrum. Despite having IQ scores well within the normal range (and sometimes reaching quite high academic levels) the majority of individuals in both the Asperger and high-functioning autism groups studied by Howlin (2003) had no close friends, remained highly dependent on their families for support and had low employment status. Larger-scale prospective studies are still required in order to clarify the extent and nature of the possible differences between these two relatively high-functioning groups. However, for the present, the weight of evidence seems to suggest that there is no marked distinction between Asperger syndrome and individuals with autism who have developed functional language and whose IQs lie within the normal range.

Many researchers have now come to the conclusion that most research in this area points firmly to a dimensional, rather than a categorical, view of autistic-spectrum disorders. As Leekham and her colleagues (2000) point out: 'It is time to move away from potentially circular attempts to differentiate Asperger syndrome and autism . . . in practice, the most useful indication of current needs and future prognosis is overall level of ability'. Certainly, there is no evidence to support the view that individuals with a diagnosis of Asperger syndrome should be deprived of the support and services that are available for those with a diagnosis of autism, or that educational and management programmes should substantially differ. Despite this, the differential diagnosis can have implications for services, with individuals with Asperger syndrome frequently being denied the level of support offered to those diagnosed as having autism. For example, in the United States, statutory educational and support services that are available for children with autism may be denied to children who are given a diagnosis of Asperger syndrome. In the United Kingdom, a recent White Paper by the Department of Health (2001), supposedly designed to improve support systems for all individuals with intellectual impairments, specifically excludes from its remit individuals with autistic-spectrum disorders 'who may be of average or even above average intelligence – such as those with Asperger syndrome'.

Despite her concerns about the Pandora's box she unwittingly opened Wing (2000) believes that the introduction of the term 'Asperger syndrome' did serve one very important purpose: that of widening prevailing concepts of autistic-spectrum disorders. She and her colleagues (Leekham *et al.* 2000) also believe that the label, if used flexibly, is of practical value in explaining the needs and problems of children and adults who have autistic features but who are of relatively high intelligence, speak grammatically and are not socially aloof. Parents of more able individuals often tend to find the diagnosis more acceptable than one of autism, and as they get older it is clear that many high-functioning individuals within the autistic spectrum prefer to use this label to describe themselves. Higher-functioning children and adults with autism have social, educational, occupational and residential needs that are often quite different to those of individuals with more severe intellectual disabilities, even though the basic principles of an autism-specific approach to intervention may apply to both groups. If the use of the 'Asperger' label enables them to gain access to appropriate support, well and good. However, it is of little value if used to discriminate against and deny services to those who need them, or to trivialize their difficulties. Asperger syndrome is often referred to as a 'mild form of autism'. Nothing could be further from the truth. For, while the cognitive impairments may be mild, the social difficulties experienced by these individuals may be just as restrictive and damaging as is the case for those who are intellectually severely impaired. Indeed, their greater awareness of their problems may lead to increased personal distress. A recent follow-up study by Gillberg and his colleagues, for example (Billstedt 2003), has indicated that quality of life ratings for more able adults with autism are actually lower than for those with moderate to severe intellectual impairments.

There is also little value in the label if used incorrectly. Parents given this diagnosis will understandably expect their son or daughter to have a much better chance of making progress than if they have been given a diagnosis of autism. It is unforgivable, therefore, for clinicians to use the term without careful consideration of the child's level of functioning, even if this is done to 'make parents feel better'. The parents of five-year-old Seth, for example, were suing the local education authority for failing to provide him with appropriate schooling. He had been diagnosed as having Asperger syndrome and hence they wanted him to go to a primary school with a particularly strong 'academic' record in an adjoining borough. The local education authority had managed to obtain a place for him in the nearby – and heavily oversubscribed – specialist autistic school. Cognitive and linguistic assessments indicated that Seth had an IQ in the severely impaired range and that his use and understanding of language was around an eighteen-month level. In no way did he meet diagnostic criteria for Asperger syndrome. However, because this label had been applied incorrectly his parents were unable to recognise that he was in need of highly specialised schooling or to accept that he would almost certainly fail in a pressurized mainstream environment, even if some additional support were to be provided.

Terminology

Because recent research provides little support for the distinction between Asperger syndrome and high-functioning autism, when describing case examples in the present book, the term 'autism' has been used for individuals across the spectrum. Asperger syndrome is not distinguished from 'high-functioning autism' or from 'more able' people with autism. In the case of accounts by other authors, the original terminology (Asperger syndrome, HFA, autism etc.) has been retained, whether or not diagnostic criteria are specified.

2 Outcome in autism

What becomes of adults with autism?

Until relatively recently, the vast majority of literature on autism has focused on children. There are numerous books exploring the causes of autism, the implications for families, therapeutic interventions, and training and educational programmes. In contrast, there has been remarkably little written about outcome in adulthood. Moreover, when autism in adults is described, the picture is often far from reassuring. Accounts of individuals with autism are frequently found in books or reports dealing with 'challenging behaviours', leaving many families to fear that all that may be expected in adulthood is the development of aggressive, self-injurious or disruptive behaviours. On the other hand, there is an increasing number of impressive personal narratives documenting how – often against tremendous odds – individuals have fought against, and to a considerable extent overcome, their early difficulties. Amongst the most prominent of these autobiographical accounts are those of Gunilla Gerland (1997), Temple Grandin (1995), Liane Holliday Willey (1999), Wendy Lawson (1998, 2002) and Donna Williams (1992, 1994). Occasionally, too, there are reports of young people who, although remaining generally disabled, may show remarkable skill in isolated areas such as art, music or calculations (Hermelin 2001, Wiltshire 1987).

Most individuals with autism, however, will fall into none of these categories, and few families know what to expect as their children grow older. Many parents dread the onset of adolescence, fearing that this is certain to bring increased difficulties. Furthermore, reports of possible links with 'schizoid' disturbances (Wolff 1991, Wolff and McGuire 1995) may conjure up the spectre of a schizophrenic illness waiting in the wings. Almost all parents will worry about the degree of independence that can be attained, or the ability of their son or daughter to cope when they are no longer there to care for them.

To make matters worse, the anxieties and uncertainties of caring for a young adult with autism must frequently be faced with little or no support. Even if families did have access to appropriate resources when their child was younger, once late adolescence is reached paediatric, psychiatric or psychological services are often summarily withdrawn. The valuable informal support systems available via schoolteachers and other parents also tend to diminish. There may be no one to whom families can turn at times of stress; no one who knows their son or daughter well; no one to offer advice or support.

Nevertheless, information does exist that may help to allay at least some of these anxieties and which can enable families to plan more effectively for the future. Much of this comes from studies that have followed up children with autism through adolescence and into adulthood. Because of the cost of long-term research, investigations of this kind are relatively few, often involve small numbers of individuals and, because they tend to ask rather different questions, may produce somewhat variable findings. Yet despite these limitations the findings do provide important data on the lives of adults with autism as well as indicating ways in which outcome might be improved.

The first descriptive studies

In the mid- to late 1950s there began to appear a number of studies reporting on the outcome for children with autistic types of disorder. However, the heterogeneity of the groups in terms of age, intellectual level, diagnosis and aetiology meant that few conclusions could be drawn about long-term prognosis. Victor Lotter, for example, in 1978, reviewed a total of twenty-five follow-up studies of 'psychotic children', but because the majority of these suffered from serious flaws, such as inadequate diagnostic criteria, subjective reporting or very mixed subject groups, findings were difficult to interpret.

One of the earliest reports focusing on children who clearly met diagnostic criteria for autism was that of Leon Eisenberg (1956), a close colleague of Leo Kanner and one of the first writers to describe the condition in detail. Although the account is largely anecdotal, with many cases being still in their early teens when assessed, Eisenberg, like many subsequent authors, noted the wide variety of possible outcomes. Most of the individuals described remained very dependent, but about one-third were found to have made 'at least a moderate social adjustment' despite the lack of any specialist provision or treatment available at that time. A minority had managed to achieve a high level of independence, although even amongst this group social impairments remained apparent, as in the case of the young man who, when called upon to speak as a student leader at a football rally, announced (with absolute accuracy) that his team was going to lose.

In a slightly later report from Britain, Mildred Creak (1963) described a hundred cases of 'childhood psychosis' (the term then often used for autism). Again, the information is very anecdotal, and includes both adults and children, so that the longer-term outcome is unclear. Although forty-three individuals were placed in institutional care, forty remained at home attending school or day centres and seventeen were coping with mainstream schooling or employment.

Among the most fascinating and detailed accounts of this period are those of Kanner himself. He kept meticulous records of what happened to the children he had diagnosed and followed up, many of them into their twenties or beyond. He, too, noted the great variability in outcome and, like Eisenberg, stressed the importance of well-developed communication skills and intellectual ability for a good prognosis. Individuals who remained mute had the least favourable outcome. Most of these remained highly dependent as they grew older, living with their parents, in sheltered communities, in state institutions for people with learning disabilities or, in a few cases, in psychiatric hospitals. Amongst cases with better communication skills outcome was rather more positive. Just over half of this group was functioning relatively well, at home or in the community, although with varying degrees of support (Kanner and Eisenberg 1956).

In 1973 Kanner published one of the first reports focusing specifically on higher-functioning individuals with autism. The eleven cases (ten men and one woman) had been seen initially in the late 1940s and early 1950s and were in their twenties and thirties when followed up. They were reported to have done remarkably well as they grew older, and were said to be 'mingling, working and maintaining themselves in society'. Kanner also noted that in the majority of these cases, 'a remarkable change took place' around their mid-teens: 'Unlike most other autistic children they became uneasily aware of their peculiarities and began to make a conscious effort to do something about them.' In particular they tried to improve their interactions with their peers, often using their obsessional preoccupations or special skills 'to open a door for contact'. As adults:

> They have not completely shed the fundamental personality structure of early infantile autism but, with increasing self-assessment in their middle to late teens, they expended considerable effort to fit themselves . . . to what they came to perceive as commonly

expected obligations. They made the compromise of being, yet not appearing alone and discovered means of interaction by joining groups in which they could make use of their preoccupations . . . as shared 'hobbies' in the company of others. In the club to which they 'belonged' they received – and enjoyed – the recognition earned by the detailed knowledge they had stored up in years of obsessive rumination of specific topics (music, mathematics, history, chemistry, astronomy, wildlife, foreign languages etc.). Rewards came to them also from their employers who remarked on their meticulousness and trustworthiness. Life among people thus lost its former menacing aspects. Nobody has shoved them forcibly through a gate which others had tried to unlock for them; it was they who, at first timidly and then more resolutely, paved their way to it and walked through.

(Kanner 1973)

The following vignettes illustrate what, for some, lay on the other side of this gate.

Kanner's 'success stories'

Thomas G.   Found recognition by teaching astronomy and playing the piano; he also joined the Boy Scouts and swimming and athletic clubs. Despite developing grand-mal epilepsy (and neglecting to take his medication) he had a series of jobs, eventually working for a charitable organisation. Owned his own house and car, but was not interested in girls 'because they cost too much money'.

George W.   Interested in languages, played the violin, and was in charge of mailing books in a library. He lived with his mother but had no friends and 'girls are not interested in him'.

Fred G.   At university; gifted in mathematics and earned the respect of his peers through his academic ability. Drove his own car, living partly at home and partly at college.

Sally S.   Utilised her good memory to achieve highly at school and college. Although she failed in her attempt to become a nurse (she would stick rigidly to rules and, for example, having been told that twenty minutes was the usual time it took for breastfeeding, would remove babies from their mothers' breasts if they exceeded this), she later succeeded as a lab technician in a hospital. She belonged to a church singing club and lived alone. She had a six-month relationship with a man but was 'frightened by any intimacies', and at school noted: 'I don't have the same interest in boys that most girls of my age have'.

Edward F. Obtained a BA degree in history, despite initially attending a class for 'retarded children'. Had an active social life involving hiking clubs and was much admired for his knowledge of plants and wildlife. Had his own apartment and car and had begun to date girls. Worked 'in a blue-collar capacity' in a horticultural research station but was disappointed at not having a higher-level post, preferring to associate with 'educated people'.

Clarence B. Obtained a master's degree in economics, but failed when employed in a supervisory capacity. Worked as an accountant and had his own apartment and car. His main hobby was collecting train timetables. He felt he ought to get married but 'can't waste money on a girl who isn't serious'. Remained socially awkward 'but can make superficial adjustments'.

Henry C. Enlisted in the army, and despite 'an uncontrollable urge to gamble' had several well-paying jobs, mostly as a general office worker. He lived alone 'with no desire to get tied down for a long time'.

Walter P. Worked in a restaurant as dishwasher, doing well there despite his communication difficulties. He lived with his mother and was helpful at home but had no voluntary conversation.

Bernard S. Had continuing difficulties at school and junior college and eventually helped to fill shelves in his father's store. His chief interest was the streetcar museum, where he would lay tracks, paint cars and go on trips; his other main interest was politics.

Donald T. Worked as bank teller, no ambitions for promotion; had trophies for golf and was described as a 'fair' bridge player, though lacking in initiative. Was a member of several clubs and secretary to a local church group.

Frederick W. Interested in music and bowling. Worked in an office on the photocopying machine. A letter from his acting director noted: 'He is an outstanding employee by any standard. Outstanding to me means dependability, reliability, thoroughness, and thoughtfulness toward fellow workers.'

Robert F.   (described in the earlier paper by Kanner and Eisenberg 1956). Worked as a meteorologist in the navy, and was married with a young son. He studied musical composition and had works performed by chamber orchestras.

Two other cases were also noted. One, formerly attending college, could no longer be traced, and another, 'a gifted student of mathematics', had been killed in a road traffic accident.

Noting that 11 to 12 per cent of his original sample had done well in the absence of any specialist intervention or support, Kanner speculated that the outcome for people with autism might well improve in future years as recognition of the disorder and knowledge about appropriate educational and therapeutic facilities progressed.

Asperger's accounts

Writing at much the same time as Kanner, Hans Asperger also noted the very variable outcome amongst the individuals he studied. The least favourable outcome was for those with learning disabilities in addition to their autism. For those more able individuals who did make progress it was, again, often their special skills or interests that eventually led to social integration. Asperger quotes examples of many individuals who had done remarkably well in later life, including mathematicians, technologists, chemists, high-ranking civil servants, a professor of astronomy and an expert in heraldry. Indeed, he suggests that:

> able autistic individuals can rise to eminent positions and perform with such outstanding success that one may even conclude that only such people are capable of certain achievements. It is as if they had compensatory abilities to counterbalance their deficiencies. Their unswerving determination and penetrating intellectual powers . . . their narrowness and singlemindedness . . . can be immensely valuable and lead to outstanding achievements in their chosen areas.
>
> (For an annotated translation of Asperger's initial paper,
> see Frith 1991)

Although Asperger also notes that 'in the majority of cases the positive aspects of autism do not outweigh the negative ones' his rather overenthusiastic views of the benefits of autism have raised concerns. As Uta Frith wisely comments: 'There is no getting round the fact that autism is a handicap. . . . It would be tragic if romantic notions of genius and unworldliness were to deprive bright autistic people of the understanding and help they need' (Frith 1991).

There is no doubt that amongst adults of high intellectual ability – especially if this is accompanied by specialist skills or interests – many do manage to function well. Nevertheless, even if they are able to develop effective coping mechanisms almost all individuals will remain affected, to some degree, by their autism throughout their lives.

Autobiographical writings

Personal accounts offer great insight into the lives of individuals with autism. Although they provide evidence of the successes of which individuals are capable, they also make clear the extent of the difficulties with which they have to contend. Donna Williams, now married and making an independent living though writing and lecturing, writes movingly of her journey from *Nobody Nowhere* (1992) to *Somebody Somewhere* (1994). Misunderstood, and often mis-treated as a youngster by her teachers, her family and her peers, in adulthood her great strength and determination, the eventual support of an understanding psychologist and her contacts with individuals similarly affected have resulted in considerable personal and professional success. Her *Somebody Somewhere* book concludes with the clarion call: 'I CAN CONTROL AUTISM . . . I WILL CONTROL IT . . . IT WILL NOT CONTROL ME.'

Yet the penultimate sentences also give some indication of the many challenges faced by someone with autism:

> Autism tries to stop me from being free to be myself. Autism tries to rob me of a life, of friendship, of caring, of sharing, of showing interest, of using my intelligence, of being affected . . . it tries to bury me alive.

Temple Grandin, a woman in her mid-forties, has carved out for herself a successful career as an animal psychologist (Grandin 1995). She travels throughout the world, designing livestock-handling facilities for zoos, farms and ranches. Many of her designs have been developed from the 'squeeze machines' that she first began to construct while at school. Although she continues to have difficulties in understanding ordinary social relationships and feelings, describing herself as in many ways like 'an anthropologist on Mars' (Sacks 1993), she has clearly come a long way from her confused, withdrawn, non-communicating early childhood.

Wendy Lawson was forty-two years of age, and had raised four children (some of whom also have an autistic spectrum disorder) before she was diagnosed as having Asperger syndrome. Prior to this she had been diagnosed as 'intellectually disabled' and then as schizophrenic, a diagnosis that persisted for over twenty-five years. Her books tell of how the correct diagnosis finally brought some understanding of, and help for, her condition. She went on to gain graduate and postgraduate degrees, and is now a successful writer and lecturer on autism. (c.f. Lawson 1998, 2002).

A somewhat similar account of the isolation and often desperation that confronts individuals with autism if they are not correctly diagnosed has been published by Liane Holliday Willey (1999, 2001). She has an academic career, specialising in psycholinguistics, but it was not until her youngest daughter was diagnosed as having Asperger syndrome that she realised that she, too, had these characteristics.

Another well-known autobiographical account is that of Gunilla Gerland (1997), whilst Clare Sainsbury, an Oxford graduate with a First in philosophy and politics (2000), has published an anthology of her own experiences and those of other children with Asperger syndrome as they attempt to cope with the demands of school life. Although all very different individuals, the common theme running through these books is the confusion and frustration, fear and anxiety they experienced in having to mix and fit in with their peers at school and college and in the workplace; and their problems in coping with the demands of family life. The titles themselves tell their own story: *Martian in the Playground, Life on the Outside, Life Behind Glass, Pretending to be Normal.*

There are many other, though less extensive, accounts of the personal experience of autism, several of which can now be accessed via Internet sites (e.g. Sinclair 1992, www.nas.org.uk). Newsletters, such as those produced by self-help or support groups, also contain many first-hand accounts of the difficulties, tribulations and achievements experienced by people with autism and Asperger syndrome. These include the National Autistic Society's publication *Communication* and newsletters produced by Asperger United and Autism Network International.

Autobiographical writings by people with autism are of course fascinating because of what they reveal about the ways in which people with autism think and feel and understand. Nevertheless, although providing us with a rich source of information, these accounts give little indication of what happens to most people with autism as they grow older. In order to investigate this larger-scale and long-term follow-up studies are required.

Early follow-up studies

Initial reports of the outcome for children with autism were, as noted above, largely anecdotal and unsystematic (Lotter 1978). However, towards the end of the 1960s Michael Rutter and his colleagues carried out a detailed assessment of sixty-three individuals, initially diagnosed as autistic at the Maudsley Hospital in London in the 1950s and early 1960s. At follow-up, thirty-eight of the group were aged sixteen years or over. Of these, two were still at school, but of the remainder only three had paid jobs. Over half were placed in long-stay hospitals, seven were still living with their parents, with no outside occupation; three were living in special communities and four attended day centres. Rutter notes that at least some of the individuals living at home or in a special community could have been capable of employment 'at least in a sheltered setting, had adequate training facilities been available'. General outcome for the adult cases in this study is not differentiated from that for the under-sixteens, but overall only fourteen per cent of the group was said to have made a good social adjustment. Nevertheless, most individuals tended to improve with age, and although a number of cases had shown some increase in behavioural difficulties over time, Rutter noted that 'it was rare to see marked remissions and relapses as in adult psychotic illnesses'. No significant sex differences were found, although girls were somewhat less likely to fall within the 'good' or 'very poor' outcome groups. (For details see Lockyer and Rutter 1969, 1970, Rutter and Lockyer 1967, Rutter *et al.* 1967).

Although a number of other follow-up studies were conducted around this time (Creak 1963, DeMyer *et al.* 1973, Mittler *et al.* 1966) most of the individuals involved were still in their early teens, so the studies contain little information about adult life. The first study to look specifically at outcome in an older age group was that of Victor Lotter (Lotter 1974 a,b). Twenty-nine young people between the ages of sixteen and eighteen, who had been diagnosed as autistic when younger, were assessed. In general, the findings were similar to those of Rutter and his colleagues. However, many more of the children (24 per cent) were still at school, reflecting the substantial improvements in educational provision that had occurred over the previous decade: fewer than half the children seen by Rutter had received as much as two years' schooling, and many had never attended school at all. Nevertheless, amongst the twenty-two individuals who had left school only one had a job, fourteen were in long-stay hospitals, two were living at home and five were attending day training centres. In terms of overall social adjustment, again, 14 per cent were described as having done well, although the majority were described as having a 'poor' or 'very poor' outcome. Overall, women did less well, with none being rated as attaining either a 'good' or 'fair' outcome.

Later follow-up studies

Although the 1980s and 1990s witnessed a steady stream of new follow-up reports, many of these involved cases who were in their teens or focused more specifically on high-functioning individuals. Thus outcome data on adults within the wider autistic spectrum remains limited.

Chung and colleagues (1990), for example, followed up sixty-six children attending a Hong Kong psychiatric clinic in the decade from 1976. As in other studies the best outcome was found for cases who had developed speech before the age of five, and who scored more highly on tests of intellectual and social functioning. However, as only nine cases were above twelve years old there is no information about longer-term outcome.

There have been a number of follow-up studies conducted in Scandinavia, where social and psychiatric databases tend to be particularly well maintained. Gillberg's Swedish group (Billstedt *et al.* 2003) have followed up eighty-three individuals aged seventeen or over (mean age twenty-five years), with a childhood diagnosis of autistic disorder. Only three people were found to be fully self-supporting as adults. Of the remainder, around a quarter was described as functioning fairly well but the majority (76 per cent) had a 'poor' or 'very poor' outcome. Three individuals had died (one, possibly two, of status epilepticus, and one in a fire accident). As in other studies, IQ at initial diagnosis was one of the most important prognostic indicators. In some cases but not all, the development of epilepsy around puberty seemed to result in a worse outcome. There was no difference in the outcomes for males and females. Another Swedish study, this time in the north of the country (von Knorring and Hägglöff 1993), examined functioning in thirty-four cases with a mean age of around nineteen years. Although details of social outcome are limited, one individual was described as having lost all autistic symptoms, three had some signs only and thirty remained clearly autistic. In Denmark, Larsen and Mouridsen (1997) completed a thirty-year follow-up of eighteen individuals, nine with autism and nine with Asperger syndrome, all in their thirties or forties. Cognitive levels ranged from below 50 to 85 and above. All had been admitted at some stage as adult psychiatric inpatients, and two had died. Nevertheless, over 40 per cent lived more or less independently, and four individuals were, or had been, married. However, only three were in paid, independent employment, three attended sheltered workshops, five were on disability pensions and the remainder attended day programmes at their local psychiatric hospital.

In the United States, a telephone survey by Ballaban-Gil and colleagues (1996) found that amongst forty-five adults initially diagnosed as children over half (53 per cent) were in residential placements and only one was living independently. Eleven per cent were in regular employment (all of them in menial jobs) and a further 16 per cent in sheltered placements. Rates of behavioural difficulties were high, and only three adults were rated as having no social deficits.

A much larger study of young adults with autism (170 male, 31 female), aged between eighteen and thirty-three, was conducted by Kobayashi and colleagues (1992) in Japan. Outcome was assessed by means of postal questionnaires to parents. The average follow-up period was fifteen years, during which time four cases, all male, had died (from encephalopathy, aged six; head injury from severe self-injury, aged sixteen; nephritic syndrome, aged twenty; and asthma, aged twenty-two). Almost half the group were reported as having 'good' or 'very good' communication skills, and over a quarter was described as having a 'good' or 'very good' outcome (i.e. as being able to live either independently or semi-independently and succeeding at work or college). Women tended to have better language outcomes than men, but there were no significant differences in social functioning between the sexes.

Forty-three individuals were employed, with a further eleven still attending school or college. Jobs were mostly in the food and service industries, but several individuals were described as having 'realised their childhood dreams' of being a bus conductor, car mechanic or cook. The highest level of jobs obtained were by a physiotherapist, a civil servant, a printer and two office workers. All but three of those in employment still lived with their parents, one was in a group home and two had their own apartments; none were married.

Approximately one-fifth of the sample had developed epilepsy (usually in their early teens) but this was well controlled in all but three cases. Seventy-three families reported a marked improvement occurring in their children between the ages of around ten to fifteen years, the period when Kanner, too, had remarked on significant change. However, in forty-seven cases, deterioration in behaviour (such as destructiveness, aggression, self-injury, obsessionality, overactivity etc.) was noted, and these changes also tended to occur around early adolescence. As in earlier studies it was found that outcome in adulthood was significantly correlated with early language abilities and intellectual functioning in males. However, there was no significant correlation with early language in females, and the correlation with IQ was also small. Generally the outcome for females was less good than for males.

Although, by virtue of its size, this is in many ways a very informative study, reliance on questionnaire data, with little or no direct contact with the autistic individuals themselves, clearly raises problems. Parents' ratings of how well their children are functioning may not always accurately reflect their true status. Moreover, diagnostic assessment of autism in the past has not always been entirely satisfactory, and hence some current confirmation of diagnosis is also required.

In a more recent study carried out at the Maudsley Hospital in London (Howlin *et al.* 2004) parents and individuals were all interviewed independently, diagnostic criteria were reconfirmed, and detailed assessments were carried out of language, cognitive, social and academic functioning. Moreover, only individuals with a childhood IQ of at least 50 were included since it is now well established that below this level outcome is almost certain to be very limited. Sixty-eight people (sixty-one male and seven female) were followed up between the ages of twenty-one and forty-eight years. As adults their average performance IQ was 75 (range 33–122).

Seven individuals were living independently or semi-independently, but a third were still with their parents and half the group lived in sheltered communities, mostly specifically for people with autism. Eight individuals were in long-stay hospital care. Despite the fact that one-fifth had obtained some formal qualifications before leaving school (five had attended college or university), employment levels were generally disappointing. Only eight individuals were in regular paid employment, and one was self-employed; twelve others worked on a supported, sheltered or voluntary basis. The remainder attended day or residential centres, where there was little scope for the development of competitive work skills.

In terms of social functioning, around one-quarter of the group was described as having some friends, with thirteen individuals having relationships that involved shared enjoyment or closer intimacy. One individual was married, although he later divorced, and two have married more recently. However, almost two-thirds had no friends at all. A composite rating of outcome, based on social interactions, level of independence and occupational status, indicated that fifteen individuals could be described as having a 'good' or 'very good' outcome. Most of these had some friends and either had a job or were undergoing training. Even if they still lived at home they had a relatively high level of independence, being largely responsible for their own finances, buying their own clothes or taking independent holidays. Thirteen remained moderately dependent on their families or other carers for support, and few in this group had any close friendships. Thirty-one people were in special residential units, which by their very nature (most were geographically isolated) severely limited individual independence, and outcome in all these individuals was considered 'poor'. The eight individuals in long-term hospital care were all rated as having a 'very poor' outcome.

Follow-up studies of high-functioning people with autism and Asperger syndrome

In addition to these more general follow-up studies, some have focused more specifically on individuals with autism or Asperger syndrome who are of normal or near-normal intellectual ability.

Rumsey and his colleagues (1985), in a very detailed study involving a five-day inpatient assessment, followed up fourteen young men aged between eighteen and thirty-nine, all of whom fulfilled DSM-III (American Psychiatric Association 1980) criteria for autism, and several of whom had initially been diagnosed by Kanner himself. Nine were described as 'high-functioning', with verbal IQs well within the normal range; in the 'lower-functioning' group, three were of normal nonverbal IQ but had continuing language impairments; two had mild intellectual impairments.

Socially, all the group continued to have marked difficulties. Most were described as 'loners'. None was married or was thought to have contemplated this; only one had friends, mostly through his church (although he was described there as 'underinhibited'); and a number, even amongst the intellectually more able group, were said still to show socially inappropriate behaviours. Half the group, including those who were high-functioning, showed peculiar use of language such as stereotyped and repetitive speech or talking to themselves.

Academically, those in the 'lower-functioning' group had needed specialist education into late adolescence, but all had developed basic reading, writing and mathematical skills commensurate with their intellectual levels. In the higher-ability group, only one had remained in specialist educational provision, five had completed high school and two had attended junior college; several showed strong ability in maths and two in foreign languages.

Nevertheless, assessment of social outcomes, as measured by the Vineland Social Maturity Scale, indicated that their scores here were often 'strikingly' low in relation to IQ. Problems amongst the more able group were generally related to deficits in the areas of self-direction, socialisation and occupational achievements. Similar difficulties were found in those who were less able, but they also had additional impairments in communication and independence of travel.

In terms of independent living, six individuals in the more able group still lived with their parents and two were in supervised apartments; only one lived entirely alone. In the less able group, none was living independently: three lived with their families, one in a group home and one in a state hospital. With the exception of one person who was unemployed, all the 'lower-ability' group were attending a sheltered workshop or special job programme. Amongst the higher-ability individuals, four were in employment (a janitor, a cab driver, a library assistant, and a key-punch operator); three were in special training or on college courses, one was in a sheltered workshop and one was unemployed. Even amongst those who had jobs, only two had found these independently and generally 'parents played a major role in finding employers willing to give their sons a chance'.

Szatmari and his colleagues (1989b) working in Toronto, studied a group of twelve males and four females with an average age of twenty-six (range 17–35 years) and an average IQ of 92 (range 68–110). Educationally, half the group had received special schooling but the other half had attended college or university, with six obtaining a degree or equivalent qualification. Two were unemployed and four in sheltered workshop schemes; three were still studying; one worked in the family business and six were in regular, full-time employment. Of the latter one was a librarian, another a physics tutor, two were salesmen with semi-managerial positions, one worked in a factory and one as a library technician. Ten of the sixteen cases still lived at home and one in a group home, but five lived independently and a further three individuals living at home were said by their parents to be completely independent. Only one individual was considered to need constant supervision at home, one required moderate care and six some minimal supervision. Socially, nine individuals had never had a sexual relationship with anyone of the opposite sex but a quarter of the group had dated regularly or had long-term relationships; one was married.

In contrast with some other studies, little or no relationship was found between early measures of language or social behaviour and later functioning (early IQ data were not available). However, there was a high and significant correlation between current IQ and social functioning as measured by the Vineland.

The authors are open about the problems related to the study, including the small sample size (compounded by a high refusal rate), and because of the group's high IQ the findings cannot be generalized to people with autism more widely. Nevertheless, it was clear that outcome could be much more positive than indicated by many earlier studies. The authors conclude: 'A small percentage of non-retarded autistic children . . . can be expected to recover to a substantial degree. It may take years to occur, and the recovery may not always be complete, but substantial improvement does occur.'

Another Canadian-based study (Venter *et al.* 1992) has also assessed outcome in more able individuals. Fifty-eight children (thirty-five males and twenty-three females) with an average full-scale IQ of 79, were given a detailed battery of tests and assessments. The results focus predominantly on intellectual and academic attainments rather than social functioning, and the authors note a marked improvement in children's academic attainments compared with the earlier follow-up studies carried out by Rutter and Bartak in the mid-1970s (Rutter and Bartak 1973, Bartak and Rutter 1973). Thus, even amongst the lower-functioning group, over half were able to read and do simple arithmetic, compared to about one-fifth in the studies conducted twenty years previously. Twenty-two individuals in the study were aged eighteen or over; of these six were competitively employed and thirteen were in sheltered employment or special training programmes. Only three had no occupation. Nevertheless, again, all those who were employed were in relatively low-level jobs and all but one had required special assistance in finding employment. Of the three individuals not involved in any adult programme two were female, and all of those in competitive employment were male. No individual was married, and only two lived alone, one of these with considerable support from his mother. Four people lived in apartments with minimal supervision.

In a further study based at the Maudsley Hospital, London (Mawhood *et al.* 2000) the outcome for nineteen young men was studied in detail, as part of a comparative follow-up study of individuals with autism and developmental language disorders. Individuals had initially been seen between the ages of four and nine years and all had a non-verbal IQ within the normal range. When followed up in their mid-twenties, the average performance IQ of the group remained well within the normal range and five individuals had attended college or university. Despite this they showed continuing problems in social relationships, and most remained very dependent. Only three individuals were living independently, one of these in sheltered accommodation; three had jobs (two of these under special arrangements); none had married and only three were described as having friends. Fifteen individuals had never had either a close friendship or a sexual relationship. Thirteen were still described as having moderate to severe behavioural difficulties associated with obsessional or ritualistic tendencies. A composite rating of outcome, based on communication skills, friendships, levels of independence and behavioural difficulties indicated that, overall, only three subjects were considered to have a good outcome, two remained moderately impaired and fourteen continued to show substantial impairments.

There is also a number of cross-sectional studies, which, although lacking the advantage of data on functioning in childhood, do provide a detailed description of status in adult life. Tantam (1991), for example, has described outcome in forty-six individuals with Asperger syndrome, with an average age of twenty-four years. Despite being of normal intellectual ability, only two had received any education after school and only four were in jobs. One individual was married, but most continued to live with their parents or in residential care. A somewhat similar group of ninety-three young adults were described by Newson and her colleagues in 1982. Unfortunately formal diagnostic and IQ data are lacking, but overall more subjects than in Tantam's study had received further education, 22 per cent were in jobs and 7 per cent were living independently. Of this group 15 per cent were said to have had heterosexual relationships, although only one was married. Nevertheless, at an average age of twenty-three years almost three-quarters still lived with their parents.

What can studies of outcome in adult life tell us?

A summary of studies that have examined outcome in adults with autism is presented in Table 2.1. Comparisons between them must, of course, be treated with caution for a number of reasons. First, the data from the later studies are much more systematic and objective than those from earlier ones. Second, several of the more recent reports have concentrated on individuals of higher ability, and therefore a more favourable outcome would be expected. Nevertheless, there were

Table 2.1 Independence and social outcomes in follow-up studies of adolescents and adults*

Study (total N)	Age (years)	IQ	% Semi-independent	% With parents	% Residential provision	% Hospital care	Married	% Some friends	Outcome summary 'Good'	% 'Fair'	% 'Poor'
Eisenberg 1956 (50)	12–35		0						6	28	67
Lockyer et al. 1970 (38)	16+	x=62	0	18	19	53			14	25	61
Kanner 1973 (96)	22–29		8				1 (1 child)	2	11		
Lotter 1973 (29)	16–18	55–90	0	28		48			14	24	62
Newson et al. 1982 (93)	x=23		7	71	16		1	15	7	77	16
Rumsey et al. 1985 (14)	18–39	55–129	21	64	7	7			35	35	28
Szatmari et al. 1989b (16)	17–34	68–110	33	63	12	0	29	21	38	31	31
Tantam 1991 (46)	x=24		3	41	53		2	1			
Kobayashi et al. 1992 (201)	18–33	23%>70	1	97		2	0		27	27	46
Venter et al. 1992 (22)	18+	x=90	21			0	0				
von Knorring and Hägglöf, 1993 (34)	x=19								3	9	88
Ballaban-Gil et al. 1996 (45)	18+	31>70	2	45	53				6	?	?
Larsen and Mouridsen 1997 (18)	32–43	78%>50	44	17	12	17	22 (2 with children)		28	28	44
Mawhood et al. 2000 (19)	21–26	70–117	16	32	47	5	5	21	26		74
Billstedt et al. 2003 (83)	25.5	53%<50	4				1		0	24	76
Howlin et al. 2004 (68)	21+	51–137	10	38	38	12	4	19	22	19	57

* Summary ratings based on authors' own classification where provided. Otherwise 'Good' = moderate to high levels of independence in living and/or job; some friends/acquaintances. 'Fair' = needing support in work and/or daily living but some limited autonomy. 'Poor' = living in residential care or hospital provision (or parental home but with close supervision in most activities). Blank cells indicate insufficient information to rate.

many individuals in the earlier reports who were of relatively high intellectual ability, and indeed the average non-verbal IQ of subjects in the Rutter and Lotter studies fell just within the normal range (i.e. above 70). Similarly there were many subjects in the later investigations who were well below average intelligence. Third, overall judgements of whether outcome is 'good', 'moderate' or 'poor' tend to be somewhat subjective, even if attempts are made to quantify what is meant by these terms. Finally, no doubt because of factors related to the variability in subject selection and assessment, there continue to be quite marked differences between studies in outcome results. Thus, 'good' ratings, for example, range from 0 per cent to 38 per cent and 'poor' ratings from 16 per cent to over 80 per cent.

The proportions living independently also remain very variable. The best outcome was reported in the Canadian study of Szatmari and his co-workers, and although this may be partly understood because of the high ability of the subjects involved, it does not explain why the findings should be considerably better than for the British subjects in the Mawhood study, who were of very similar intellectual levels. It may well be that cultural factors play an important role here, since schemes involving supported employment or semi-sheltered living are generally much better established in Canada and the United States than in Britain. The small number of subjects who were living independently in the Japanese study is also likely to be related to cultural factors.

Despite these qualifications, improvements do appear to be taking place. Figure 2.1 summarises the results of studies conducted over the last three decades (1980–2001), with those appearing in the 1950s to 1970s, in terms of general outcome. Whereas the mean percentage of those rated as having a 'good' outcome in follow-up studies conducted before 1980 was around 11 per cent, over the following two decades the proportion had risen to almost 20 per cent. 'Poor' outcome ratings declined from an average of 65 per cent to around 50 per cent over the same period. 'Fair' ratings remained around 25 per cent to 30 per cent. However, the proportion still living with their families or in specialist residential provision remains high: often around 30 per cent or more. One particularly noticeable change has been in the frequency of admissions to long-stay hospital care. Around 40–50 per cent of individuals in the earlier studies moved into such placements as adults, but there was a marked decline from the 1980s onwards, with the average being around 6 per cent and in many cases far less. However, despite the general trend towards the closure of large residential institutions, for some individuals it has proved extremely difficult to find an alternative

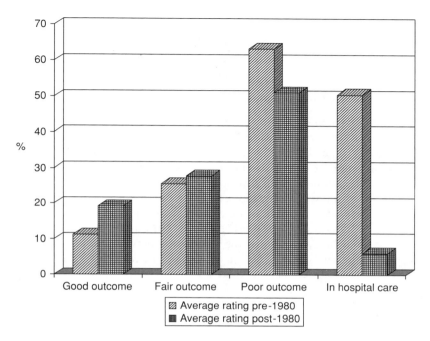

Figure 2.1 Adult outcomes in follow-up studies published pre- and post-1980

to hospital care. This is because their behavioural problems, and especially their lack of social understanding, greatly limit their ability to settle into community-based provision. Nevertheless, there has been a substantial increase in the numbers of those living in their own homes or apartments, either independently or with some minimal supervision. Apart from the individuals described by Kanner in his follow-up, none of the earlier studies mentions subjects living independently. However, in the post-1980 studies an average of around 12 per cent had their own homes. This may not be a particularly high figure, but is certainly a great improvement compared with earlier years.

Although the quality of relationships has generally not been studied in great detail, from the few investigations to have looked at this crucial aspect of adult life it appears that some individuals are capable of making close relationships. Whilst there are few recorded marriages, both Howlin *et al.* (2004) and Mawhood *et al.* (2000) found that around 15–20 per cent of their participants were described as having friendships that involved both selectivity and shared enjoyment. A quarter of the individuals studied by Szatmari also had close relationships, and over 40 per cent had had some relationships with members of the opposite sex. Heterosexual relationships were also reported by 15 per cent of subjects studied by Newson and her colleagues.

Factors related to outcome

The variability in outcome amongst individuals with autism has been noted since the very earliest follow-up studies of Eisenberg and Kanner (Eisenberg 1956, Kanner and Eisenberg 1956), and there have been many attempts to try to isolate the variables that best predict later functioning. Kanner, in his follow-up (1973), noted that lack of appropriate education was highly damaging and that admission into hospital care, as opposed to a school placement, was 'tantamount to a death sentence'. Subsequent studies (e.g. Lotter 1974 a and b, Lockyer and Rutter 1969, 1970) also noted the association between years of schooling and later outcome. The most positive outcomes were generally reported for individuals who had attended mainstream schools, but since this is directly affected by pupils' linguistic and cognitive levels the influence of schooling per se on long-term functioning remains obscure.

The relationship between later outcome and severity of autistic symptomatology in early childhood is also unclear. Rutter and colleagues (Lockyer and Rutter 1969, 1970, Rutter and Lockyer 1967) found no significant correlation between individual symptoms in childhood (other than lack of speech) and adult outcome, although there was a significant relationship with the total number of major symptoms rated. De Meyer *et al.* (1973) also reported a relationship between overall severity of autistic symptoms and later progress. In contrast, Lord and Venter (1992) found no association between prognosis and total number of early symptoms as rated on the ADI. Of greater predictive value were the degree of language *abnormality* and the level of disruption caused by stereotyped and repetitive behaviours. Tolbert and colleagues (2001) also failed to find any relationship between age of onset of symptoms and later autistic symptomatology.

The possible impact of many other variables remains uncertain. In almost every follow-up study in which women have been involved – many studies are exclusively male – outcome has been poorer for females than males. However, the number of women participants has generally been very small and the differences found rarely reach significance; the tendency for females with autism to be of lower IQ also complicates the issue (Lord and Schopler 1985). In some studies, the presence of epilepsy has been associated with a poorer outcome but, again, epilepsy is more likely to occur in individuals with more severe cognitive impairments. Socio-economic factors and ratings of family adequacy have also been correlated with prognosis in some studies, (DeMyer *et al.* 1973, Lotter 1974 a and b), but there is little evidence of a direct causal relationship between adult outcome and an impoverished or disruptive family background, although, as with any other condition, disruption at home may well result in an increase in problems generally.

The two factors that have been consistently associated with later prognosis are early language development and IQ. Very few children who have not developed some useful speech by the age of five to six years are reported to have a positive outcome, although occasionally older children may develop relatively good communication skills. The relationship between long-term outcome and cognitive ability in childhood has also been noted in many follow-up studies (Gillberg and Steffenberg 1987, Lotter 1974 a and b, Lockyer and Rutter 1969, 1970 and Rutter, Greenfield and Lockyer, 1967). Thus, individuals who were either untestable as children, or who had non-verbal IQ scores below 50 are almost invariably reported as remaining highly dependent. However, more recent studies suggest that a minimum childhood IQ of 70 is necessary for a positive outcome in adulthood. Howlin *et al.* (2004) found that on virtually every adult measure (academic attainments, communication skills, reading and spelling, employment status, social independence) individuals with a childhood IQ below 70 were significantly more impaired than those with an initial IQ of 70 or above. Only one individual with an IQ between 50 and 69 obtained a 'good' outcome rating in adulthood. Nevertheless, even amongst the forty-five individuals in this study with an initial IQ above 70, outcome was very mixed. Thus, although almost one-third of this subgroup was rated as having a 'good' or 'very good' outcome, 22 per cent were rated as only 'fair' and 44 per cent obtained ratings of 'poor' or 'very poor'. Moreover, those individuals with an IQ above 100 did no better as a group than those with an IQ in the 70–99 range. Indeed, several individuals in this lower range achieved considerably more highly as adults than many with a childhood IQ of above 100.

It is clear that childhood performance on non-verbal tests of intelligence, whilst being a *relatively* good predictor of outcome, is by no means perfect, and Lord and Bailey (2002) have proposed that childhood *verbal* IQ is a far more reliable indicator of later functioning. However, in the Howlin *et al.* study, although correlations between child and adult verbal IQ were high, there was a sizeable subgroup of individuals who, despite being unable to score at all on verbal tests when younger, subsequently made considerable improvement in this area. Over a third of individuals who were initially 'untestable' on verbal measures obtained a verbal IQ equivalent of at least 70 at follow-up, and several of these children were subsequently rated as having a 'good' or 'very good' outcome as adults. In the case of other children, who *were* able to obtain a verbal IQ score when first assessed, the relationship with adult outcome was also very variable. Whilst a third of those who scored above 50 on verbal IQ tests as children obtained an outcome ratings of 'good' or 'very good' in adulthood; one third were rated as 'fair' and a further third as having a 'poor' or 'very poor' outcome. Even amongst the few children who scored above 70 on a verbal IQ when first assessed, less than half was rated as having a 'good/very good' outcome as adults. Thus, although statistically there is a positive correlation between early verbal IQ and later prognosis, from an individual, clinical perspective, this variable has only limited predictive value.

Lord and Bailey (2002) have also suggested that the presence of useful speech by the age of five is highly predictive of later outcome. Certainly, for many young children it is much easier to obtain information of this kind than to obtain a verbal IQ score, although there may be some problems of recall if interviewing parents of older individuals. However, in the Howlin *et al.* study even this variable was only weakly associated with adult outcome. Over 40 per cent of children who had little or no language when first diagnosed had developed useful language subsequently, and the higher their linguistic levels as adults the more likely were they to do well on a range of other outcome measures. Other research has pointed to the impact that improvements in language may have on the developmental trajectory of children with autism (Szatmari 2000), but as yet we have little information on what is associated with such improvement or by what age language should have emerged in order to indicate a better prognosis.

To some extent it may prove easier to identify correlates of 'poor' outcome than the variables predictive of good prognosis. In the Howlin *et al.* study, as already noted, most individuals with an initial performance IQ below 70 remained highly dependent as adults. Moreover, *no one* with a childhood performance IQ below 70 *and* a verbal IQ below 30 achieved even a 'fair' rating in adulthood and only one individual with a performance IQ below 70 coupled with a verbal IQ below 50 did so.

Identifying the reasons why some individuals make significant improvements in their general levels of functioning over time whilst others show little or no change has major implications for our understanding of autism and of the factors influencing the trajectory from childhood to adulthood. It may be, as Kanner postulated, that the presence of *additional* skills or interests (such as specialised knowledge in particular areas, or competence in mathematics, music or computing etc.), which allow individuals to find their own 'niche' in life and thus enable them to be more easily integrated into society, is of crucial importance. Alternatively, the ability to function adequately in adult life may depend as much on the degree of support offered (by families, educational, employment and social services) as much as basic intelligence (Lord and Venter 1992, Mawhood and Howlin 1999).

Whatever factors are involved, however, it is essential that from the earliest years children with autism are offered every opportunity to develop their social, cognitive and linguistic abilities. As Kanner, Eisenberg and Rutter all proposed many years ago, appropriate and adequate educational provision, and encouragement to develop skills that may lead to later acceptance, are vital. Moreover, especially for those who are more able, it would seem more profitable in the long term for educational programmes to concentrate on those areas in which the individual with autism already demonstrates potential rather than focusing solely on areas of major deficit.

How great is the risk of deterioration in adulthood?

The transition to adulthood can be a time of upheaval and difficulties for many young people and their families. It is not surprising therefore that parents of children with autism approach this life stage with considerable trepidation and anxiety. In a number of long-term studies there have been accounts of an increase in disruptive behaviours in adolescence, and these can undoubtedly prove very difficult for families to deal with. Rutter *et al.* (1970), for example, noted that five individuals (out of a total of sixty-four) in their follow-up study showed a marked deterioration in communication together with progressive inertia and general cognitive decline. Three of these cases had also developed epilepsy. In the adult follow-up by Gillberg's research group (Billstedt *et al.* 2003) 18 per cent had shown a marked deterioration at puberty, and the majority of these never really recovered, subsequently. There was no difference between males and females. Gillberg and Steffenberg (1987) in an earlier study also reported increases in hyperactivity, aggressiveness, destructiveness and ritualistic behaviours, inertia, loss of language skills and slow intellectual decline. Von Knorring and Hägglöf (1993) noted that of the four individuals in their sample of thirty-four who showed a 'mildly deteriorating course' three were women. Ballaban-Gil *et al.* (1996) reported that ratings of problem behaviours had increased in almost 50 per cent of their adult sample, although the nature of these difficulties is not defined. In the Japanese follow-up of 201 young adults, Kobayashi and his colleagues (1992) found that 31 per cent showed a worsening of symptoms, mainly after the age of ten years, but there was no difference in the proportions of males and females who experienced a loss of skills. Larsen and Mouridsen (1997), in a comparative study of autism and Asperger syndrome, reported that three of the nine cases with Asperger syndrome and two of the nine with autism had shown deterioration, mostly occurring in late puberty. In both these latter studies the pattern of deterioration described was very similar to that outlined by Rutter *et al.* (1970) and Gillberg and Steffenberg (1987).

In one of the very few systematic investigations of deterioration over time, Hutton (1998) examined data on the emergence of problems in adulthood for 125 individuals. Over a third were reported to have developed new behavioural or psychiatric difficulties including psychosis, obsessional compulsive disorder, anxiety, depression, tics, social withdrawal, phobias and aggression. The average age when these symptoms developed was twenty-six years, with most people developing symptoms prior to the age of thirty. 'Periodicity' – that is episodes of disturbance occurring at fairly regular and frequent intervals – was noted in eight individuals. The increase in problems of this nature was not associated with epilepsy, cognitive decline or residential placement. However, women were more likely to show an increase in problems than men, and individuals with a lower verbal IQ in childhood were also at greater risk of developing new problems in adulthood. A marked deterioration in cognitive abilities occurred mostly among individuals in long-stay hospital placements.

Although it is clear that some individuals with autism do show an increase in problems as they grow older, it is also important to note that in many studies tracing progress from childhood to adulthood the overriding picture is one of *improvement* over time. This was reported in the early follow-up studies of Rutter and his group, and by Kanner himself, who noted that for some individuals, particularly those who become more aware of their difficulties, mid-adolescence was often a period of 'remarkable improvement and change' (Kanner 1973). Although a third of the individuals in the Japanese study of Kobayashi *et al.* (1992) had shown some increase in problems during adolescence, rather more (over 40 per cent) were rated as showing marked improvement, generally between the ages of ten and fifteen years. Similarly

Billstedt *et al.* (2003) noted that although 18 per cent of their sample showed a marked deterioration in adolescence, 38 per cent had 'a remarkably problem-free adolescent period'. Even in the Ballaban-Gil study (1996), where increases in ratings of behavioural disturbance were higher than in other groups, 16 per cent had improved, and 35 per cent had shown no deterioration in behaviour from childhood to adulthood. Many other studies, both retrospective and prospective, indicate that change over time is more likely to be positive rather than negative. Howlin *et al.* (2004), for example, report many improvements in social, linguistic and cognitive functioning amongst their sample of young adults, especially those with a childhood IQ of 70 or above.

Retrospective studies using standardised assessment instruments such as the Autism Diagnostic Interview-Revised (ADI-R; Lord *et al.* 1994) or the Autism Diagnostic Observation Schedule-Generic (ADOS-G; Lord *et al.* 2000) have also documented a decrease in the severity and frequency of many symptoms over time (Gilchrist *et al.* 2001, Howlin 2003, Piven *et al.* 1996). In a study of over 400 individuals with autism aged from ten to fifty-three years, Seltzer *et al.* (2003) found clear evidence of improvement on ADI-R scores from childhood to adolescence and adulthood. Verbal and non-verbal communication had improved, as had scores on the Reciprocal Social Interaction domain. Scores on *all* the items in the Restricted, Repetitive Behaviors/Interests Domain had also decreased from childhood to adulthood. Similar improvements have been reported even in individuals with severe learning disabilities. Thus, Beadle-Brown and her colleagues (2000) reported changes in scores on the Handicaps, Behaviours and Skills schedule (HBS, Wing and Gould 1979) for 146 young adults with severe learning disabilities and/or autism over a period of twelve years (age at initial assessment two to eighteen years, age at follow-up thirteen to thirty years). Although there was no marked change in IQ, self-care skills (toileting, feeding, grooming, washing and dressing etc) had improved significantly, and there had also been progress in certain areas related to educational achievement (e.g. reading, writing, numbers, money and time). There were fewer significant changes in communication skills as measured by the HBS, although both expressive and receptive scores on the Reynell Developmental Language scale had increased significantly. Improvements were related to initial IQ level, with those individuals with an IQ below 55 (or who were untestable) as children showing less improvement than those with an IQ of 55 or above.

Follow-up studies with a focus on more able individuals have also documented steady improvements over time. For example, in the studies of Mawhood and her colleagues (2000) of nineteen young men followed up from seven to twenty-three years of age, verbal ability on formal IQ tests had increased significantly, and in terms of general social competence almost one-third of the group had moved from a rating of 'poor' functioning in childhood to a 'good' rating as adults. There was relatively little change, however, in ratings of friendship quality.

In summary, whilst it is evident that skills may be lost or problem behaviours increase in adolescence or early adulthood, it is also essential to get the picture into perspective. Conclusions about 'improvement' or 'deterioration' may depend on the particular measures used, and whereas individuals may fail to make progress in certain areas (for example, in the ability to form close friendships), other skills, notably those related to communication, may show positive and significant change. The numbers of adults who show marked deterioration in all aspects of their functioning are, fortunately, very small and overall regression appears to be the exception, not the rule.

Conclusions

Writing in 1973, Kanner commented:

> Over (the last) 30 years . . . there has been a hodge-podge of theories, hypotheses and explanations . . . yet no-one has succeeded in finding a therapeutic setting, drug, method or technique that has yielded the same or lasting results for all children. It is expected that a next 30- or 20-year follow-up will be able to present a report of . . . a more hopeful prognosis.

Would Kanner have considered that the findings from recent follow-up studies fulfil the 'better expectations' he was hoping for, as therapeutic and educational provision for individuals with autism have improved? We shall never know. Yet it is clear that many, although continuing to be affected by their autism, are able to find work, live independently, and possibly develop close relationships with others. These achievements do not come easily, however. Jobs are often found only with the support of families; opportunities to live independently seem to depend heavily on local provision; and friendships are often forged through special interests and skills rather than via spontaneous contacts. Nevertheless, as admissions to hospital care have fallen, and expectations about the future for people with disabilities generally have risen over the years, the outlook now seems far less bleak than was once assumed. At least for those individuals who are of relatively high intelligence, and who develop effective communication skills, appropriate education is able to offer them a chance of being accepted – if never quite completely integrated – into society. In particular, those who view their autism as a challenge to be overcome seem to make most progress, although the extent to which they are able to succeed is likely to depend heavily on the assistance offered by families, schools and other support systems.

3 Interventions for autism

Historical background

The first published accounts of treatments for autism began to appear in the 1950s, when the condition was viewed primarily as an early form of schizophrenia. Indeed, Szurek and Berlin (1956) suggested that it was 'clinically fruitless, even unnecessary, to draw any sharp dividing lines between psychosis, autism, atypical development, or schizophrenia'. Kanner (1951), too, although initially suggesting that autism was a developmental disorder ('We must assume that these children come into the world with an innate inability to form the usual biologically provided affective contact with people'), was influenced by contemporary views of the link between autism and schizophrenia. Consequently, throughout the 1950s and 60s autism was viewed as a psychiatric disorder with a psychogenic basis, and psychoanalysis, together with drugs and other treatments (including ECT) used for schizophrenia, tended to be the treatment of choice (Campbell 1978).

In the mid- to late 1960s autism began to be viewed as a behavioural disorder, with many studies demonstrating the effectiveness of operant approaches (Bandura 1969, Ullman and Krasner 1965). Such interventions were generally clinic-based, with children frequently being treated as long-term inpatients. Parents were only minimally – if at all – involved in treatment, and the focus of therapy tended to be on the elimination of 'undesirable' behaviours, notably tantrums, aggression or self-injury. The procedures used to increase skills such as social interactions or communication were often highly prescriptive and inflexible, and took little note of individual factors such as the child's developmental level or the family situation. There was a heavy reliance on food-based rewards and frequent use of aversive procedures, including electric shock (see Howlin and Rutter 1987).

During the 1970s, largely due to the influential work of Michael Rutter (1972), recognition of the fundamental cognitive, social and communication deficits underlying the disorder led to a shift to more individually based treatment programmes in addition to an acknowledgement of the importance of structured educational approaches and of the crucial role of parents in therapy. As problems of generalization and maintenance became evident, home-based interventions began to replace inpatient programmes and there was much wider use of naturalistic teaching and reinforcement strategies.

The 1980s witnessed increasing integration of home- and school-based programmes, greater involvement of typically developing peers in therapy and a steady movement towards more inclusive education. There was growing recognition, too, of the need for early intervention and of the role played by communication deficits in causing many of the 'challenging behaviours' frequently associated with autism. Reactions against abuses arising from the uncontrolled use of aversive procedures led to a focus on the development of more positive treatment strategies. However, in some quarters, the use of any form of behavioural intervention (including extinction or 'time out' procedures) was condemned (McGee *et al.* 1987), with the result that teachers or support workers were sometimes deprived of some of their most effective management techniques.

It was in the 1980s, too, thanks to the work of Lorna Wing (1981), that the needs of more able people with autism and Asperger syndrome began to be better understood. And despite the fact that, as noted in Chapter 1, there is considerable disagreement about the relationship between autism and Asperger syndrome, clinicians have become increasingly aware that high-functioning individuals within the autistic spectrum are also in need of specialist intervention.

In the last decade, therapeutic work in the field of autism has been characterized by a number of both positive and less positive trends. On the positive side there have been many attempts to extend functional analytic approaches to intervention, and recognition that communication deficits are frequently at the root of many problem behaviours (Durand and Merges 2001, Greenspan and Wieder 1999; see Chapter 4). Other positive trends have included the increased focus on developmentally based approaches; an awareness of the importance of enhancing generalized communication skills in young children (Prizant *et al.* 1997); the emphasis on teaching 'pivotal' responses related to social and communicative interactions (Koegel and Koegel 1995, Koegel *et al.* 1999); a greater reliance on naturalistic reinforcers, and recognition of the need to encourage self-initiation and self-motivation

(Prizant and Rubin 1999). There have also been a number of attempts to improve the fundamental deficits associated with autism, such as impairments in social understanding more generally (cf. Bauminger 2002) or specific impairments in 'theory of mind' (Howlin *et al.* 1998). Whilst such programmes have their limitations (principally because of a lack of generalisation to more naturalistic settings) they do provide teachers, parents and others with strategies and guidelines that can be adapted for use in many different settings

Pharmacological Interventions

Despite the growth of individually based approaches to the treatment of autism, there is still, particularly in the United States, considerable use of medication even for very young children (Gringras 2000, McDougle 1997). Among the many different pharmacological agents used are the 'one size fits all' type (such as fenfluramine) that have been claimed to have a positive impact on almost all aspects of children's functioning. Then there are more specific agents including SSRIs (fluoxitine, fluvoxamine); other antidepressants, such as clomipramine; stimulants (mainly methylphenidate); anti-hypertensive agents (clonidine); antipsychotics (haloperidol); opioid antagonists (naltrexone) to treat self-injurious behaviour; mood stabilisers, such as lithium, and anticonvulsants. Many other agents have also been recommended, including melatonin, megavitamins – even the use of a thirty-six ingredient vitamin/mineral/anti-oxidant supplement – and procedures to reduce mercury levels in the body (cf. Rimland 2000a).

Pharmacological treatments are not limited to children with more severe behavioural problems, and rates of medication even amongst older, more able individuals with autism are high. For example, in a sample of 109 high-functioning patients (adults and children), Martin *et al.* (1999) found that 32 per cent had been prescribed antidepressant medication (mostly SSRIs); 20 per cent had taken some form of neuroleptic and the same proportion had received stimulant medication. Over half the sample was currently receiving psychotropic treatment: 26 per cent were on one drug, 23 per cent on two and 6 per cent on three or more. Two-thirds (69 per cent) had received psychotropic medication at some time in their lives. Despite such high rates of prescribing there are few adequate randomised control trials of the use of psychotropic medications in autism and little if any information about the long-term effects, especially when given to young children. However, fenfluramine, which throughout much of the 1980s was widely used as a treatment of choice for many children with autism in the

United States, has now been largely withdrawn because of concerns about serious side effects and potential long-term damage (see Campbell *et al.* 1996 for review). Another recent treatment, extensively publicised by the media, involves injections with secretin (a gastro-intestinal peptide hormone). This has been claimed to have almost 'miraculous' effects (Horvath *et al.* 1998, Rimland 1998), with rapid improvements in behaviour and language being cited. Nevertheless, an increasing number of parents are now beginning to report severe, adverse side-effects, and initial control trials (Carey *et al.* 2002, Chez *et al.* 2000, Kern *et al.* 2002, Sandler *et al.* 1999) indicate no advantages over placebo. There may be a small subgroup of children with chronic, severe diarrhoea and autism who show a reduction in behaviour difficulties when treated with secretin (Kern *et al.* 2002), although this improvement may be attributable to relief from the diarrhoea, rather than being a direct impact of the treatment on children's behaviour.

Dietary and vitamin treatments have also increased in popularity and are widely recommended on numerous Internet websites. However, as is the case with many interventions given Internet publicity, there is almost no controlled experimental evaluation of these treatments. The Autism Network for Dietary Intervention (www.autismndi.com), for example, recently listed nearly a hundred studies relating to food allergy and autism, and it is claimed that there is 'significant scientific evidence to support a trial period of careful elimination of these proteins for the diet of children on the autistic spectrum'. However, many of these studies are not actually directly related to autism, and there is a dearth of double-blind trials – which are the only sure way of establishing whether intervention is actually successful. Similarly, in a recent Cochrane review of eighteen studies of vitamin B6 and magnesium treatments for autism Nye and Brice (2003) found that only one (Findling *et al.* 1997) involved randomised, double-blind allocation to treatment or control conditions. This study showed no benefit of magnesium and B6 compared to placebo. Moreover, there is very little consideration of the possible dangers of removing basic foodstuffs such as gluten, milk or wheat without ensuring that any resulting dietary deficiencies are adequately compensated for. The potential risks of adding vitamins or other supplements also tend to be almost completely ignored. The argument is, essentially, that vitamins are good and therefore more can only mean better, but there is no room for complacency in such matters. It should be remembered that in the 1960s a similar argument was applied to the use of extra oxygen for neonates with breathing problems – a treatment that was later found to result in irreversible brain damage for some.

Other specific interventions for autism

There is no shortage of claims for other therapies that are said significantly to improve outcome, some even resulting in cures or 'recovery' from autism. Listed below, in alphabetical order, are just some of the approaches that have received widespread (if sometimes short-lived) media publicity over recent years.

Auditory Integration Training (AIT)

This involves listening to electronically processed music through headphones for a total of ten hours, (usually in two thirty-minute sessions over a ten-day period). The training device uses filters to dampen peak frequencies to which the participants are said to be 'hypersensitive'. AIT is claimed to result in a dramatic reduction in autistic symptomatology (cf. *'The Sound of a Miracle: A Child's Triumph over Autism'*, Stehli 1992) and was widely promoted in Australia, Europe and the United States during the late 1980s/early 90s (Rimland and Edelson 1994, 1995).

Cranial osteopathy

This involves very gentle manipulation of various parts of the body, particularly the head. It is claimed that a disturbed pattern of motion in the frontal lobes of the brain can sometimes be identified, or that the whole head is tight and unyielding. Treatment may last for several months, and the effects are said to range from minor reductions in hyperactivity to major improvements in communication (NAS 1997).

Daily Life therapy and the Higashi schools

'Daily Life therapy', as practised in the Japanese-run Higashi schools, has been claimed to produce unprecedented progress in children with autism (Kitahara 1983, 1984 a and b). The focus of the curriculum is on group activities, with a vigorous physical education programme, much music, art and drama. The high anxiety levels of many children with autism are said to be reduced by physical exercise, which releases the endorphins controlling anxiety and frustration. There is rigorous control of challenging and inappropriate behaviours, but individuality is not encouraged and there is relatively little emphasis on the development of spontaneous communication skills.

Facilitated communication

A facilitator supports the client's hand, wrist or arm whilst he or she uses a keyboard or letter board to spell out words, phrases or sentences. The use of facilitated communication with people with autism is based on the theory that many of their difficulties result from a physical inability to express themselves rather than more fundamental social or communication deficits. The facilitator should presume that the client possesses unrecognised literacy skills and the provision of physical support can then lead to 'Communication Unbound' (Biklen 1990).

Gentle teaching

'Gentle teaching' is defined as 'a non-aversive method of reducing challenging behaviour that aims to teach bonding and interdependence through gentleness, respect and solidarity'. Emphasis is placed on 'the importance of unconditional valuing in the caregiving and therapeutic process'(Jones and McCaughey 1992). The approach was claimed to be successful for all individuals with learning difficulties and challenging behaviours (McGee 1985) and rose to popularity in the wake of growing concerns about the use of aversive procedures in the treatment of people with autism or other learning disabilities.

Holding therapy

'Holding' was initially promoted in the United States by Martha Welch (1988), who claimed it was effective for a wide range of problems, from autism to marital difficulties. It was also publicised widely in Germany (Prekop 1984), Italy (Zappella 1988) and the United Kingdom (Richer and Zappella 1989). The therapy involves holding the child tightly until he or she accepts comfort. Central to this is the requirement to provoke a state of distress in order that the child will need to be comforted. Richer and Zapella (1989) claimed that this approach 'had a major contribution to make to the treatment of autistic children' and that it could result in their becoming 'entirely normal'.

Movement therapies

Conductive education which involves 'patterning' or systematic exercising of autistic children by their parents, and usually teams of volunteers, has also been advocated as a potential cure for autism (Delacato 1974, Cummins 1988). The stimulation of muscle activity in a controlled way, often throughout many hours of the day, is claimed to repair damaged or non-functional neural networks.

Vigorous exercise

This has been reported in a number of studies to have a positive effect on behavioural problems and is a crucial component in Daily Life Therapy (see above) There are also suggestions that it may play a role in the effectiveness of holding therapy (Welch 1988). Parents have reported various behavioural improvements following physical exercise (Rimland 1988), and reductions in stereotyped, disruptive and hyperactive behaviours, sleep disturbance, aggression, anxiety, self-injury and depression have been noted in other studies. Vigorous exercise has also been claimed to improve attention span, social skills, work performance and cognitive functioning, and to reduce self-stimulatory behaviours in subjects with autism, as well as other forms of learning disability (see Elliott *et al.* 1994, Rosenthal-Malek and Mitchell 1997).

Music therapy

Although mostly used as one component of a broader educational programme for children with autism, there are claims that music therapy alone can play 'a significant role in developing . . . emotional, integrative and self organisational experiences' (Trevarthen *et al.* 1998). However, the term covers a wide variety of different techniques, and reports of its effectiveness often incorporate additional interventions such as psychoanalysis or play therapy.

Pet therapies

Claims of apparently dramatic improvements in behaviour after exposure to pet therapy of various kinds make occasional appearances in the media, and the positive effects of swimming with dolphins have received particular publicity. However, there is now a growing movement in California to protect dolphins from being used for the benefit of human beings, and the specific or long-term benefit of these approaches for people with autism have never been assessed.

Psychoanalytic psychotherapy

Kanner's comments (1943) on the lack of warmth shown by parents of children with autism and their tendency towards a 'mechanization of human contacts' led many to view the condition as being predominantly psychogenic in origin. It was variously suggested that autism was due to a lack of stimulation, parental rejection, lack of warmth, or deviant family interactions (Bettelheim 1967, Boatman and Szurek 1960, O'Gorman 1970). Such theories had a profound and widespread influence on therapeutic practice, and for many years individual psychotherapy (mainly in the form of psychoanalytically oriented non-directive play therapy) was considered the treatment of choice (Szurek and Berlin 1956, Goldfarb 1961). Although Campbell *et al.* (1996), in a general view of interventions, concluded that psychoanalysis is of 'limited value', the approach is still viewed as beneficial by some (e.g. Hobson 2002).

The Son Rise Programme (formerly the Options method)

This approach is based on the premise that the child with autism finds the world confusing and distressing and hence attempts to shut it out. This then starves the brain of the stimuli needed to develop social interaction skills, thereby further increasing confusion and reinforcing the desire for isolation. The essential principle is to make social interactions pleasurable, and to ensure that involvement with *people* becomes more attractive than involvement in obsessional or ritualistic behaviours. Problem behaviours should be viewed as an understandable reaction to children's difficulties in making sense of or controlling their world (Kaufman 1977, 1981). In order to 'reach' the child with autism, adults must be prepared to join in with and enjoy the activities that the child finds pleasurable (very often his or her obsessional activities). Parents are taught to become more aware of the cues given by their own children and to respond more effectively to these. After 9,000 hours of such treatment the Kaufmans' own son is said to have progressed from being 'a severely autistic child . . . with an IQ of about 30' to a completely normal young man with 'a near-genius IQ' (cf. *A Miracle to Believe In* 1981).

Scotopic sensitivity training

Scotopic sensitivity, or sensitivity to certain wave lengths of light is said to result in many different symptoms, including reading and communication difficulties, spatial and perceptual deficits, and attentional problems. Special spectacles, incorporating lenses of a variety of different colours, can be designed to provide the 'optimum' tint for each individual and are reported to bring about improvements in body and spatial awareness, eye contact, communication and self-control in many different disorders, including autism (Irlen 1995). Donna Williams is claimed to have found the results 'close to miraculous . . . she was able to listen and concentrate better; her speech became more fluent and spontaneous'.

Sensory integration therapy

Many children with autism have problems in dealing with complex sensory stimuli (Minshew *et al.* 1997). Sensory integration therapy aims to improve sensory processing and increase sensory awareness and responsivity by using a variety of stimuli such as swings, balls, trampolines, soft brushes and cloths for rubbing the skin, perfume, massage, coloured lights or objects with unusual textures (Ayres 1979). 'Deep pressure therapy' (rolling children up tightly in mats or mattresses) may also be involved. Rimland (1995) reported that around a quarter of programmes for autistic children in the United States were utilising this approach.

Unfortunately, despite the impressive claims, few of these methods have been subject to any form of experimental investigation; there are no randomised comparison trials or even well-controlled single-case or small-group studies. Instead, information on outcome tends to be based on a few, mostly anecdotal, single-case reports; there is no information on long-term effectiveness, and publicity is rarely afforded to families for whom the treatments did not work. Thus, for most of the procedures described above, there is neither any evidence that the treatment is effective – nor that it is not!

Facilitated Communication (FC), Auditory Integration Training (AIT) and Sensory-Integration programmes are amongst the very few therapies that have been subject to experimental evaluation. Because of its widespread use in the United States, and an increasing number of legal cases in which false accusations of (mostly sexual) abuse were made during facilitated sessions, Facilitated Communication has now been the focus of at least fifty studies involving several hundred subjects (see reviews by Green 1994, Jacobsen, Mulick and Schwartz 1995, Mostert 2001, Simpson and Myles 1993). These have clearly demonstrated that there is virtually no evidence of independent communication. Instead all the evidence points to the fact that the communications are directed by the facilitator, not the client with autism. Moreover, so extensive have been the concerns over abuses arising from the use of this technique that, in 1994, the American Psychological Association adopted the resolution that: 'Facilitated Communication is a controversial and unproved procedure with no scientifically demonstrated support for its efficacy'. Similarly, the American Academy of Pediatrics Committee on Children with Disabilities (1998) concluded that 'there are good scientific data showing (FC) to be ineffective. Moreover ... the potential for harm does exist, particularly if unsubstantiated accusations of abuse occur using FC'. However, although the method is now widely discredited among researchers, its occasional use within schools continues (*The Times*, Court Report, July 13 2000).

There are also a few evaluative studies of Auditory Integration Therapy (see Dawson and Watling 2000 for review), although most of these have involved very small numbers of subjects. In general there is no evidence that AIT produces any greater benefits than placebo or control conditions (Dawson and Watling 2000, Mudford *et al.* 2000, Zollweg *et al.* 1997), and the American Academy of Pediatrics Committee (1998) concluded, 'there are no good controlled studies to support its use'. This committee also recommended that the use of either Facilitated Communication or Auditory Integration Training 'does not appear warranted at this time, except within research protocols'.

Sensory–Integration procedures have been the focus of much more limited research, despite their widespread use within many educational settings. In a recent review, Dawson and Watling (2000) were able to identify only four evaluative studies, involving twenty-six children in total. Although some positive outcomes were reported, the fact that no study involved a comparison group meant that no conclusions could be drawn concerning effectiveness.

Interpreting treatment claims

Whilst professional researchers in this area bemoan the lack of randomised control treatment trials, parents themselves may find it almost impossible to make sense of the many claims and counter-claims with which they are continually bombarded. After all, who can easily turn their back on a treatment that could change the course of their child's life for ever? As one parent with a twenty-two-year-old son writes:

> Nobody wants to give up without a good fight. ... We weren't so much searching for a miracle. Really, we were just looking for something – anything – because to do nothing had become intolerable. Perhaps that is the case for all parents. If you had a child like this you would try everything. For one mother 'everything' means to go into debt, fly to a foreign country, put her child into a tank with dolphins ...
>
> For our family it meant different things at different times: pounds of bitter-tasting vitamins, rigid behavior modification, spinning in a suspended net, doing what the doctor didn't say, travelling

2,500 miles across the country to a new home, keeping him at home, giving him over into the care of others.

I try not to think too much about what would or would not have happened had we tried or not tried a particular treatment. But each time I hear of something new – often a therapy we could not even have imagined – a little spark inside my brain briefly ignites and I wonder once again, what if . . . ?

(Muller 1993)

Professional dismissal of unproven treatments as 'garbage science' (Rimland 2000a), although possibly quite correct, may simply provoke parents into seeking alternative therapies. Instead, it may prove more productive to encourage families to seek basic facts on the results of therapy for themselves. Any effective programme should be able to provide some information on longer-term outcome (not just immediately after intervention). It should be made clear what assessments are carried out on individual children prior to treatment, what are the criteria for acceptance into treatment, and what are the exclusion criteria. Information should also be provided on the types of children or families for whom the programme is most effective (is it more successful, for example, for those of high or low ability; for those with good language or poor communication skills; does it work better with younger or older children; are there any family factors that seem to be related to outcome?). If possible, parents should also try to establish whether any independent evaluation methods have been used to assess the outcome of treatment and whether evidence exists to demonstrate its superiority over other programmes. Media reports of the latest miracle cure, or glowing testimonials on office walls *do not* constitute satisfactory evidence of treatment effectiveness. Parents also need to be clear about the economic and other hidden costs of treatment. How much time will be involved? What is likely to be the impact on siblings and family relationships generally and can it be fitted into regular family/school/social life? Moreover, parents are less likely to be seduced by claims for the latest 'miracle therapy' if they are provided with sound practical advice by local services, from the earliest years on ways of dealing with difficulties at home.

Educational programmes

In contrast to the paucity of data on most of the treatment approaches described above, educational approaches for children with autism have been studied in considerable detail. The importance of structured educational programmes has been recognised for many years, since research by Rutter and Bartak (1973) confirmed that autistic children exposed to structured, task-oriented, 'academic' programmes made significantly better educational and social progress than children in less structured environments. The TEACCH programme, (Schopler and Mesibov 1995, Schopler 1997) provides a framework for teaching that emphasises the need for structure, appropriate environmental organisation and the use of clear visual cues to circumvent communication difficulties. The programme also takes account of developmental levels and the importance of individually based teaching, as well as incorporating behavioural and cognitive approaches. A recent controlled study by Ozonoff and Cathcart (1998) reported significant short-term gains in pre-school children with autism following the introduction of a daily TEACCH session into their daily home programme, although no large-scale controlled school-based comparisons have been conducted.

A number of other, mostly United States based, models exist. Among the best evaluated of these are the Denver model (Rogers *et al.* 1987), the Douglass Centre programme (Harris *et al.* 1995), the Individualized Support Programme (Dunlap and Fox 1999) and the LEAP programme (Strain and Hoyson 2000) (see National Research Council 2001 for review). In the United Kingdom, the National Autistic Society promotes the SPELL (Structure, Positive, Empathy, Low Arousal, Links) approach. Other programmes focus on the encouragement of play and pleasurable interactions between pre-school children with autism and their parents or peers. These include the Developmental Intervention Model (Greenspan and Wieder 1999), the Waldon Program (McGee *et al.* 2002), the Hanen approach (Sussman 1999) and the Early Bird Project (Shields 2001). However, there have been few independent evaluations of these interventions.

Many other approaches to education focusing specifically on strategies to overcome the fundamental impairments in autism have been reported, although, again, evaluative studies are sparse. Quill (1995a) provides detailed information on programmes designed to improve social and communication functioning. The Picture Exchange Communication System, (PECS, Bondy and Frost 1996) uses symbols, pictures or objects to enhance communication skills in the classroom. The 'Bright Start Programme' (Butera and Haywood 1995) focuses on the development of cognitive and meta-cognitive abilities. Koegel and Koegel (1995) illustrate how traditional behavioural techniques can be successfully adapted for use in more naturalistic school settings. There is also an increasing number of studies documenting the potential value of computer-based teaching (Chen and Bernard-Opitz 1993, Powell and Jordan 1997, Tjus *et al.* 2001).

Early intervention programmes

In recent years there has been a steady growth in early intervention programmes for toddlers and pre-school children with autism. These are designed to help parents and teachers develop appropriately structured and consistent management strategies during the child's early years, which, in principle, should enhance developmental progress and minimise later behavioural problems (see Rogers 1996). A variety of developmental, educational and behavioural approaches has been found to have positive effects, with significant improvements being reported in language and social behaviours, self-care, motor and academic skills. (Dawson and Osterling 1997, Rogers 1998a). When control groups have been involved (which is by no means always the case) the gains made by the experimental children have generally been greater, with more children in the treatment groups subsequently being accepted into mainstream school. Nevertheless, although children's overall level of functioning appears to be enhanced by programmes of this kind, there is less evidence of a marked reduction in autistic symptomatology. This conclusion holds even for the very early, intensive behavioural interventions of Lovaas and his colleagues (Lovaas 1996). These have been reported as bringing about major changes in children's cognitive ability (sometimes as much as thirty IQ points or more), and it is claimed that around 40 per cent of the children involved become 'indistinguishable' from their normally developing peers. However, such claims have been disputed, and it is evident that the way in which IQ is measured, both prior to and following intervention, can have a significant impact on results (Magiati and Howlin 2001). The restricted range of the outcome measures used in these early interventions studies has also been criticised (Gresham and MacMillan 1998).

Generally, the number of cases involved in evaluative studies of early behavioural/educational interventions remains very small, and blind, randomised control trials are virtually non-existent (Lord 2000). Many other questions remain to be answered concerning the *specific* effects of these early programmes, since the content is often very eclectic and the relative importance of the different components of treatment is unknown. There are also questions about the comparative merits of one-to-one versus group teaching, or home-based versus school-based programmes. Similarly, surprisingly little is known about the characteristics of the children who appear to respond best to programmes of this kind. Thus, although several studies indicate that IQ and language levels are important predictive variables (Harris and Handleman 2000), with the most able children generally making most progress, this is not invariably the case (Koegel 2000). The optimal length of time in therapy is another issue. Lovaas (1996) has proposed that forty hours a week of therapy, over two years or more, is required, although positive results have been reported for less intensive behavioural programmes (Gabriels and Hill 2001). On the whole, the more successful early intervention programmes appear to involve a minimum of around fifteen to twenty hours a week, last at least six months, and require a relatively high adult-child ratio (Rogers 1996). The active participation of parents in therapy is also important (Schreibman 2000). Finally – but perhaps most importantly – longer-term evaluations, covering many different aspects of functioning are required in order to evaluate the true effectiveness of early intervention programmes.

The recent New York Health State Department Review (1999) of interventions for pre-school children with autism highlights the poor quality of much of the research in this area (see Tables 3.1–3.4). Of the several hundred published papers reviewed only a minority met the basic criteria for experimental research. It was concluded that there was no evidence for the effectiveness of many therapies, including sensory integration, touch therapy or auditory integration. The use of facilitated communication was 'strongly discouraged'. Of the various medical or dietary interventions reviewed (secretin, immunoglobulin injections, anti-yeast treatments, vitamin or dietary manipulations)

Table 3.1 New York State Department review of interventions for children with autism (1999). Number of studies reviewed meeting basic research criteria

Type of intervention	(N Studies reviewed)[1]	% meeting basic experimental criteria[2]
Behavioural/educational	300	8%
Other (auditory integration; facilitated communication etc.)	63	5%
Drugs	99	12%
Vitamins/diet etc.	44	7%

1 Includes only studies providing adequate description of techniques and participants involved
2 I.e. non-biased assignment of cases; employing appropriate single-case/case-series research design or comparison groups

Table 3.2 New York State Department review of interventions for children with autism (1999). Conclusions re effectiveness of miscellaneous programmes

Type of intervention	General conclusions
Sensory integration	No evidence of effectiveness
Auditory integration	No evidence of effectiveness; use not recommended
Facilitated communication	No evidence of effectiveness; use strongly discouraged
Music therapy	No evidence of effectiveness as 'stand-alone' therapy
Touch therapy	No evidence of effectiveness

Table 3.3 New York State Department review of interventions for children with autism (1999). Conclusions re effectiveness of dietary and medical treatments

Type of intervention	General conclusions
Medication	Some benefits but trials small-scale; concerns about long-term effects for very young children
Hormone injections (including secretin)	No evidence of effectiveness; serious concerns about long term effects
Immunologic interventions (e.g. intravenous immune globulin)	No evidence of effectiveness; serious concerns about long term effects
Anti-yeast	No evidence of effectiveness; serious concerns re possible side effects
Vitamins	No evidence of effectiveness unless child is vitamin-deficient
Diet	No evidence of effectiveness; not recommended

again there was little if any evidence of effectiveness, and on the whole, because of serious concerns about side effects or long-term sequelae, these were not recommended. There was more evidence in favour of pharmacological treatments, but little information on the likely benefits and disadvantages for specific subgroups of children, and serious

Table 3.4 New York State Department review of interventions for children with autism (1999). Conclusions re effectiveness of behavioural/educational programmes

Type of intervention	General conclusions
Intensive behavioural programmes	20+ hours of intensive ABA per week appears to convey some advantages compared with no/briefer interventions
Specific behavioural programmes	ABA techniques effective (though most studies small scale); no evidence for superiority of any one specific approach
General behavioural programmes (to reduce behaviour problems, increase social and communication skills etc.)	Appear to be useful in combination with parent training and/or other educational programmes. Various strategies effective

concerns were raised about the long-term effects, particularly when used with very young children. The most positive findings related to behavioural and educational programmes, but although applied behavioural analysis techniques were deemed to be useful, as in previous reviews it was concluded that there was no evidence for any one specific approach. It was concluded that interventions of moderate intensity (i.e. around twenty hours a week) produce better results than shorter programmes, but there was no evidence that programmes of forty hours or more a week provided greater benefits. The involvement of parents in therapy was viewed as important and programmes with a focus on reducing behavioural problems, improving communication or enhancing social interaction showed positive outcomes. However, there were no data to support the use of any one particular behavioural programme. The findings of the New York State Health Department report are generally endorsed by other reviews of this area. Thus Sheinkopf and Siegel (1998) concluded that early behavioural/ educational interventions are a good option for children with autism and certainly far better than no intervention or non-specialist school placements. However, they found no evidence in favour of any one approach, any one level of intensity or any particular degree of structure. Similarly, Prizant and Rubin (1999) note that, given the current state of research in the field, no one approach has been demonstrated to be superior to all others or to be equally effective for all children.

Evidence in support of the value of early intervention?

Whilst the relative effectiveness of different treatments for children with autism has generated much empirical research, there have been few investigations of the long-term benefits of early intervention per se. It is widely accepted that early intervention is vital in helping children with autism to develop essential skills in the earliest years, and in preventing the escalation of later behavioural difficulties. The claims, particularly by Lovaas and his colleagues, that intervention is most effective if it can begin between the ages of two to four years has led to a push towards earlier and earlier educational and behavioural programmes. Indeed, in order to ensure access to pre-school intervention, much research over the last decade has concentrated on improving facilities and techniques to ensure early identification and diagnosis (Lord 1995). However, what, in fact is the evidence that early intervention, particularly in the pre-school years, does confer advantages compared with later therapy? Although several studies report positive outcomes for children enrolled in intervention programmes prior to four years of age (Anderson *et al.* 1987, Birnbrauer and Leach 1993, Sheinkopf and Siegel 1998), these have not conducted systematic comparisons between children of different ages. Lovaas (1993) noted that the younger children in his intervention studies did much better than those who were older, but again there was no direct comparison between children who began therapy at the recommended age, (i.e. around two) and those who started later, at around four or five years. Fenske *et al.* (1985) conducted a small-scale comparative study of eighteen children, nine aged under five years, and nine aged over five when therapy began. Despite the fact that they were actually in therapy for less time, two children in the early treatment group went on to mainstream school, compared with only one child in the later intervention group. However, school placement was the only outcome measure utilised, and – more importantly – the children in the two groups were not matched prior to the onset of treatment. Recent findings by Stone and Yoder (2001), in showing that the amount of time in language therapy from the age of two tends to predict outcome at four, might also be cited in support of the argument that 'earlier equals better'. Similarly, Harris and Handleman (2000) found that children admitted to a specialist pre-school programme before the age of three and a half were more likely subsequently to be placed in a regular educational classroom than those who were aged on average four and a half when pre-school intervention began. However, outcome, in terms of later educational placement, was also significantly related to pre-school IQ measures, and the relative importance of IQ versus age was not explored.

Rogers (1998a) notes that 'the hypothesis that age at start of treatment is an important variable in determining outcome has tremendous implications for the field and needs to be tested with methodologically rigorous designs'. Unfortunately, no such designs have yet been employed.

In the absence of any evidence to the contrary, it would seem to make common sense (and in reality that is all we have to go on) to ensure that families of young children with autism are offered appropriate help as soon as possible after diagnosis. Given the rigid behaviour patterns of children with autism, it is clear that once problem behaviours are established it can be very difficult to change these. Thus the earlier effective management strategies can be put into place, and appropriate patterns of behaviour established, the less are the chances of problem behaviours developing in the future. It is also evident that certain behaviours, whilst entirely acceptable in very young children, become increasingly less so as individuals grow older. Informed advice to parents concerning the types of behaviour that may lead to potential problems with age can also have important preventative effects (Howlin 1998b). There is a danger, however, that a single-minded focus on the importance of early pre-school intervention could have a negative impact on older children with autism. Despite improvements in the age of diagnosis over recent years, many children, particularly those who are more able, do not receive a definitive diagnosis until they reach junior school, or even later (Howlin and Asgharian 1999). For them, or for the thousands of children who for a variety of other reasons have no access to early intervention, an assumption of 'better late than never' is more appropriate than 'early intervention or nothing'. Harris and Handleman (2000), for example, noted that even the older children in their study made important progress and they are explicit that their data should 'not be taken to suggest that children four years of age and older should be denied intensive treatment'. Whatever the age at which an individual's problems are recognized, appropriate strategies can and should be put into place to help deal with these. After all, there is nothing inherent in behavioural principles to suggest they are only effective up to a certain age. In addition, there is considerable research indicating that many individuals with autism continue to make considerable improvements as they grow older (Gilchrist *et al.* 2001, Howlin 2003, Howlin *et al.* 2004, Mawhood *et al.* 2000, Mesibov *et al.* 1989, Piven *et al.* 1996, Seltzer *et al.* 2003). Indeed, for some

– particularly those who are more able – adolescence can often be a period of remarkable improvement and change (Kanner 1973). This is an age at which some children, at least, become more aware of their difficulties and of how they can moderate their behaviours in order to improve social interactions. Unfortunately, there are very few intervention programmes geared specifically to the needs of this age group, and this may mean that they, their families and the professionals involved in their care are missing out on a crucial opportunity for change.

Interventions for adults

In comparison with the vast amount of research on interventions for children with autism there are very few studies of special therapeutic programmes for older individuals. Moreover, there is little if any evidence, even from the most rigorously evaluated programmes designed for children, that these have any significant long-term impact on outcome in adulthood. Much of the literature on adult-focused programmes relates to the reduction of very challenging behaviours or the acquisition of basic life skills by those with severe or profound intellectual disabilities. However, as previously noted, outcome studies suggest that most individuals tend to improve with age, and there are indications that progress can be enhanced if adequate social support structures are in place (Lord and Venter 1992). Programmes to enhance social understanding and improve interpersonal behaviours in adults have also been found to have positive effects (Howlin and Yates 1999, Mesibov 1992, Attwood 2000). Much wider provision of social skills programmes, and social support networks more generally for adolescents and young adults could help to minimise the many problems they face in daily interactions at school and work. Many others might profit from cognitive–behavioural programmes, to help them cope more effectively with emotional or practical difficulties (Bauminger 2002, Hare *et al.* 1999, Reaven and Hepburn 2003, Stoddart 1999). Success in the job market can also be significantly improved by supported employment schemes that focus on teaching appropriate work and social skills. Even individuals with moderate to severe intellectual impairments have been helped to find and maintain employment by these means (Keel *et al.* 1997, Smith, Belcher and Juhrs 1995). For those who are more able such schemes can significantly increase the chances of clients finding employment, and lead to much higher and better-paid levels of work (Mawhood and Howlin 1999, see Chapter 9 for further details).

Research-based evidence for effective approaches to intervention

It is clear, given the current state of research in the field of autism, that no single approach has been demonstrated to be superior to all others or to be equally effective for all individuals. Prizant and Rubin (1999) note that the knowledge base for intervention programmes should derive from a combination of different sources, including theory (developmental, learning, family systems etc.), clinical and educational data, knowledge about best practice, and empirical data from well designed small group and single case studies. Such information can then be used to indicate *components* of treatment that are likely to be beneficial.

1   There is evidence of the advantages of individually designed intervention programmes (Anderson and Romanczyk 1999, Prizant and Rubin 1999). These will need to take account of the individual's cognitive level, the severity of autistic symptomatology, and overall developmental level.

2   Many studies attest to the importance of structured educational/daily living programmes, with a particular emphasis on visually based cues. These provide the individual with autism with a predictable and readily understandable environment, which helps to minimize confusion and distress (Jordan and Powell 1995, Quill 1995a, Schopler and Mesibov 1995, Wetherby and Prizant 1999).

3   Effective treatments must take account of the core deficits of autism. Thus, although profound communication deficits – which are found at all levels of intellectual ability – may never be fundamentally altered, much can be done by ensuring that the communication used by others is appropriate for the individual's *comprehension* level and that verbal messages are augmented as much as possible by visual or other means (Howlin 1998a). Beneficial effects have been demonstrated for interventions that focus on the social-communication deficits associated with autism (see Rogers 2000). Thus, specialist training programmes, for example to improve 'mind-reading' skills (Howlin *et al.* 1998, Ozonoff and Miller 1995, Swettenham 1995) or social understanding (Bauminger 2002, Gray 1995, Mesibov 1984, Williams 1989) may prove of value for both adults and children. Stereotyped and ritualistic tendencies, too, may often be the underlying cause of many behaviour problems, and as these frequently become progressively more unacceptable with age it is important to ensure that they are effectively managed from early childhood (Howlin 1998b, Schopler 1995).

4   It is now well established that many so-called undesirable or challenging behaviours are frequently a reflection of limited behavioural repertoires or poor communication skills. A focus on skill enhancement, and the establishment of more effective communication strategies is, therefore, often the most successful means of reducing difficult or disruptive behaviours (Durand and Merges 2001, Koegel 2000, Prizant *et al.* 1997).

5   The implementation of treatment approaches that are family-centred appears to ensure more effective generalization and maintenance of skills (Marcus *et al.* 1997). The development of management strategies, which can be implemented consistently but in ways that do not demand extensive sacrifice in terms of time, money or other aspects of family life, seems most likely to offer benefits for all involved.

In the following chapters examples of how these principles may be put into practice with adults with autism are described.

4 Problems of communication

Follow-up studies have consistently indicated that the development of language is a crucial indicator of later outcome in autism. Unless some useful speech is acquired by around the age of six years, future development is likely to be severely limited. Very few individuals who fail to achieve spoken language by this age later develop complex speech, although there are of course occasional exceptions to this. Cases have been reported of individuals who did not begin to speak until their teens, and Jim Sinclair (1992), for example, notes that he did not learn to use speech to communicate until the age of twelve. Howlin *et al.* (2004) also found that several individuals who were using little or no speech when assessed around the age of five, six or seven later went on to become very fluent speakers. On the whole, however, the level of language acquired after this stage is generally very limited. Overall, approximately 30 per cent of individuals with autism remain without useful speech but, even amongst those who do learn to talk, significant impairments may continue throughout adulthood.

These difficulties are not confined to individuals of lower intellectual ability. Thus, Szatmari and his colleagues (1989a) found almost two-thirds of their sample of young adults continued to have problems related to verbal inflection or over-formal language; one-third had impoverished speech and had difficulties in making sense of conversations. Rumsey *et al.* (1985) reported that 50 per cent of their cases continued to demonstrate, 'peculiar language usage' and the same proportion showed perseverative and repetitive speech patterns. Over 40 per cent still had little spontaneous speech, and abnormal intonation was common. Mawhood *et al.* (2000) also found that only a third of the sample of young adults whom they followed-up could be regarded as having good communication skills ('good' was defined as having good comprehension, using mature grammatical structures and being able to take part in reciprocal conversations). Almost two-thirds were rated as having, 'poor' or 'very poor' verbal skills: that is, they had immature grammar, were unable to take part in even simple conversations and had very limited comprehension of speech.

These difficulties are brought to life even more vividly in the personal accounts of people with autism. Therese Jolliffe, a young woman with autism who also has a Ph.D. in psychology, recalls:

> It was ages before I realised that people speaking might be demanding my attention. But I sometimes got annoyed when I realised that I was expected to attend . . . because my quietness was being disturbed. . . . Speaking for me is still often difficult and sometimes impossible. . . . I sometimes know in my head what the words are but they do not always come out . . . sometimes when they do come out they are incorrect. Sometimes when I really need to speak and I just cannot, the frustration is terrible. I want to kick out at people and objects, throw things . . . scream. People's names are difficult to remember . . . and I still get the names of similar objects confused (e.g. knives and forks, dresses and skirts). . . . It is hard to understand words that are similar in sound. . . . You do not seem to be aware that words can be put across using all different kinds of voices and that there are alternative ways of saying things. It was only from my academic work that I picked up the fact that there is more than one way of saying things. . . . Sometimes I used to repeat the same words over again as this made me feel safer . . . when I first started repeating back phrases exactly as I had heard them. I think I did this as I was only able to come out with one or two words for myself.
>
> (Jolliffe *et al.* 1992)

In the following sections some of the most common problems associated with the use and understanding of speech by young people with autism are discussed.

Comprehension difficulties

Discrepancies between the use and understanding of language

For the majority of individuals with language impairments, the comprehension of language is generally at a higher level than their expressive abilities. In autism, this is frequently not the case. Superficially, spoken language can seem well developed, with many individuals possessing good vocabulary and syntax. However, there may be profound comprehension difficulties, particularly within a social context. Problems are further compounded by the fact that on formal tests of language many individuals may perform relatively well, as their understanding of individual words may be better developed than their ability to decode more complex instructions or concepts. Because of this very uneven profile of linguistic functioning it is often difficult for other people to appreciate the true extent of the language impairment. In consequence, the failure of someone with autism to respond appropriately to instructions may be variously misinterpreted as uncooperative, rude, or mere 'stupidity'. Paradoxically, problems of this nature may actually increase with age as expectations of their competence increase. Thus, although it is widely recognised that children with autism have comprehension difficulties, as such individuals grow older, often showing marked improvements in *spoken* language, deficits in understanding may be less apparent.

Ros Blackburn is a woman with autism who lectures widely on such problems. She has a particular fascination with words and describes herself (quite accurately) as having a 'phenomenal' expressive vocabulary. However, *understanding* is very different. For example, when attending a meeting she is likely to be asked 'Would you like to sign in?' and later 'Would you like a cup of coffee or tea?' The latter is a genuine request – to which acceptance or refusal is equally acceptable. The former is actually an order; there is no choice. However, for Ros interpreting the very different underlying meanings of the phase 'Would you like' is virtually impossible. She also tells of the day the vicar rang. 'Is your mother there?' he asked Ros, who had picked up the phone. 'Yes,' she said, immediately replacing the receiver. 'I thought he was just interested in where you were' was her explanation to her mother for such apparently rude behaviour.

Colin, a young man with mild learning difficulties, had not been diagnosed as having autism until he was over eighteen. Relationships within the family were greatly strained because 'he never did anything he was told'. For example, if asked to take a towel (clearly meant for the bathroom) upstairs, he would infuriate the family by simply leaving it on the top stair; if told to get something from the kitchen he would go and find it but then fail to return to the person needing it; if sent to ask his mother if she wanted a cup of tea he would deliver the message but not the answer. On one occasion, when asked to post a letter to a family friend, he spent all day travelling across London to take the letter to the friend's house. Whilst his mother was much distressed by what seemed to be deliberate provocation, his father openly ridiculed him for his 'stupidity' and 'ignorance'.

Literalness

A further difficulty associated with poor comprehension – and one that continues to cause problems well into adulthood – is the tendency to interpret what is said very literally. Take, for example, the incident cited by Wendy Lawson (1998): ' "Hop on the couch for a minute while I talk to mum," says the doctor. After hopping up and down on the couch for exactly one minute, I tell the doctor his time is up!'

Sama got into trouble on her first day at college for venturing onto a nearby building site. Students had been explicitly told not to go there alone because it was potentially very dangerous. However, as Sama had seen workmen on the site she assumed that she was not alone and that therefore her presence there was allowed. On a more serous note, Chris, a young man who had also just started college, became so distressed when one of the other students, obviously joking, threatened to 'kill him' after a slight argument that he refused to return. Eleanor, on being taken to London for the first time by her parents, began screaming and throwing herself on the floor at the bottom of a store escalator. Her parents could not understand this as she usually loved escalators, and she was very keen to get up to the toy department. Unfortunately the sign at the bottom of the escalator read 'Prams must be carried', and Eleanor did not have a pram! David, who was on a work experience placement was warned by his exasperated boss: 'You do that once again . . . !' and promptly repeated his action. Similarly, when Jake accidentally dropped and broke a cup his father remarked sarcastically 'Why don't you smash the lot' – which Jake immediately did. One young woman, Faith, who had been attending a special class in art at her local college, was asked not to come back after allegedly deliberately destroying a floral display. Knowing that she was usually extremely careful and reliable, her key worker investigated further. It appeared that the tutor had instructed the class to paint the flowers on display, and Faith had done exactly that! Another young man, attending a long- awaited interview for a residential placement, was clearly unhappy with the seating arrangements. When the principal suggested 'You can have my chair if you like', he sat down in it immediately, although the occupant had not yet had time to move. In Chapter 7 the example is also given of a young teenager who got into serious trouble at school for refusing to cooperate in maths lessons. In particular, he had become very upset at being asked to measure the area of tarmac in the playground. His reason for not doing so was that tarmac could only be measured by its *volume*. Lorna Wing recounts the tale of her daughter, who was told that, on their next holiday to

France, she would be 'going to sleep on the train'. Thinking that she would be delighted by such a novel experience no one could understand her distress at this news. It was only when they rephrased the explanation to 'going to *bed in* the train' that they realised the original message had been totally misinterpreted.

This literal response to language can also make individuals sound very abrupt or even rude at times. Eric, having just enrolled in college, was asked by his new tutor when his birthday was. He looked at her with incomprehension and replied with scorn, 'Well, every year of course!'

Problems with spoken language

Although many aspects of spoken language improve as individuals grow older – especially in the case of those of higher intellectual ability – other, more subtle, deficits tend to persist and may continue to pervade many aspects of linguistic functioning.

Intonation and delivery

In many cases the very stilted, mechanical, almost robotic quality of speech that characterises the delivery of younger children diminishes somewhat with time. However, there is considerable variation here, and some people continue to have poorly modulated speech which can be difficult to understand or interpret. Neville is a forty-year-old man living in semi-sheltered accommodation who, because of staffing problems, has taken on a considerable amount of responsibility in the organisation of the house where he lives. Many of his views on how the other residents can make their lives more comfortable or get a better deal from the housing association involved have proved very constructive. The problem is that his tone of voice is unremittingly querulous and somewhat aggressive. This frequently leads to resentment amongst both residents and care workers – and to the rejection of his often sensible proposals.

A 'flat', poorly modulated voice can also give other people a mistaken impression of an individual's general level of competence. Peter, for example, is a young man of normal intellectual ability who has obtained a number of GCSE qualifications over the years. Through his attendance on a part-time art history course he also has interesting and informative views on art and drawing. However, the slowness of his delivery, and the time he takes to find the 'right' words to express himself, tends to make him sound both unintelligent and boring, although in fact he is neither. Even his mother admits, 'You have to drag everything out of him' and 'It's like watching the cogs go round in his head, seeing him trying to come up with the right answer.'

Even the accents acquired by people with autism can lead to difficulties. Many never seem to recognise the importance of 'fitting in' with their peer group, and may continue to speak in a very difficult style or accent regardless of the social pressures. This can be a particular problem for adolescents, who fail to appreciate that not adopting the same style of speech as their peers is very likely to result in bullying, teasing or rejection.

Semantic problems

Although the vocabulary of some people with autism continues to remain limited, many do show considerable improvements in their expressive skills over time. Nevertheless they may continue to experience problems in finding the correct form of words to express their ideas so that what is said can appear slightly 'odd' or out of place. Jenny, for example, had once been told by a teacher that she should try to avoid repetition and use more variety in her written work. She then adapted this to her spoken language, and would never use a simple word if a more unusual one existed. Events would be described as 'melancholy' rather than 'sad'; people as 'amicable' rather than 'friendly'; places as 'repellent' rather than 'nasty'. Although the words were not incorrect, they made her speech sound slightly absurd and certainly far too formal. Johnny, whose use of English had also been corrected at school, began to correct others in the same way, becoming extremely agitated if anyone used 'me' instead of 'I' or 'should' instead of 'would' etc., and would continually interrupt conversations with his corrections.

The way in which words are used may also be out of keeping with an individual's age, social group or family background. Giles was frequently taunted by his brothers and peers for his use of terms such as 'spiffing' or 'jolly good show'. He appeared to have picked these up from boys' comics produced in the 1950s and early 1960s, but he had no awareness of the fact that they now belonged to a totally different era. Similarly, Asperger (see Frith 1991) described one individual as sounding like 'a caricature of a degenerate aristocrat' because of his over-formal and pedantic style of speech and his 'high, slightly nasal, and drawn-out' voice. Such problems are not necessarily restricted to those of higher ability. Gareth, a young man of seventeen with mild to moderate learning difficulties, was asked what he did with his small amount of weekly pocket money. Somewhat disconcertingly he replied solemnly: 'I spend all my allowance on confectionery or comestibles.'

Whilst having a superior vocabulary might, on the surface, appear to be an advantage rather than a handicap, for individuals who already have difficulties in 'fitting in' or being accepted any unusual aspects to the way in which they speak can easily exacerbate existing problems. Josh, a young teenager who had moved to a new comprehensive school, was so bullied and teased by his peers for his 'posh voice and big words' that teachers actually became anxious for his physical safety. Moreover, whilst an unusual vocabulary is often a sign of superior intelligence in the general population, in autism this is not necessarily the case, and may again give a deceptive impression of an individual's true level of understanding.

Echolalic speech

Echolalia, both immediate and delayed, is a common characteristic of the language of people with autism. Although it is often viewed as inappropriate and non-communicative, studies by Barry Prizant and his co-workers (Rydell and Prizant 1995, Rydell and Mirenda 1994) have been influential in illustrating the functional nature of much echolalia. They have shown that echoing, particularly in older and less cognitively impaired individuals, frequently serves identifiable and important functions. Thus, it may be used to indicate a lack of comprehension, for self-regulation and rehearsal, or as a direct but simplified form of communication. Echolalia is also more likely to occur when individuals are stressed, anxious or in highly constraining situations. In many cases, too, echolalia is an important precursor to more creative and rule-governed language. As with any other 'autistic' behaviour, therefore, it is crucial to assess the role that the echolalia plays for the individual concerned before any attempts are made to modify it.

A particular problem associated with echolalia is that speech copied from other people may lead to serious overestimates of an individual's true level of competence. Although some adults may continue to echo at a very simple level, others develop much more complex and in many ways contextually appropriate forms of repetitive speech. Micky, for example, who had left school some months earlier, was asked by a visitor if he had heard anything of his former headmaster. There then ensued a lengthy monologue, which the questioner eventually recognised as the repetition of a radio interview in which the headmaster had been speaking about the problems of children with autism. The interviewer's questions and the head's replies were all faithfully reproduced. Micky had certainly replied to the question, but not in quite the way expected nor in the most efficient manner. Sarah, when asked if she had any problems conversing with those she met socially (she was an avid swimmer and met many people in this context), said this was no problem for her. When she was a teenager her parents had deliberately coached her in the most appropriate ways to engage visitors in conversation, and since the family entertained a great deal she received considerable practice in this. However, difficulties arose when the early stages of the conversation had passed and she was then expected to develop, or expand on, more socially complex themes for which rote leaning was of little use. Adrian, who was seen by an occupational psychologist for a job skills assessment, so impressed her by his sophisticated use of language that she became convinced that earlier reports of his social and learning difficulties must be mistaken. Despite warnings from his school teachers of the problems that could occur if his abilities were overestimated, he was sent on a work experience placement that demanded far greater social and intellectual competence than he was capable of.

Repetitive use of language

Repetitive language may occur for a variety of reasons: it may be the individual's only effective way of making contact with others; it may be deliberately attention-seeking; it may be caused by anxiety or insecurity; it may be linked to an individual's obsessions and routines; or it may be associated with a combination of these factors. Whatever the underlying origins, however, speech of this kind can lead to considerable problems either because it tends to disrupt ordinary social exchanges or because of the annoyance it causes to others.

Dominic, a young man attending a day centre, had very limited-phrase speech, but nevertheless caused considerable disruption there by repeating certain phrases to other clients or members of staff. None of these was particularly offensive: he might say one client's name in a certain way, repeat the title of a television serial to another, accuse another of liking a particular politician or TV star or tell another that they would be having semolina for lunch. The use of these phrases, no matter how innocuous they may have appeared to outsiders, was clearly deliberately calculated to irritate the individuals concerned. Even staff admitted to 'getting very wound up' by this, and several of the clients had actually hit him, but the attention he received was more than enough to ensure that the behaviour persisted.

Other people with autism, especially those whose language skills are poor, show high levels of repetitive speech in situations in which they are unsure or anxious. Any potential changes, or the occurrence of situations that they do not like, can provoke persistent questions, repetitions or even self-admonishments: 'Not going to go swimming on Thursday?', 'Not going to kick grandma', 'Going to see mummy and daddy?' are typical of the types of utterances that may be repeated over and over again and which, though harmless in themselves, can be very wearing for people living or working with them. Lydia constantly asked everyone she met throughout the day if she could go in the minivan to fetch petrol on Friday. If the answer were 'No' or 'Don't know' she would become very distressed. If it were 'Yes' she would continually ask when she could go. Persistent questioning about birthdays, makes of cars or bus and train routes can also become very tedious, as can constant seeking reassurance. Carol had been on numerous work experience placements, all of which had broken down because of her need for continuous guidance. A simple task, such as sealing envelopes, would require repeated assurances that she had done it correctly and even the most sympathetic of supervisors rapidly became exasperated.

Even if direct questioning is not involved, constant repetition of the same phrases can prove very irritating for listeners. Maria, a young woman in her mid-twenties, goes through phases of using particular utterances which are said to 'drive her family mad', the current one being, for some reason, 'unsecured floating-rate loan stock'.

Repetitive speech can also disrupt attempts to foster more normal conversation. Chris, a young man with a history of placement breakdowns, proved very difficult to help because his conversation was entirely dominated by complaints about the wrong done to him during the previous placement, interspersed with questions about the relative sizes of London hospitals.

Lydia, an outgoing and chatty woman who longed for friends, would start off conversations well enough but then launch into lengthy monologues about her favourite topic – potatoes. Even if the topic of interest seems to be rather more socially 'promising' it can still prove difficult to develop the conversation much further. Owen, for example, was a young man who appeared to know everything possible about Welsh rugby teams. He knew all the important players, past and present; the positions they played; and the scores of previous matches. However, if asked a simple question about which teams would be playing the next weekend he was often quite unable to answer and insisted instead on talking about games gone by.

As they grow older some individuals are able to learn to control this constant repetition or questioning, particularly if they realise that it is likely to reduce their chances of making friends or can lead to teasing or bullying. Nineteen-year-old Sally had had an obsession with the singer Edith Piaf since she was very young, but had gradually learned to talk less and less about her. She knew the topic tended to irritate other students at college, and although she admitted that she 'still really wanted to talk about her all the time' had learned to suppress her obsession as far as possible. Nevertheless, certain triggers continued to set her off, despite her good intentions. In particular, any mention of the number forty-nine (the age at which Piaf died) would result in an explosion of questions again, often to individuals who had never even heard of the singer.

Neologisms

Idiosyncratic or made-up words generally seem to be less in evidence in adulthood than they are in younger children. As they grow older many people come to recognise the 'silliness' of these words or phrases and may become quite embarrassed if other people mention them. If neologisms are maintained these are often kept as a sort of 'family joke' and tend to be rarely used in public. Ros Blackburn, mentioned above, now jokes about the time when she used the phrase 'little glacien jars' to describe anything made from glass. The utterance had originally arisen from a little glass jar in which she kept a small piece of her toy tiger's tail! As a child she used numerous convoluted utterances of this kind, but now the only one remaining is 'flappy' which is used to describe the pieces of paper or cardboard that she continues to hoard.

'Bluntness'

A major problem for many people with autism as they grow older results not so much from the actual words they use as from the ways in which they use them. This is closely interwoven with their lack of appreciation of social rules and their failure to understand the impact of what they say on others. For people with a knowledge of autism such remarks are unlikely to give offence. However, for strangers, particularly if the individual concerned possesses a good vocabulary and has no obvious learning difficulties, such remarks can appear at the very least insensitive and at worst extremely offensive. A few examples here should suffice to illustrate these problems.

In the course of my own clinical work, patients often remark on my somewhat small stature. Indeed, one young woman always refers to me simply as 'Little Doctor'. Another individual, who had grown considerably since I had last seen him, announced: 'I think your desk has shrunk since I was last here . . . and I think you may have too.' Another young woman said nothing about my size during my interview with her, although I knew she was particularly interested in people's weights and heights. As she left she remarked loudly, 'I think I must have grown taller today,' and then announced proudly to her key worker: 'There, I didn't say anything about how little she is!'

Similar comments in other circumstances may be viewed with less approval. Notions of political correctness, in particular, are often difficult for people with autism to grasp. Damien, attending an employment preparation course, was soon under threat of suspension because of comments about his supervisor. Having previously been taught by men, he was obviously surprised to find that his new supervisor was a young Asian woman. He was constantly remarking on her colour, race and gender, and although this was not done in any negative way, his remarks were considered totally unacceptable. Jason, a young man in his late teens, alienated all his sister's friends after one of them had a baby by someone she had met on holiday in Jamaica. Jason was fascinated by the child's skin colouring and repeatedly questioned its mother about whether or not she had realised that she would have 'a half-white baby' as well as lecturing her on the perils of single motherhood. He also kept urging her to have the baby checked 'as it probably has AIDS'. Jonas, another young man who was usually very well mannered, horrified his mother at a large social gathering by approaching a very small, elderly, white-haired woman with large ears and protruding teeth and asking politely 'Excuse me, but are you a rabbit?'

Dealing with abstract concepts

Talking about the future

Abstract or hypothetical concepts are frequently a source of particular difficulty for people with autism. Even vague or uncertain responses to questions, such as 'Soon', 'Perhaps' or 'I'll think about it' can give rise to immense anxiety, since the individual has no real information on whether or when something will happen. Irony, too, can give rise to major problems and will almost certainly result in confusion and misunderstandings.

The ability to deal with events that are due to happen in the future is also affected. Even if the individual seems to understand the explanations given, or appears to comply with plans for his or her future, a real understanding of what is to happen may be woefully lacking. David, a young man with autism and severe learning difficulties, was to be transferred to a new group home in the community. Great efforts had been made by his key worker to explain what would be happening; he had been involved in the plans for decorating his new bedroom and he had visited the house on a number of occasions, spending increasing periods of time there. However, when the day of the move came it was clear that he still had little understanding that this was to be his permanent home, After several hours he re-packed his case and attempted to leave, becoming terribly distressed when prevented from doing so. Max, who had agreed to a divorce from his wife after several years of unhappy marriage, went through all the legal procedures quite calmly. However, it was only when the decree finally came through that he realised he actually had to leave the house and could no longer continue living there.

Talking about feelings or emotions

The failure to understand abstract concepts also affects the ability to talk about feelings or emotions, or even physical pain. A number of cases have been reported of individuals with autism who have become seriously ill with tooth abscesses, infections, even appendicitis, without being able to indicate that they were in pain. This inability to explain how they are feeling, coupled with a possible lowered sensitivity to pain (Biersdorff 1994), can have serious implications. The problem is obviously most marked in individuals who have severe learning difficulties and little or no speech. For example, in a study by Gunsett and colleagues (1989), nine out of twelve residents living in an institution who had developed severe behavioural problems in adulthood were found to have undiagnosed medical conditions including fractures, urinary tract infections and toxic levels of anticonvulsants.

Emotional or psychiatric disturbance may be even more difficult to convey, and the ways in which language difficulties can disrupt normal diagnostic processes or lead to a failure to obtain appropriate help are described in further detail in Chapter 10.

Humour

Perhaps surprisingly, given their concrete language and thought processes, humour is something that can be enjoyed by many people with autism. Admittedly, their sense of humour may be somewhat unsubtle, and appreciation of comedy is often restricted to the slapstick, but jokes, puns and riddles can also be enjoyed. Werth *et al.* (2001), for example, describe the case of a young woman with autism called Grace living in a residential home for people with intellectual impairments. She made frequent use of puns, word play, neologisms, nonsense naming, jokes and riddles to entertain those around her. These devices were also used to tease other people or to 'get her own back' on someone who had annoyed her. In addition, she used them as a surreptitious outlet for her obsessional interest in war and weaponry (which she was otherwise discouraged from talking about). For example: 'Tank you very much', 'What weather we have had here! It is so strong the air it is an air force'. What happens if a boa constrictor argues with another boa constrictor? You get a boar war.' 'I was glad to get back ack ack flack.' Van Bourgondien and Mesibov (1987), in their studies of the humorous responses of adults with autism also report frequent use of riddles and simple jokes, which clearly resulted in considerable enjoyment for all concerned. Indeed, the TEACCH social skills programme incorporates joke sessions into the timetable, and these are considered to play an important role in encouraging positive social interactions. Autistic humour may give rise to difficulties, however, if jokes are socially zinappropriate or so repetitive that they become a source of irritation to others.

Lack of reciprocity

Although people with autism may exhibit many of the problems noted above to a greater or lesser degree, the overriding problem, for almost everyone, and at whatever linguistic level they function, is the lack of reciprocity in their language: their failure to engage in normal conversations, to listen to other people's points of view, or to 'chat' simply for the pleasure of doing so. This does not mean that they do not wish to take part in conversations. On the contrary, as they grow older, many people with autism become almost desperately keen to interact with others and to be accepted by them. However, they are rarely able to engage in the often inconsequential 'chit-chat' that is so important for normal social interactions; they often have little or no interest in the other person's views and may be quite unaware of cues indicating that they are becoming boring, disrupting ongoing discussions or dominating the conversation in an unacceptable way. This lack of reciprocity, and the failure to appreciate the 'two-way' nature of conversation, is very evident in more intellectually handicapped individuals, who may tend to bombard almost anyone they meet with stereotyped questions or phrases, frequently regardless of the answers they receive.

However, the problems can be equally disruptive in individuals who are verbally and intellectually much more able. Stephen, a young man with superficially good language skills, would launch into lengthy diatribes on the potential dangers of the Channel Tunnel whenever the opportunity arose, often disrupting family gatherings or outings because of this. Fred, a twenty-year-old whose family entertained a lot, prided himself on his conversational skills and claimed that he had no problems meeting people or making friends. His parents had tried to stop him from 'barging into conversations' by persuading him not to speak until someone introduced a topic relevant to his overriding interest in computers. This helped to make his comments rather more relevant, but even so he would often misinterpret what had been said. Someone's innocent comment about fish and chips, for example, could launch him into intricate descriptions about the internal workings of the latest computers. Even if the ongoing discussion were related to computers he would then completely dominate the conversation until people moved off in boredom or embarrassment. However, because he did manage to talk to lots of different people in this way, and because no one wanted to be directly rude to him, he remained convinced of his excellent conversational skills.

What can be done to help?

As is apparent from the follow-up studies reviewed in Chapter 2, difficulties related to speech and understanding generally persist throughout adulthood, even in the most able of individuals. Other research also indicates that impairments in communication are both central and fundamental to the disorder. Hence any approaches to intervention in this area are likely to have their limitations. Nevertheless there are many different strategies that can be used to enhance communicative functioning in adulthood, even in individuals who have little or no spoken language, and intervention can be crucial in helping them to develop more effective ways of expressing their needs or to better understand what is happening around them. (For useful reviews of communication interventions in autism – though mostly involving young children – see Goldstein 2002, Koegel 2000, Lord 2000, Schuler and Fletcher 2002.)

Increasing understanding and decreasing inappropriate speech

As with any successful intervention programme, the development of appropriate strategies relies on understanding the underlying reasons for the behaviours involved and recognition of the functions that they may serve for the individual concerned. Thus many of the communication problems described above, such as apparent lack of cooperation or repetitive and stereotyped questioning, may result from a failure to understand what is required, a misinterpretation or anxieties about what is likely to happen.

Helping to improve others' communication skills

In many instances cooperation can be significantly improved if the individual is given greater help to understand what is required. However, this may well require a change of focus onto the ways in which *other people* communicate rather than on the person with autism. The situation between Colin and his father, described above, was greatly helped, firstly, by the family's realisation that his understanding was much more limited than had been previously thought and, secondly, by his father being given advice on how to make his own speech much more specific and in particular to avoid complex, abstract or ambiguous instructions. For example, it was often necessary to split apparently simple commands into separate components. Thus asking him to 'Take the towel upstairs and then put it in the bathroom' avoided the possibility of Colin simply dumping the towel on the top stair. Telling him to 'Ask your mother if she wants a cup of tea and then come and tell me what she said' improved his ability to take messages. Instructions such as: 'Go to the kitchen, look for a knife in the drawer and then bring it back here to me' significantly increased the chances of family members obtaining the items they needed.

Similarly, if anger or distress occur when new activities or events are suggested, then it may well be that the intended message is being misinterpreted in some way and will need to be conveyed in a different form. Sometimes this can be relatively easy, and may simply require a restructuring of what has been said. Explaining to someone that he or she is to go 'to bed in the train' rather than 'sleep on the train' may remove any number of unknown and frightening images. Many unforeseen problems can arise over the literal interpretation of what is said, and hence care needs to be taken to establish what the source of the confusion is and then to remedy this. Peter's mother began to have great trouble with him when they were out in the car, as he would attack her whenever they stopped. Eventually it was realised that the problems occurred because if she said 'We're going to see Auntie Jean' he would expect to go straight there and became very angry if they had to stop en route for traffic lights, pedestrians or other drivers. The problem was dealt with by helping him first to tolerate brief and predictable stops and later with more frequent and unpredictable ones. Thus she began by saying, before they set off: 'We are going to Auntie Jean's, but we will stop at the traffic lights on the way' (though she would stop at the lights even if they were green). Peter accepted this without difficulty, and his mother then began to predict more stops (e.g. at the corner by the pub or opposite the paper shop), which again were readily tolerated. The next stage was to tell him, before they left, that they would stop somewhere on the way but that she would not tell him where. He would then have to try and guess where this would be. Turning the trips into a guessing game in this way, and at the same time making it clear that a specified trip would require additional stops, quickly reduced his 'aggressive' behaviour.

Removing uncertainty

As noted above, lack of understanding may be a primary cause of obsessional speech. Asking questions is a natural way to gain information, but if the answers supplied are not understood then the questioning will tend to continue. Sometimes rephrasing the reply may be enough, but more often information may need to be supplied in an alternative and non-verbal form. Visual information is often far more powerful than verbal messages alone. Thus photographs of places that are to be visited, people who are to be met, activities that are to be followed, can prove much more effective than words alone (Krantz and McClannahan 1998). In many instances, once the information is understood, repetitive questioning can be greatly reduced. Moreover, if an individual continues to seek reassurance in this way, they can be guided to look at the pictures (or written instructions etc.) for information rather than remaining dependent on direct, verbal assurance.

Again, although particularly important when dealing with less able or non-verbal individuals, such aids can prove surprisingly effective in helping those of higher ability to deal with complex or abstract situations. Patrick became very anxious when he started a college placement and was constantly asking his parents, the college staff, other students or whoever happened to be close by where he should be at every hour of the day. This behaviour was a source of considerable irritation, and Patrick's anxiety was not lessened by the answers he received as he then worried that his informant 'could have got it wrong'. Eventually he was supplied with a Filofax diary, and with the help of the special needs tutor this was filled in on an hourly basis, with each entry indicating where he should be at any time of the day. He was reminded to look in his diary every time the anxious questioning began and eventually his reliance on the written information reduced his need for verbal reassurance and guidance.

Reducing attention for inappropriate speech

Although repetitive and obsessional speech is frequently used to gain attention, and although traditional behavioural techniques, such as time out or extinction, can usually be very successful in reducing attention-seeking behaviours, this is often not the case with verbal routines. Ignoring someone who is spinning a piece of cloth, lining up bricks or making long trails of coins around the house is relatively simple and, if carried out consistently, can prove remarkably effective. However, with verbal obsessions it is all too easy for other people to become part of the repetitive pattern without their even realising that this is happening.

Richard's principal obsession was with quiz games, and he was able, with quite remarkable skill to turn around almost any question asked of him into a response related to quiz games. A remark about his new jumper would elicit a reply about its similarity to one worn by a recent quiz contestant; a comment on the weather would be immediately associated with a question he had been able to answer the previous week; even if he were told off for doing something unacceptable at home he would begin to talk of the 'rules' of various programmes and how contestants sometimes flouted these. His obsession was thus being constantly and unwittingly reinforced by others, despite their attempts to try to reduce it.

Even if family members are able to avoid responding to obsessional themes themselves, visitors may well act differently, and the intermittent reinforcement of behaviours in this way is a particularly powerful way of maintaining them. Jeff, for example, had a passion for politics and in brief interactions could actually be very interesting and informative. Constant exposure to political debate, however, became increasingly irritating for his family, and eventually they decided that the only way to cope was to ignore his political comments totally. Although this resulted in a reduction of the behaviour at home, whenever visitors came, or when he met people outside, his favourite topic of conversation would be unwittingly reinforced once more.

In another case, Jerry's mother had managed to reduce his swearing at home to a reasonably low level by ensuring that she, her husband and his sister ignore it. Although this had proved very difficult for them initially, over the years they had become quite expert and established firm control over the problem. However, whenever his grandmother came to the house the swearing would instantly increase. She refused to tolerate this behaviour, gave him lengthy lectures whenever it occurred, scolded her son and daughter-in-law for allowing it and generally afforded Jerry great satisfaction. The only other situation in which the problem was just as difficult to control was on the bus, whenever he sat within earshot of other elderly women!

Setting rules

A more effective approach – but one which needs to be established from the earliest years – is to lay down explicit 'rules' as to when, where, how often or with whom such speech can be used. If children can be taught, from an early age, that talk about particular topics is only allowed with certain people, in certain situations, at a certain time of day, or for a specified period, it is much easier to minimise the disruption that it can cause. At the same time, knowledge that such talk will be allowed, at least at certain times or in particular situations, reduces the anxiety that tends to erupt if the behaviours are banned altogether. Although it is possible to impose such limitations on older people, if the habit has been well established for many years it will be much more difficult to deal with than if appropriate steps had been taken in childhood. However, this requires that parents be given early help, by the professionals involved in their child's care, to identify the stage at which behaviours may be becoming a problem and, most importantly, that they be provided with practical advice and support to enable them to intervene effectively.

It is also necessary to be aware that communication patterns that are acceptable in childhood may become less acceptable as the individual grows older. Repetitive questioning about Thomas the Tank Engine, for example, may not seem too inappropriate for a five-year-old but would certainly be considered very abnormal for someone in late adolescence. Similarly, whilst informing complete strangers all about one's private life, or asking them intimate personal questions, can seem quite amusing in a three-year-old, in a thirteen-year-old it may sound impertinent and in a thirty-year-old quite threatening. Thus, intervention may be needed even before the behaviour becomes a problem – a balance that, without adequate support, may be very difficult for families to achieve.

Moreover, although the need to establish consistent rules regarding appropriate and inappropriate topics of conversation cannot be over-emphasised, rules of this kind can also have their drawbacks. Normal social communication is regulated by highly subtle, complex and ill-defined influences and attempts to apply concrete (and hence often inflexible) guidelines, although helpful in certain situations, may backfire in others. Ronnie's parents decided, as he grew older, that they must stop him from approaching strangers and asking them questions (usually about distances or directions). He was told firmly that he must never talk to people whom he did not know in the street and, on the whole, this rule proved very effective. As he grew more independent, however, he began to travel about on his own, and on one occasion failed to return after a train journey. When he finally arrived home, late at night and obviously very distressed, it emerged that he had accidentally got off at the wrong stop and become hopelessly lost. When his parents asked why he had not asked anyone the way, he replied: 'Because you told me not to!'.

Rules can also backfire for other reasons. Laurie was a young man working in a voluntary capacity for a large charity. He was a calendrical calculator, able to work out accurately, within seconds, on what day of the year any date would fall (see also Hermelin 2001). His favourite pastime was to ask people when their birthday was and then tell them what day of the week it fell on and announce how old they were. Although amusing initially, his constant questioning soon became a source of irritation for the people at work, and it was agreed that he should restrict his questions about birthdays to one per day. Usually he would ask the first person he met in the morning when their birthday was, but on one day, when the charity's royal patron was visiting, Laurie was unusually silent. Finally the royal visitor arrived, and Laurie had been chosen as one of the people to greet her. After politely shaking her hand, he immediately asked his daily question!

Recognising the importance of obsessional speech

Whatever strategies are implemented, it should be recognised that repetitive or obsessional speech may be one of the few resources that someone with autism may have to occupy his or her time, to fill in the many hours of solitude, to reduce anxiety or deal with potentially troubling situations; it may, too, be the individual's only way of making verbal contact with other people. To deny someone the opportunity of talking about their special topics at all, unless these can somehow be replaced with alternative and more socially effective conversational skills, is not acceptable. Indeed, attempts to do so may well prove counterproductive, leading to an upsurge in anxiety and, in turn, to

even higher levels of repetitive speech. As with other ritualistic behaviours, therefore, the aim should be to modify such talk to the extent
to which it is no longer disruptive whilst at the same time retaining
any potential benefits.

Repetitive and stereotyped speech patterns may, of course, stem
from a variety of other causes. First, it should be remembered that in
early language learning, repetition and echolalia play a crucial role in
helping children to consolidate what they hear and, as well as enhancing understanding, provide the opportunity to practise new words or
expressions. For adults with limited language skills, repetition may
continue to serve an important function and should not automatically
be discouraged.

Second, repetition is, for all of us, an important factor in rehearsing
potentially worrying situations, in dealing with feelings of anger or in
helping to allay anxiety. How many of us will repeatedly practise what
we are going to say to someone the next day if we know that a difficult
situation is likely to occur or a personal problem needs to be resolved?
If things do not go as planned, who has not gone over and over what
they should have said, or rehearsed cutting and witty remarks that
could have been used to devastate an opponent? In fearful situations,
who has not continually reassured themself that their fears are ground-
less; or tried to persuade themself, for example, that the noises heard
on the stairs in the dead of night are caused by the cat or a creaking
floorboard, rather than admitting to their real fears? Stuck in a traffic
jam while the deadline for arriving at the station or airport draws
perilously close, are we not likely to check the time repeatedly, even
though we know this only too well? Autistic people also do all these
things. Their problem is not that the behaviours are unusual but that
they are not carried out silently, in their heads, as is usually the case for
the rest of us. Understanding *why* such behaviours may occur, recognising the normality – indeed the importance – of them, may well help
others to be more accepting. Greater understanding may also suggest
alternative intervention strategies. For example, desensitisation to feared
situations or the teaching of relaxation techniques may be a more
appropriate way of dealing with the problem of constant repetition than
ignoring or 'time out', which might well exacerbate the situation. Help
with anger management may also be more productive, and techniques
developed for use with individuals with other forms of learning disabilities may prove useful here (Clements and Zarkowska 2000). Alternatively, allowing the individual concerned to rehearse and practise the
most effective ways of dealing with anxiety-provoking situations – but
in a controlled way, facilitated by others – can also prove effective.

Finally, as indicated below, providing permanent and concrete information through pictures, written instructions or other cues may also help to clarify situations when verbal instructions alone are inadequate, again reducing the need for stereotyped speech or repetitive questioning.

Teaching alternative skills

One of the particular advantages of ritualistic or stereotyped forms of speech is that they avoid the need to develop different ways of greeting people and, in turn, cause others' responses to be much more predictable. Asking someone about the make of car they drive, for example, results in a much more restricted set of responses than open questions about his or her health, job or family. Stereotyped questions of this nature can reduce uncertainty and the risk of being questioned about unfamiliar topics. Thus, whilst offering the opportunity to indulge in obsessional interests, they also allow the individual to maintain much greater control over social interactions.

If ritualistic or inappropriate conversational routines are to be reduced, the autistic person will need additional help to develop more effective strategies. Role play, social skills groups and drama classes can all be helpful in teaching more appropriate conversational skills, and research indicates that such interventions can be helpful for people of very different levels of ability (Mesibov 1984). For the more handicapped, learning how to shake someone's hand, to say hello and to introduce themselves by name may have a great impact on how they are perceived by others. Teaching at higher levels of ability is obviously much more complex, since attention needs to be directed towards so many different social issues. Once the early stages of introduction are over, the scope for conversational development becomes so wide that it can be very difficult to offer detailed guidelines on how to proceed. However, helping individuals to develop better listening skills and the ability to pick up obvious signs of interest or boredom in others, helping them to develop conversational strategies around the news, films, TV programmes, sport, music etc., can all be valuable. The TEACCH programme of Gary Mesibov and his colleagues offers helpful advice in this area, and there are a number of other social communication programmes available that can be used to guide teaching. The social skills manual of Spence (1991) or the visual strategies recommended by Hodgdon (1996), though devised for children, can be readily adapted to enhance communication skills in adults. Whatever programmes are used, instructions needs to be very basic, concrete and highly specific and visually based strategies are particularly important (Klin *et al.* 2000). Role-play techniques can prove very effective, and feedback from audio or video recordings can help to improve conversational exchanges generally or more specific behaviours, such as tone of voice or speed of delivery (Howlin and Yates 1999).

The appropriate generalisation of newly taught skills, however, may give rise to problems. Ina van Berckelaer-Onnes, who conducts social skills training in Holland, recounts how she had been encouraging one of her students to use compliments when talking to other people. Learning how to comment positively on the colour or style of people's clothes or hair were skills much practised. Finally, one student reported excitedly that he had met a girl at a dance and had put the lessons to good use. 'What did you say to her?' asked his tutor. 'I told her how much I liked her dress and what a lovely colour it was'. 'Great . . . and what next?' prompted the tutor. 'Well, then I told her how it exactly matched her gums' was the disarming reply.

Talking about emotions and dealing with abstract concepts

A major problem for almost everyone with autism is the ability to talk about or fully to understand abstract concepts, such as feelings or emotions or even pain. Even individuals of normal intellectual and verbal ability continue to show specific deficits in areas related to the deciphering and labelling of emotions (Hobson 2002, Stanford 2003). Unless help can be provided to improve these skills, coping with physical, emotional or psychiatric problems in later life can present many difficulties. Again, the best solution seems to be to start young. Simon Baron-Cohen and colleagues (see Howlin *et al.* 1998) have shown that after only a few sessions of teaching, children with autism aged between four and nine years of age can be taught to understand and use mental-state terms related to other people's beliefs and emotions. Whilst this work was restricted to largely experimental settings, the fact that even brief training was effective suggests that more prolonged input might well result in substantial improvements in this area of communication and understanding. More recently Baron-Cohen has produced an interactive DVD that focuses on talking about and 'reading' emotions, and this can be very helpful across the age range – from young children to adults (including university students).

Work with more severely disabled individuals also indicates that, even within this group, people can learn to express simple emotional concepts if given appropriate help. Pictures, photographs, audio or video tapes have all been used to help people decipher emotional states and to explain why certain situations arouse different feelings (Quirk-Hodgson 1995). Teaching people to label emotions in structured, albeit somewhat artificial settings, may then help when they need to express their own feelings. Lorraine, a young woman with cerebral palsy as well as autism, was confined to a wheelchair throughout the day. Although generally relaxed, at times she would come to her day centre clearly feeling frustrated, angry or miserable. Beginning initially with photographs of happy, sad or angry faces, she has learned to identify these emotions and to match them to situations that might provoke them. Subsequently, using a picture board portraying a wider variety of expressions, she has been taught to label emotions in different contexts, taken from photographs or stories in books. She is also encouraged to point each day to the face that best expresses her current mood and appears to do this with some reliability. It is now hoped to introduce a more complex set of 'emotional faces' in order to allow greater scope for expression. Figure 4.1 shows an example of the types of 'emotion boards' that have been used in other situations to enable people with learning disabilities to express their moods and

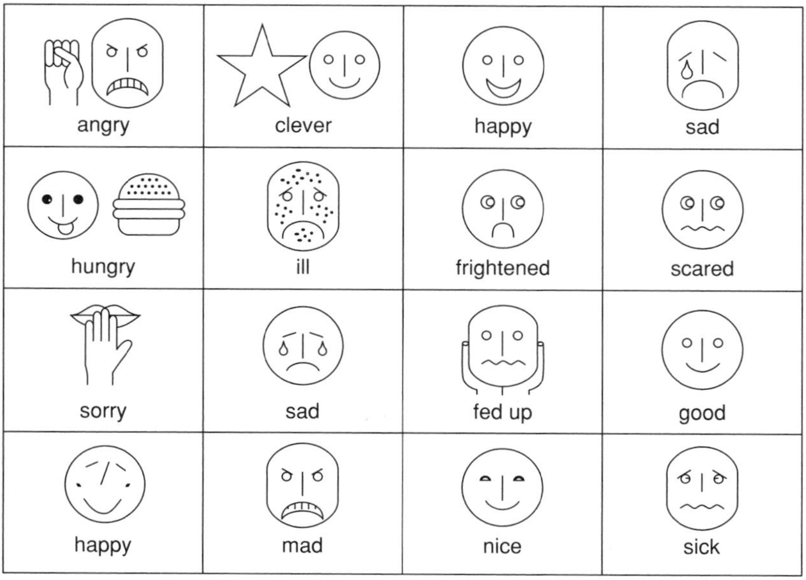

Figure 4.1 Communication board for identifying emotions
Source: Gaboney 1993

feelings more effectively. Although this may be too complex for some people with autism, it can be modified to suit a range of different abilities. There are now also many computerised programmes available to aid emotional labelling and recognition that can be used with individuals with intellectual impairments.

Unfortunately, help of this kind is often provided much too late in life for it to have a significant impact on people's ability to understand and express their emotions effectively. More attention to helping young children with autism in these areas could greatly improve their social-communication skills as adults and offer much greater chances of success. Many autistic children, for example, will spend hours watching videos of Disney cartoons or stories such as Thomas the Tank Engine, in which the characters tend to be highly stereotyped and actions and responses very repetitive and predictable. Because they relate in a very simplified way to specific events and situations, such materials can be extremely effective in helping children with autism to appreciate that there are such things as emotions, to learn the names of these, and to help them talk about feelings of happiness, anger, sadness, pain or jealousy themselves.

Developing communication skills in less able individuals

Although there are many texts available on the teaching of communication skills to people with autism (see Quill 1995a) the majority of these have focused on young children rather than adults. In adulthood the acquisition of novel, complex and spontaneous communication skills tends to be limited. This is hardly surprising, since anyone who has managed to cope with only minimal communicative ability for many years will hardly be greatly motivated to acquire new skills later in life. Although programmes designed to increase the communicative use of signs or pictures have had some degree of success, the spontaneous generalization of such skills to untrained settings is often poor. And, even if alternative skills such as signing are acquired, they tend to be used in the same stereotyped, non-communicative and ritualistic way that typifies spoken language in autism (Attwood *et al.* 1988).

In recent years, some of the most promising results in improving communication skills have stemmed from studies examining the communicative functions (or 'functional equivalence') of so-called 'challenging behaviours' (see Carr *et al.* 1999, Durand and Merges 2001 for detailed accounts of this approach). It is apparent that many such behaviours, far from being *inappropriate*, may be the only way in which someone with very limited communication skills can rapidly, effectively and predictably gain control over his or her environment. Indeed, analysis of the function of these behaviours frequently indicates that so-called 'maladaptive behaviours' may be extremely *adaptive* and effective if an individual is unable to express his or her needs, feelings or emotions in any other way. Head-banging, throwing the television across the room, pulling someone's hair, are all likely to result in rapid and usually predictable responses from others. An unwanted activity may be stopped, boredom may be relieved, and certainly attention will be received. Analysis of the possible reasons underlying these behaviours and their replacement by other means of communicating feelings of distress, frustration, neglect or anxiety can help greatly to decrease aggressive, self-injurious or stereotyped behaviours. In other words, if people can be taught alternative ways of communicating the same message, whether verbally, by gestures, tokens, signs, touch, or even by pressing a micro-switch, then appropriate communication is likely to increase, whilst challenging behaviours decline (Oliver 1995). Carr and his colleagues have demonstrated, in a number of different studies, that teaching individuals to express their need for assistance by means of a simple word, phrase, sign or picture indicating 'Help me', or enabling them to obtain attention or desired objects, or to escape unwanted situations by similar means has rapid and positive effects (Carr *et al.* 1999). Thus, as the communicative behaviours increase there is a concomitant decline in previously existing 'disruptive behaviours'.

Nevertheless it is important to recognise that much of this work, although clearly very effective, has been conducted in highly intensive experimental settings. Detailed analyses of the possible functions of undesirable behaviours may require considerable time, expertise and technology and are often impracticable within mainstream settings (Owens and MacKinnon 1993). In an attempt to overcome these practical difficulties, Durand and Crimmins produced a 'Motivation Assessment Scale' (1988) which can be used by carers to classify the main functions of disruptive behaviours. They suggest that the majority of such behaviours can be categorised as attention-seeking, self-stimulatory, escape or avoidance, or as indicating the need for help or assistance. Once the primary function of a behaviour has been identified in this way, the individual can be provided with alternative forms of communication (signs, words, simple phrases, pictures, symbols or gestures) to obtain the same ends.

Despite its potential value, the Motivation Assessment Scale has received some criticism (Sigafoos *et al.* 1994a). In particular, agreement between different raters may be poor and the four summary categories cannot encompass all the possible reasons for disruptive behaviours. Nevertheless, by helping carers to appreciate that such behaviours may be a function of poor *communication* skills, rather than being 'deliberate' acts of aggression or provocation, it can have a positive effect on both attitudes and approaches to intervention.

A similar but less complex form of assessment is the schedule devised by Schuler and colleagues (Schuler *et al.* 1989, Schuler and Fletcher 2002). Although designed primarily for children with autism, there is no reason why a schedule of this kind should not be adapted for use with adults (see Table 4.1). By systematically questioning how an individual expresses their need to do something (sit by someone, obtain food or some other object, protest if something is taken away etc.), this process can again help to indicate how behaviours that may be viewed as 'inappropriate' (screaming, self-injury, tantrums, aggression etc.) can have important communicative functions. This information can then be used to plan ways in which alternative and more acceptable responses might be established.

Increasing general communicative ability

The need to increase communicative skills is not, of course, restricted to individuals who exhibit challenging behaviours. Often, once they leave school and are relieved of the daily pressure on them to communicate, the language of less able people with autism ceases to improve and may even decrease in frequency or complexity. Because care staff working in adult units may be unaware of the previous capabilities of the individual concerned they may accept relatively impoverished language levels as being quite typical. Utterances may also become very abbreviated, so much so that their meaning can be quite obscure to people who do not know them well. Peter, for example, on moving to a new adolescent unit confused all the staff there by repeating constantly the phrase 'Morris Mummy, Morris Mummy', becoming very distressed when no one responded. Enquiries to staff at his previous school revealed that the phrase had originated many years earlier when the family lived in the country and an old Morris car was his mother's only source of transport. Many years (and cars) later, the same phrase was still used to indicate his wish to go out. Only when staff at the new unit began systematically to prompt and encourage more appropriate requests did his use of language begin to improve.

In other cases it is crucial that new staff or carers are made fully aware of an individual's potential ability and ensure that an appropriate level

Table 4.1 Establishing a communication profile (adapted from Schuler et al. 1989)

Communication profile

What does x usually do if he or she wants:

	Cries	Screams/attacks	Tantrums	Self injures	Just looks	Moves to person	Pulls other's hand	Touches/moves other's face	Grabs/reaches	Does it/gets it by self	Goes away	Changes facial expression	Makes sound	Changes tone of voice	Looks at person/object	Gives object	Points/uses simple gestures	Uses pictures/symbols	Uses signs (e.g. Makaton)	Echoes	Uses single words	Uses phrases/sentences	No indication of needs
Adult attention																							
Help with dressing/washing etc.																							
To be read to																							
To play a game																							
To go outside																							
To go shopping etc.																							
An object out of reach																							
A door/container opened																							
A favourite food/drink																							
Music/tv/video																							
Games/books etc.																							
Other special object																							
What happens if:																							
Usual routine is stopped																							
Favourite object etc. removed/lost																							
Made to go somewhere s/he doesn't want to go																							
Made to do something s/he doesn't want to do																							
Someone stops an activity with him/her																							
Wants to show you something																							
Wants you to look at something																							
Wants to request a break																							
Wants to indicate 'No' or 'Yes' to something																							

of skill is maintained. In the long term it will not be helpful if people with spoken language are allowed to take whatever they need without asking, or to communicate simply by means of signs or gesture. Similarly, if non-speaking individuals possess even very rudimentary signs or gestures, staff should make sure that they are familiar with and respond to these; otherwise they are likely rapidly to disappear. If existing signs are not adequate within the new environment, then new and more appropriate ones may need to be taught. This may require staff themselves becoming trained in sign or symbol systems such as Makaton (Walker 1980), but if this can be achieved the results can be very positive for all concerned.

For some individuals, even simple sign or symbol systems may be too complex. Layton and Watson (1995) provide a useful breakdown of the different skills required for using signs, pictures or written words with children who are non-verbal, and a similar strategy may be helpful in choosing alternative communication systems for adults. On the whole, a system using pictures or photographs makes least demands on cognitive, linguistic or memory skills, although it is essential that the pictures used reflect the individual's particular interests or needs if they are to be used successfully. The PECS (Picture Exchange Communication System) programme of Bondy and Frost (1994) stresses the need for active participation and initiation in using pictures or objects to communicate, and there is now a wide range of PECS materials and resources to encourage spontaneous communication, both non-verbal and verbal. Although evaluation studies are limited, and tend to focus only on young children (Magiati and Howlin 2001, Charlop-Christy *et al.* 2002, Kravitz *et al.* 2002), there is no reason why this approach should not be adapted for adults too. See Figure 4.2 for examples.

Commercially produced equipment is not the only option. Homemade wall charts with photographs indicating the daily timetable, the staff who will be on duty or the food on offer at mealtimes can be just as effective in increasing understanding or in enabling people to indicate their own choices more effectively. Individuals can be provided with their own personal set of photographs or pictures to enable them to indicate basic needs or wishes (for example, to leave the building, have a drink, go to the toilet etc.). These must be easily accessible for both the staff and the individual, and might be attached to a key ring on a belt or on a clipboard or even a long neck-chain (the sort that is often used for identity badges at work) – anything that is age-appropriate. Digital cameras are an invaluable source of almost instant visual cues. A 'triple print' film-processing system (which provides one

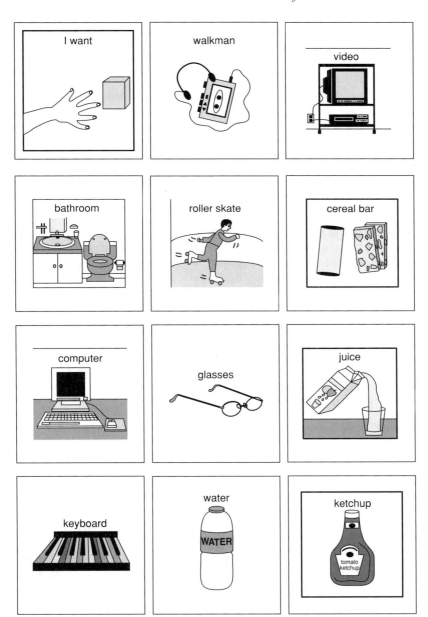

Figure 4.2 Examples of PECS pictures that can be used to indicate needs/wishes

large photo and two smaller copies for every negative) is also useful, providing identical pictures for staff and clients as well as for a central display. Picture cards should be updated or replaced as necessary and be properly protected, preferably on laminated board. Even if there is little spontaneous use by the individual concerned, consistent prompting can be effective in gradually establishing the link between the picture and the resulting activity. Cards of this type also have the advantage, particularly in large or busy units, of being readily understood or used by new staff, whereas signs or more complex symbols may require prior knowledge or training.

The growing market in computerised communicative aids has been of great value to many non-verbal adults with autism, and some equipment is now specifically designed for this group. Interchangeable and increasingly complex keyboards make it possible for individuals to proceed gradually from single-symbol boards (with, for example, a large red square or circle that will emit a sound to attract attention) to multi-symbol displays, indicating a wide variety of stimuli, that can be personally tailored to the individual's own environment, needs or interests.

The use of specialist equipment of this kind, which also incorporates prompting and shaping procedures to build up *independent* communication skills, should not be confused with the use of 'facilitated communication', discussed in Chapter 3, in which clients remain heavily dependent on the physical support of facilitators to type out messages. Here, experimental studies have constantly demonstrated communication to be under the control of the facilitator, not the person with autism (Mostert 2001).

Alternative, or augmentative, forms of communication may also be of help for individuals who are able to talk but for some reason are reluctant to do so. Stuart, who had developed speech late in his childhood, had never been a fluent speaker, but during a period of severe depression refused to utter anything other than an occasional 'Yes', 'No', 'Hello' or 'Goodbye.' When his depression finally responded to treatment he continued to resist speaking, becoming virtually non-communicating. In the past he had seemed to enjoy reading and writing, and so, rather than insisting that he speak – which resulted in much anxiety and even aggression – his parents and day-care staff encouraged him to communicate in writing. This he was able to do quite effectively, and after several years of expressing himself mainly in this way he eventually began to use speech fluently once more. Recently he wrote a long letter to the BBC pointing out an obscure mistake in the rules of one of their quiz programmes (quiz games being his main obsession in life). He was delighted when they read this out to viewers and changed the rules accordingly!

Written communication, in a simpler form, may also be effective in helping other individuals to communicate their needs by single words. Computers, too, can be used to develop written ability in more able individuals, although care needs to be taken to ensure that their use also involves interactive skills; otherwise communication may be with the machine, and no one else!

5   Social functioning in adulthood

Autism is associated with many different impairments in social functioning, and social deficits are at the core of all diagnostic systems, such as DSM-IV/DSM-IV TR (American Psychiatric Association 1994, 2000), or ICD-10 (WHO 1992). Amongst the specific deficits noted are the failure to understand or respond appropriately to others' feelings or emotions, the lack of ability to share emotions or experiences, and poor integration of social, emotional and communicative behaviours within an interpersonal context (Bauminger and Kasari 2000, Sigman and Ruskin 1999, Volkmar *et al.* 1997).

Difficulties in these areas tend to persist over time, even in the most able of individuals, and the pervasiveness and profundity of the social impairment continues to have a marked impact on almost every aspect of adult life. Nevertheless, as individuals approach adulthood many of the grosser social abnormalities evident in young children become less apparent. No longer are they likely to shrink away from all physical or social contact, or remain happiest left alone in a corner to indulge in ritualistic or obsessional behaviours. Problems lie instead in the understanding of social rules, in the ability to comprehend why others behave as they do, and in the interpretation of even the simplest of social situations.

The analogy of being like a stranger from outer space occurs in a number of personal accounts of autism. Therese Jolliffe, a woman with autism and a doctorate in psychology, writes:

> Normal people, finding themselves on a planet with alien creatures on it would probably feel frightened, would not know how to fit in and would certainly have difficulties in understanding what the aliens were thinking, feeling and wanting, and how to respond correctly to these things. That's what autism is like . . . Life is bewildering, a confusing, interacting mass of people, events,

places and things with no boundaries. Social life is hard because it does not seem to follow a set pattern . . . I find it as difficult to understand the things I see as I do in trying to understand the things I hear. Looking at people's faces, particularly into their eyes, is one of the hardest things for me to do . . . People do not appreciate how unbearably difficult it is for me to look at a person . . . It disturbs my quietness and is terribly frightening.

(Jolliffe *et al.* 1992)

In Oliver Sacks's (1993) interview with Temple Grandin in *The New Yorker*, the notion of alien beings crops up again:

She said she could understand 'simple, strong, universal' emotions but was stumped by the more complex emotions and the games people play. . . . She was bewildered, she said, by Romeo and Juliet ('I never knew what they were up to'). . . . 'Much of the time . . . I feel like an anthropologist on Mars'.

Jim Sinclair (1992), a young man with autism, comments in a similar vein: 'I didn't need a cattle shute [referring to the support this offered Temple when she was younger]; I needed an orientation manual for extraterrestrials'.

Social Interactions in those who are less able

Social behaviours in those who are less able, of course, also continue to give rise to many difficulties. In this group there may continue to be avoidance of contact with others, and this, together with their lack of understanding of group situations, can make integration into community settings very difficult. In small group homes individuals may become very unhappy and distressed because of the social demands made on them. In social education centres or other forms of day provision, they may be equally out of place. Activities that other clients, students or residents particularly enjoy, such as holidays, special treats, birthdays or Christmas, may incorporate the very things that someone with autism finds most difficult: change, noise, unpredictability, novelty, crowds. Having to live or work in large groups or in close proximity to people with whom they are unfamiliar can cause much distress and may well produce aggressive and other disturbed behaviours. For those caring for them, their inability to take part in community or group activities, their failure to relate to other clients and often their need for one-to-one staff input can produce intense strains on staffing.

Many of these problems are described by Hugh Morgan (1996) in his book on working with adults with autism in day and residential settings, and carers involved with this group should find much valuable information there to advise them. In the following chapter, therefore, the focus will be on individuals with autism who are more able. For them, making friends, talking to people and being engaged in social activities may become of supreme importance. In their case it is not avoidance of social interactions that poses problems, but the *quality* of these interactions. It is the desire for friendship, without the necessary social competence, that leads to many difficulties.

Qualitative impairments in social interactions

Problems with peer relationships

The inability of young autistic children to engage in social play, to join in with the activities of their peer group, or to form close friendships is well documented (Lord and Bailey 2002, Tanguay *et al.* 1998;) As infants they tend to lack automated social responses, such as orienting to their names or to a parent's voice across the room. Later, they may avoid contact with others of their own age, preferring adult company, or, if they play at all, may try to join in the games of much younger children. Aggression towards other children may also be a problem. Often, young children with autism have so few appropriate social skills that they attempt to make contact with others simply by hitting them or taking their belongings. As they grow older, difficulties with peer relationships persist but whereas in the case of young children there may be an active attempt to avoid contact with peers, later individuals may become much more anxious to be accepted, to join in with others and to make friends. The problem is that often they are not sufficiently aware of their own social difficulties and have little idea of the very complex sequences of interactions that are involved simply to enter into a social group.

Donna Williams (1992) remembers trying to make friends with a young girl in her neighbourhood:

> I did not know how to make friends, so I would stand there calling this girl every four-letter word I knew. . . . Eventually [she] would take to her feet and chase me for several blocks. . . . One day she caught me. She was about to 'smash my face in' when she decided at least to ask me why I had tormented her so persistently for so long 'I wanted to be your friend,' I blurted out furiously.

Appreciation of the many complex and intertwined factors involved in the development of more intimate relationships is often entirely lacking. However, this is perhaps hardly surprising in that the skills necessary for forming and maintaining close friendships are so subtle and complicated that even most social scientists would admit to only partial and limited understanding of the 'rules' involved. Most human beings are born with a fundamental ability that enables them to understand why others feel or respond as they do and what their own responses, in turn, should be. Without this inborn understanding, and in the absence of any formal rules to guide social interactions, the simplest of personal contacts can, for someone with autism, become a frightening and confusing experience.

Wendy Lawson (1998) recalls:

> As I approached my teenage years I began to want friends, to share my life with others. I understood friendship was valuable and I did not want to be different anymore. However, I lacked social skills and the 'know-how' of friendship building.
>
> Most people felt uncomfortable with my egocentric and eccentric behaviour. I wanted things to go by the rules – and my rules at that! My clumsy efforts usually ended in trauma – an experience common to most Asperger's teenagers.

Even in more structured activities, such as games or sports, where rules are more explicit than in other social settings, people with autism can experience many problems, which again hamper integration. Christopher's mother reported that as a child he had loved to play hide-and-seek but always accused other children of cheating when he was discovered. On one occasion he had had a loud attack of coughing in the wardrobe where he had been hiding but completely failed to understand how the other children could possibly have found him. As he grew older he was still only half able to grasp the rules of other games. In cricket he tended to run away from the ball if it came near him, and in football would always aim the ball for the nearer goal regardless of team positions. Gradually he became vaguely aware that other pupils objected to having him in their teams, but he had no idea why this was the case. Similarly, although George was a very able cross-country runner, having a remarkable memory for routes and directions, he could never be relied on to win a race, because once he got near the finishing line he would wait to see who was coming next, often losing his place. Eventually, when he started work, his colleagues realised he would make a good member of their orienteering team, and this proved much more successful since there was then no need for him to come first.

Understanding friendship

Definitions of friendship vary, but the qualities of closeness, sharing, helping, sympathy and empathy are fundamental to almost all descriptions. A real understanding of such abstract and elusive concepts, however, may be almost impossible for many people with autism. They may well realise that friendships exist, and indeed be aware that they should have friends, but without any true appreciation of the complexity of the relationships involved. Thus, whereas many adults with autism will describe themselves as having friends, detailed questioning generally reveals that although they have acquaintances to whom they can talk, much less frequently is there evidence of shared experiences or mutual understanding.

Considerable problems can arise because of naive assumptions of what constitutes a friend. If someone speaks in a friendly tone, or wishes them good morning on a daily basis, this may be mistaken as a token of much greater intimacy. Individuals who were simply being kind or polite may become the focus of the autistic person's wish to have a friend and may be pursued unremittingly because of this.

Susie took the bus to her special college course every morning, and another young woman who waited at the bus stop, recognising her difficulties, always made the effort to say 'Hello'. Susie asked where she lived and what time she got back from work and, eventually, somehow, also managed to get her telephone number. As time went on she began to wait for the young woman's return from work and would follow her home, or telephone her as soon as she knew she was in the house. The woman involved became more and more upset by this intrusion and eventually contacted the college authorities. Although the tutors tried to explain that this behaviour must stop, Susie insisted that the woman was her friend and showed no appreciation of the distress she was causing.

Phillip, who lived in semi-sheltered accommodation, was allotted a support worker living in the same complex to help him in case of difficulties. He became more and more attached to this young woman, following her to work each morning and waiting for her to come home. If she were late he would become very distressed and would stay up until two or three in the morning waiting for her. On one occasion he telephoned her elderly parents in the early hours of the morning to tell them she had not yet come home.

Stanley, who had just begun a college course, was allotted a 'buddy' – a volunteer student who would keep a check on him and ensure that all was going well. On one occasion, feeling sorry for his isolation, the student suggested that Stan came along to the pub with him to meet some of his friends. Once he realised that the group met every Friday night, Stan would appear there without fail, despite their obvious annoyance at this intrusion.

Danny went to his local pub regularly once a week and would try to engage any young women there in conversation. On one occasion he was threatened with being beaten up after he had moved into their boyfriends' seats during a darts match. After some weeks the barman asked him not to return because of complaints that he was 'harassing' women customers. Danny could not accept this, insisting that the women enjoyed his company and conversation (mostly concerning 1960s pop music). Because they had not wished to be offensive they had not complained to him directly, and he remained oblivious to indications of irritation and annoyance. He refused to obey the barman's instructions, and when he attempted to return to the pub as usual the following week the police had to be called to eject him.

Even the tolerance of individuals with a specific goal of helping others can be stretched to the limit by the uncomprehending demands of someone with autism. Gerry, a young man in his early twenties, had become involved with a small religious organisation after members had called at his house. Delighted by the attention and 'friendship' offered by people of his own age, Gerry enthusiastically joined in the group's activities. He was constantly at the house of one member or another, and when a vacancy arose in the flat shared by some of them Gerry immediately moved in. The group members seemed to have a sincere desire to help people in difficulties and they offered Gerry much support over several years. Eventually, however, even they found the constant demands on their time and attention too much, and reluctantly they had to ask Gerry's father to take him back home. Gerry himself could not understand this 'betrayal' and was left confused, saddened and embittered by his experience.

*Understanding who is **not** a friend*

Not only do people with autism have innate difficulties in understanding the nature of friendship, they may also have profound problems in interpreting whether someone is being unkind or even malicious. As is evident from the scenarios above, if someone simply speaks to the individual he or she may interpret this as a sign of great friendship.

Similarly, if asked to do something for another person he or she may feel obliged to comply because 'that's what friends are for'. Such misunderstandings can make the person with autism highly vulnerable to the demands of others. In mainstream schools it is not uncommon for children with autism to be deliberately led into trouble by other pupils who take a delight in exploiting this vulnerability. As the child with autism is frequently unable to appreciate the difference between other pupils laughing with them or laughing *at* them, they can be easily led into all sorts of outrageous behaviours. Attempts to 'buy friendship' with money, sweets or other goods are also common.

Other people with autism may fall prey to the wiles of others simply because they do not know how else to behave. Mark was a young man in his mid-twenties whose main activity was cycling. On his fixed cycling route he frequently passed a group of youngsters belonging to the local 'gang'. One day one of them stopped him and asked for a ride on his bike; another asked if he would lend them some money. Mark handed over his bike and wallet and only when he returned home without either several hours later did his parents realise what had happened. Having a good idea who had taken his belongings, his parents managed to get the bike and his wallet (now empty) returned. However, despite warnings to avoid the gang in future, or at least to protect himself by hiding his money, Mark took no such precautions, and much to his parents' exasperation similar incidents continued at regular intervals. His only explanation was that since the boys talked to him they must be his 'friends' and therefore he should not refuse their requests.

This fear of displeasing people is a powerful factor in the lives of many able people with autism. Margaret Dewey's autistic son, Jack, is quoted by his mother (1991) as saying:

> It has always been one of the worst traumas for me to feel I have displeased somebody. I tend to remember it years afterwards. It hurts more than I can bear, practically. One thing I do is day dream about how I can be reconciled with people I have displeased, and change their opinion of me.

This obvious vulnerability may lead to increasing anxieties for parents as their children grow older and demand greater independence. Owen had always had a fascination for Welsh rugby, and had been known to the players in his local club since he was a young child. Before a match he would wander into their dressing rooms for a chat, and was much liked and accepted there. As he grew older, however, he began travelling alone to matches around the country, and it was only when his father accompanied him one day that he realised he was still wandering into changing rooms and talking to players. He showed no awareness that this behaviour might result in real difficulties.

Failure to understand or respond appropriately to others' feelings or emotions

Over recent years there have been many studies exploring the problems faced by individuals with autism in understanding and relating to other people's emotions (cf. Capps *et al.* 1995, Loveland *et al.* 1997, Sigman 1998), and the impact of these problems on social interactions more generally. In an attempt to explain how pervasive and devastating such difficulties can be Wendy Lawson (1998) writes:

> One of the best ways of understanding what autism is like is to imagine yourself as a perpetual onlooker. Much of the time life is like a video, a moving film I can observe but cannot reach. The world passes in front of me shielded by glass.
>
> I find emotions interchangeable and confusing. Growing up I was not able to distinguish between anger, fear, anxiety, frustration, or disappointment. . . . I could tell the difference between a comfortable feeling and an uncomfortable one, but I didn't know what to do with it.
>
> (With age) I have learned to recognise the subtle differences between anger, frustration and disappointment, and understand why I feel these things. When emotions are more subtle. . . . I find it helpful to ask the other person how they are feeling.
>
> Growing up, I was not aware of how I responded to others, nor they to me. Now I have a greater understanding of social interaction and usually the ability to choose whether I live in my own world or whether I join the 'world' of those around me.
>
> Even my mother could not understand my disability and disconnection and she took my inappropriate behaviour personally. 'Wendy,' she would moan, 'you don't care about your own mother. Why are you doing this to me?'
>
> Today much of that misunderstanding and discomfort has gone. . . . I have been able to talk to my family about why I appear so 'distant,' 'scatty', 'forgetful' and 'unemotional'. I explained it is not that I do not have emotions but rather that I connect with them differently and for different reasons than they do.

As Lawson makes clear, even within family settings, where there may be much greater understanding of the individual's difficulties, the lack of empathy and social understanding can continue to cause hurt and distress.

From the earliest weeks of life young infants spontaneously show their delight at seeing familiar adults, and they rapidly learn to respond in socially appropriate and effective ways. As time goes on they learn to be more discriminating in their greeting behaviours: whom to hug and kiss, with whom to share more intimate information, with whom to remain more restrained. Even as infants, however, individuals with autism often lack this natural ability to respond to others appropriately, or to differentiate between interactions with familiar and unfamiliar adults. (Dawson *et al.* 2000, Wimpory *et al.* 2000) Often, they may fail to show any clear response to people unless they are directly addressed. As children, few will rush to greet their parents returning from work or even a prolonged trip away, and this apparent 'coldness' or 'insensitivity' may continue into adulthood.

Jack, for example, has a father who is a deep-sea diver. He can be away for long and unpredictable periods of time, but Jack always insists on being given an exact time and date for his return. When his father comes home his only comments relate to whether his return is too early, too late or on time. His father recounts with some sadness that 'he has never once just said "Hello".' Robbie's mother admits her mistake in once asking him whom he loved best, her or the Hotpoint washing machine (his particular obsession). His reply was unequivocal, but not the one she had hoped to hear! Jim's parents, on the other hand, were delighted when he came to meet them at the airport after they had been abroad for some weeks. He did not say 'Hello' or ask them if they had had a good trip, and as soon as they got in the car he began telling them of the new records he had bought. However, his presence in itself was enough to reassure his mother that he did indeed love them: 'He just doesn't know how to say it.'

Even if individuals with autism do recognise the need for greetings, or other expressions of emotion, this is often done in a highly form-alised and hence inappropriate way. Ben, a young man now living independently, writes frequently to his mother and sister, of whom he is clearly very fond. Since his sister's marriage he always writes to her as 'Dear Mrs Brown', and he always concludes his letters to both of them with: 'Yours Sincerely, Ben Smith (Mr)'. He cannot understand why his mother and his sister find this formality strange, and despite their suggestions has continued to insist that this is the 'correct' way to write a letter.

Even strong emotions such as grief may be very difficult to express appropriately. When Joe's father was dying, everyone in the family was distraught. Joe himself was unable to talk directly about his sorrow or anxiety but instead dealt with his feelings by constantly asking his mother for details of why his father was dying, what parts of his body were affected, exactly when he would die and how much he would leave him in his will.

Joshua's father was a news cameraman on war assignment during the Bosnian/Serbian conflicts. When he went missing for several days Josh never once tried to comfort his mother or sister, but constantly asked them instead how many heavy weapons each side had and how many people they thought would be killed. When his father finally returned, all he did was question him about how many dead bodies he had photographed. Some time later Josh was asked whether he had felt anxiety about his father at the time. He replied that of course he had, and that he had been aware that his mother and sister were upset. But he did not know what to say to them or how to explain his own feelings, and he thought that if he talked about dead bodies they would know he was upset. He also said that he was unable to reassure them that his father was fine as he had no idea what had happened to him and therefore did not want to tell a lie. His mother and sister reported that although, deep down, they understand Joshua's difficulties and knew that he was not being deliberately callous, at the time they had not been able to feel otherwise than very hurt and angry at the way he was behaving.

Sometimes, this apparent lack of feeling can prove the final straw for carers. Kenny's mother, who had looked after him with patience and understanding throughout his fifteen years, resorted to calling social services late one night, saying that she could no longer cope with him at home. The duty social worker quickly managed to calm things down, and it transpired that the crisis had arisen after mother's late return from work. She had had a particularly difficult week, but had nevertheless stopped to do the weekly shopping at the super-market that stocked Kenny's favourite brands. On the way home her car had broken down and it was some hours later that she was eventually towed home. Kenny helped her unload the shopping as he usually did, although complaining about the lateness of the evening meal. How-ever, when he realised that she had not got his favourite brand of orange juice, he returned with her coat, telling her that if she hurried she could just get to a delicatessen some miles away before it closed. His mother, normally a quiet and gentle woman, had responded by throwing the rest of the shopping at him and then, in desperation, ringing social services. The next day she was very abashed by her response, knowing that he had not acted out of deliberate malice. However, Kenny was totally incapable of understanding why his mother should have reacted in this way to such a 'reasonable' request, and he still refers to it, rather patronisingly, as the time when his mother 'went a little bit mad'.

Accurate recognition of others' emotions, unless these are very extreme, is often seriously impaired. Signs of irritation or annoyance in other people often go unheeded; then, when they finally give full vent to their feelings, the person with autism is often genuinely surprised, having no prior understanding that anything had been the matter. Moreover, even if problems are recognised, what to do about them presents major difficulties. David, a young man in his twenties, has finally learned to bring his mother a box of tissues if she is upset. He will still not attempt to comfort her, but stands poised with the tissue box until she takes one, then quickly goes away. Ruth, a woman of normal intelligence now in her twenties, is pleased that she has finally learned to recognise when her mother is upset or ill (although she still fails to recognise signs in other family members). Her mother, who is a frequent migraine sufferer, confirms that this is the case. The problem is that once Ruth realises her mother is unwell she will constantly question her about where it hurts, why it has occurred or what she might do to help, when the last thing her mother wants to do is talk to anyone.

Knowledge that different emotions exist may also be limited. Justin, in his mid-twenties, who had suddenly begun reading fiction instead of his usual books on astronomy, admitted that he had not known about people having feelings of love or hatred or jealousy until he actually read about such things. Because of this failure to understand how others think or feel, even the most ordinary of social interactions presents enormous difficulties. Temple Grandin, in her interview with Oliver Sacks, is reported as believing, when a child, that other children must be telepathic because of their ability to communicate together in ways she totally failed to follow or comprehend. Howlin and Rutter (1987a) also quote the example of a man in his late thirties who had come for their advice on 'how to read people's minds'. He was working in an office, and was astute enough to recognise that he was having problems in interpreting what was said to him. Told sarcastically 'You just do that again . . .' after he had done something particularly foolish, he would obediently do so! Because other people in the office seemed to know when it was not appropriate to follow instructions, and because of his interest in science fiction, he had concluded that the others had learned to read minds; hence his request for help. Of course, what they were reading was not minds but the shrug of a shoulder, the raising of an eyebrow, the inflection of the voice – things about which he knew, or had read, nothing.

Another aspect of the failure to empathise with other people's feelings is reflected in the inability to assess the impact of one's own actions on other people. Robert, an eighteen-year-old whose obsessional behaviour and constant questioning at home continually intrudes into family life, is unable to understand why these behaviours are unacceptable. He claims that his parents are just trying to 'treat him like a child' and that they should realise he is now an adult. To him, being an adult means doing exactly what he wants, and as he has no recognition of the needs or indeed rights of other family members he views any attempts to modify his behaviour as unreasonably restrictive.

The failure to share emotions or experiences

A lack of 'shared attention', or the failure to participate in the activities or enjoyment of others, has been highlighted as a particular deficit of children with autism and is a problem that tends to mark them out clearly from children with other developmental or communication disorders (Sigman 1998). Few children with autism try to share their own enjoyment with others; nor do they seem able to share in other people's feelings of pleasure or happiness. Rarely will they attempt spontaneously to point out things of interest to others. And if they are ever invited to parties (an uncommon event for many), they are usually unable to participate in the group enjoyment in a normal way. Either they will remove themselves from the situation altogether or, alternatively, 'go over the top', becoming far too excited and overactive, often ruining everyone else's enjoyment. Danny, now in his late teens, remembers hiding under beds or tables whenever he went to a party, and says 'I never could understand what all the fuss was about.' Charles is described by his mother as always hating Christmas when he was a child. However, as he grew older he began to take a more active role in the yearly ritual, and now rather enjoys it. Unfortunately, 'ritual' is exactly what it has become. The family still has to eat, open presents, and play games exactly as they did when he was a child. He now spends a lot of money buying them presents, but in turn is very concerned about the cost of the gifts they give him. After wishing everyone 'Happy Christmas' he will quiz them on how much they spent on his presents, becoming very upset if he feels they have not spent enough.

Spontaneous pleasure in other people's happiness or excitement seems to be rare, and although some may try to share interests or activities with others this is often done in a rather stereotyped way. Danny, who is now in his twenties and still living at home, claims that he always tells his parents about things in which he thinks they will be interested. Although his mother and father admit that he does this, the problem is that he has no real understanding of what does interest them. If they are watching a favourite programme on television, he will interrupt to tell them about an exciting computer or computer program he has just heard about or try to get them to read something in his computer magazine. When they appear less than enthusiastic he complains that they never take any notice of him.

Just as they are often unable to share pleasurable experiences, many people with autism are unable to share pain and distress in the normal way. Examples of inappropriate responses to other people's distress are described above, but people with autism are just as likely to have problems talking about their own feelings or experiences. In discussions with young adults with autism, it is often apparent that they were badly teased and bullied at school, sometimes by teachers as well as other pupils. However, very often they were quite unable to explain to their families what was happening, or to seek help. For example, although Leonard attended normal school and seemed to have adequate language skills, the only way his parents knew if he was upset by events or people at school was when he bit the teachers. Even years later, when he was experiencing problems with a supervisor at work, he resorted to threats to bite her and remained unable to resolve the situation by talking over his difficulties.

Poor integration of social behaviours

In many cases, it is not that what the person with autism does is wrong in itself, but that it is inappropriate within a particular social setting or context. Understanding where, when and how it is appropriate to act in a particular way requires much more subtle and complex social understanding than is often available to someone with autism.

Sharon, a woman in her thirties, had always had great difficulty in talking about personal issues, but over the years and with the help of a very supportive social worker she has learned to express herself much more effectively. What she has never learned to do is discriminate *when* or *with whom* such personal revelations are appropriate.

Gerry, as a young child, was very aloof and remote and was deliberately encouraged by his parents to tolerate being hugged and kissed by visitors or friends. Now, a much more outgoing individual in his early twenties, he hugs almost everyone he meets, calling them 'Darling' or 'My lovely'. Whilst some of his mother's older female friends are rather gratified by such behaviour, other women find it much less acceptable, and men are even less sure how to respond.

The potential drawbacks of allowing behaviours that may be quite socially acceptable in a young child to continue into adulthood are often overlooked, but they can have serious implications. Sarah, when younger, had a very poor appetite and in order to get her to eat her mother used to encourage her to take tempting items from other people's plates. Now a relatively socially competent student attending college, she is still likely to lean over and remove food from her neighbour's plate without warning.

Another example is Laurie, who had always been fascinated by earrings. As a young child his mother had often been able to calm his tantrums or distress by encouraging him to play with her earrings, and certain teachers at school had also allowed this. By the time he was twenty, being allowed to touch earrings was still a very effective way of calming him down. However, when he began attending a local social education centre, problems quickly arose when he started to fondle the earrings, or sometimes the ears, of other students and staff members, both male and female.

Other problems occur because of the poor ability of someone with autism to integrate different modes of communication in socially or contextually appropriate ways. The problems of inappropriate or poorly modulated intonation in speech have been described in the previous chapter, but many other aspects of non-verbal communication may also be impaired. Gestures, if used at all, may be very stiff and stilted or, alternatively, far too dramatic and exaggerated. Eye contact, facial expression or smiles may also be affected. Many autistic children go through a stage of actively avoiding eye contact with others, or else they may have a very limited range of facial expressions. As they grow older such skills do emerge, but often with impairments in timing or sequencing. Janet had, from the time she was little, been instructed to 'Look at people when you're talking to them.' This she now does, but lacking any innate awareness of the subtle and complex rules governing eye contact, her direct and unremitting gaze is far more disconcerting and socially disruptive than if she were to look away. Being prompted to 'look at people' also led to Stuart's developing a very fixed stare. As an adult this has led to frequent problems when people have challenged him to explain 'Wot you looking at?'

Jonah, now in his thirties, had also been told at one stage to 'smile' when talking to people. This he now does, but frequently with incongruous effects. When his favourite cat died, he recounted the sad story with a large grin on his face and – more seriously – when he became depressed it proved very difficult for an unfamiliar psychiatrist to assess his mental state, as he smiled unwaveringly throughout the interview.

Problems in the appropriate use of facial or vocal expression have also been illustrated in a number of experimental studies. Work with children has indicated that they have difficulties in expressing even simple emotions such as happiness and sadness correctly and that their range of gesture or facial expressiveness is also limited (Attwood *et al.* 1988, Snow *et al.* 1987). Macdonald and colleagues (1989) found that adults with autism, all of whom were of normal intelligence, showed many more unusual aspects in their expression of emotion than did controls. The appropriateness of their facial expression, as related to different social situations, was also significantly more impaired.

Failure to interpret cues

These problems in emotional and social expression are paralleled by difficulties in recognising or responding appropriately to the emotional expressions of others. Hobson, in a series of studies, has explored the problems shown by children with autism in identifying and recognising emotions, or in matching emotional states to social contexts (Hobson 2002). Other research has documented the difficulties of adults with autism in interpreting how others are feeling from their facial expression or tone of voice (e.g. Macdonald and colleagues 1989, Rutherford *et al.* 2002). There are also problems in correctly matching vocal cues to photographs of facial emotion (Loveland *et al.* 1997).

Although many high-functioning people with autism are well aware that smiles, gesture, touch, facial expression and eye contact play a crucial role in social interactions, it may still be very difficult for them to use or interpret these correctly. Jeanette, for example, is a science student at university studying for a doctoral degree. She is fully aware of the importance of social behaviours such as eye contact and smiles, but admits that she lacks the ability to understand such cues and is painfully aware of her own difficulties in expressing emotions in an appropriate way. She describes her situation as being similar to that of someone who is blind. 'It's like knowing that other people can see, but not understanding what it's like to be able to do so. It's like that for me when it comes to understanding what other people are thinking or feeling.' Gareth describes his difficulties as being akin to 'Social Dyslexia'. He can see facial expressions or hear changes in tone of voice but cannot interpret these, just as someone with dyslexia can see the letters but cannot put them together to make words.

Rules, 'morality' and deception

A further and paradoxical twist to this inability to understand or follow normal social rules, is that once a rule is acquired, it may be adhered to rigidly and inflexibly, regardless of the social context. When someone with autism knows something is 'right' or 'wrong' they may often cling avidly to this view, whatever the circumstances. Lorna Wing cites the example of someone in the police force who, on finding that the parking meter where he had left his car had expired whilst he was on a case, immediately wrote himself a parking ticket! As described in more detail in Chapter 7, pupils with autism in mainstream schools can encounter many difficulties because of their insistence on sticking rigidly to rules, and trying to ensure that others do the same. Correcting other children for talking in class or informing the head if any are seen smoking is not usually done out of any sense of malice but because of the belief that if a rule is being broken those in charge should be made aware of this. In work situations, too, strict adherence to working practices can result in conflict with both staff and employers (see Chapter 9).

At home, as well, it can produce problems. Johnny's mother had told him *never* to open the door unless she or his father were in the house and, because of his vulnerability, she had deliberately practised this with him on several occasions, pretending to be a stranger asking for admittance. When one day she returned home without her key, he refused to open the door and despite her protestations she had to wait outside until her husband returned. Oliver, who lived with foster parents, had been told that he must always come in quietly at night in order not to wake the younger children. One evening he returned from his social club without his key. Although the lights were still on in the house, he made no attempt to rouse anyone. When found next morning, sleeping in the large rabbit hutch in the garden, he explained that ringing the bell would have woken the other children and he had been told never to do this. His only complaint was that the rabbits 'had moved about a lot in the night' and kept him awake.

David had a much younger brother with whom he enjoyed playing chess and computer games. However, he invariably won such games, and when his mother suggested that he should let his little brother 'win' from time to time he became very upset, insisting this would be a form of cheating. There was no appreciation of the fact that no harm could come from acting in this way and that it would help to encourage his young sibling. Indeed, understanding that there are rules but that in some circumstances rules need to be broken is for many people with autism a perplexing and confusing concept that they may never fully grasp.

Deception, too, is a skill that may never be acquired. Deception involves understanding not only one's own actions but the impact of what is done or said on other people's behaviour. This complex sequence of events is likely to be beyond the scope of many individuals with autism. While the notion of innocence may have its attractions, in a world that is far from innocent, the vulnerability and honesty of people with autism can be too easily exploited or abused. They are the ones left holding the brick outside the video centre whilst the other youths have made off with the goods; it is they who may be used to shoplift, or even to drive a stolen car whilst other people wait in the background. Though such incidents are rare, they do occur, and again reflect the inability of people with autism to understand what is in other people's minds.

'Mindblindness'

The belief that other people must be able to 'mind-read' in order to interpret social situations, as expressed by one of the individuals described above, gives some indication of the profundity of the deficits in this area. Possible reasons for this failure to understand how other people think or feel, or why they respond in the way they do have been explored in much detail (Hobson 2002, Baron-Cohen *et al.* 2001a). It is clear that many individuals with autism, whatever their intellectual ability, are seriously impaired in their ability to understand other people's beliefs, knowledge, emotions, desires, intentions or feelings. This ability to attribute mental states to oneself or other people is crucial for social understanding, and in normal child development is well established from the age of three to four years. In autism, however, although the ability to 'understand minds' improves to some extent with age, difficulties in this area tend to remain throughout life. Simon Baron-Cohen (1995) coined the term 'Mindblindness' in an attempt to convey the enormity of the problem.

'Theory of mind' is not, of course, actually a theory as such, nor does it help to explain *why* individuals with autism suffer from this particular deficit. (For a discussion of possible mechanisms involved see Baron-Cohen 2001). Nevertheless, it provides a crucial framework for understanding the extent of the social impairment in autism. Without the ability to comprehend the meaning behind what someone is saying, without the realisation that other people have different beliefs, or emotions, or feelings, or share different backgrounds or experiences, almost every social interaction is likely to result in difficulties and misunderstandings.

At the most fundamental level, even superficial social encounters will be marred by the inability to appreciate the need for basic contextual information. Thus the individual with autism is likely to embark on detailed monologues referring to his or her special interests, without any attempt to ensure that the listener has any background knowledge or interest in the topics raised. When more complex social interactions are involved the pervasiveness of the deficit may be even more apparent. A characteristic example is the case of Arthur, who was a very competent computer analyst. His particular role at work was to identify the bugs in other people's computer programs, a task at which he was remarkably skilled. Unfortunately, his inability to understand that they could not understand what was wrong made it almost impossible for him to explain the problems or help people to correct their errors. Many other examples, taken from clinical practice, of the impact of the failure to understand mental states on social interactions are described by Baron-Cohen and Howlin (1993).

What can be done to improve social functioning?

Although the previous section has concentrated on the profundity and pervasiveness of the social deficits in autism, this should not be taken as an indication that there is little that can be done to improve the lives of people with autism or their families. It is true that intervention is unlikely to 'cure' the fundamental deficits in social understanding, but nevertheless much can be done to minimise difficulties, and, in particular, to prevent the occurrence of secondary problems arising from social impairments.

Begin at the beginning

Probably, the most crucial component of any social intervention programme is the need to provide clear, simple and concise guidelines of what is and what is not acceptable from as early an age as possible. The natural social awareness of normal children means that they readily learn to modify their behaviour according to social context almost from infancy. Behaviours indulged in at home, such as baby talk, object attachments, immature patterns of interaction, are all rapidly dispensed with when the child enters the world of other children and adults. Few, if indeed any, explicit rules exist on *how* or *when* behaviours should change, nor are there guidelines on how to assess the complex (and often conflicting) requirements of differing social settings. Nevertheless, most children have no need of such guidelines: they are born with an innate sense that enables them to recognise unwritten social rules, to appreciate subtle changes in social interactions and to adapt their behaviours appropriately. In autism, not only is recognition of these implicit rules impaired but so too is the ability to change behaviours accordingly. Thus patterns of behaviour that are accepted, perhaps even encouraged, when they are children will remain part of the social repertoire as they grow older, no matter how socially unacceptable these may become. A-year-old child who enjoys running his hands up and down women's legs because he likes the feel of their tights, or one who enjoys putting his hands down the front of women's jumpers because they feel soft and warm inside is likely to be viewed with amused tolerance; a twelve-year-old who does the same is unlikely to be treated so indulgently and a twenty-year-old will find himself in serious trouble. However, many individuals with autism have little ability to recognise when or why a previously accepted behaviour suddenly becomes unacceptable. The onus is thus firmly on carers to ensure that behaviours that are likely to give rise to problems in the longer term are discouraged from an early age. Unfortunately, this is a counsel of perfection that is not easy to follow. It is not difficult to understand why the parents of a previously withdrawn child should praise and encourage him when, eventually, he begins to talk to, greet, or even hug and kiss everyone he meets. However, it is subsequently extremely difficult for an autistic teenager to understand why such behaviours are suddenly discouraged, and he or she may understandably resent such apparent inconsistency. The ability of parents to see into the future, and to predict the possibility of later problems, can be a crucial factor in preventing or at least minimising social difficulties, but this may be at on the cost of placing restrictions on the child's social behaviours earlier on.

At about the age of seven Harry began to copy his older sister's habit of hugging and kissing all her friends, much to the amusement of the family and the entertainment of visitors. However, his mother, aware of his tendency to become fixed in routines, worried that this behaviour could lead to problems in other settings as he grew older. Much against the wishes of her daughter and her friends she insisted that Harry should not be allowed to respond in this way. Instead, he was taught to shake hands and say 'Hello, how are you?', a much less spontaneous and natural response but one which his mother recognised would stand him in better stead in years to come.

A similar dilemma was faced by Kieren's mother. Because of his behaviour problems she had great difficulty in finding babysitters for him. The only reason she was able to retain one or two was that, no matter how much trouble he caused during their stay, as they left he would always tell them how much he loved them and give them a great hug and kiss. By the time he was twelve, she realised that it was time to discourage these behaviours, and rather reluctantly placed an embargo on physical interactions of this kind. Other behaviours, such as removing clothing, revealing intimate personal or family details, approaching strangers, wandering into other people's houses or gardens, whilst acceptable, if not always desirable, in a three- or four-year-old, may become a source of embarrassment, rejection or even personal danger in later years. Thus, basic rules of behaviour must be established from as early an age as possible.

Learning the rules of social behaviour

Unfortunately, the fundamental problem in attempting to formulate rules to guide social interactions is that, in the majority of cases, such behaviours are not governed by formal or explicit rules. Normally, there is an inborn sense of what is or is not acceptable in different situations and an innate ability to recognise when social demands change, even though the setting and the people involved are apparently the same. Even if rules do exist, these are so complex, and so dependent on innate social sensitivities, that there is rarely any point in trying to put them into operation. However, without this innate understanding, rules will be all that the person with autism has to guide his or her behaviour, and, imperfect as they are, they will be crucial for acceptable social development.

Individuals may also need to be given specific guidance on when, how often or how to carry out tasks that are necessary for social acceptance. Maurice, as a teenager, had many problems because of his ritualistic washing habits. He would only shave every three days, bath once a week and wash his hair once a fortnight. This routine was strictly adhered to whatever activities he had been involved in. Over the years his parents had slowly managed to increase the frequency of his washing, but they were worried that he might develop equally unhelpful routines when he moved into semi-sheltered accommodation. In collaboration with Maurice and his care workers a daily timetable was drawn up specifying what activities should be done on each day of the week. In order to avoid the routine becoming too rigid, a slightly different timetable was organised for each week. Eventually, provided with a list of tasks that had to be completed on a daily or regular weekly basis, Maurice was able to design his own monthly 'personal care' timetable without help from others.

Often, even for very intelligent individuals, there is little point in offering detailed explanations of why certain behaviours are unacceptable. This may have no impact on the behaviour, and may lead to prolonged and futile arguments. Gerald's parents, for example, tried to stop him walking around the streets at night whenever he could not sleep. The problem was made worse by the fact that they lived on the edge of a very rough area of East London, and although Gerald did not actually go out in his pyjamas he would don any item close to hand, including on one occasion his mother's pink tracksuit and on another occasion a black plastic bin-liner. When they tried to explain to him the potential danger of this behaviour he immediately produced detailed and lengthy statistics on the relatively low risks of a sixteen-year-old such as himself being 'mugged' in that particular area.

Unsuspected difficulties of course may arise when it becomes necessary to *bend or break* established rules. It may be essential to take off one's clothes or to talk about intimate personal details, for example, when visiting the doctor or if in hospital; it may be necessary to approach strangers if one is lost or needs help; similarly it may be acceptable to take off most of one's clothes on a beach, or, as relationships develop, to begin to reveal more about personal feelings. In such circumstances established rules may well prove counterproductive.

Daniel's parents experienced difficulties when he was a small child because of his tendency to take off all his clothes whenever he could. From his early teens, therefore, they made a rule that he could strip down to his underpants or shorts *only* in the house (and then only if there were no visitors there), *or* in the swimming pool, *or* in the gym at school, *or* if he was examined by a nurse or doctor. Daniel stuck rigidly to these rules and in other circumstances it could be very difficult to persuade him to dispense with even a single garment. As they lived in the north of England they felt they could cope with occasional visits to the beach, where his insistence on remaining fully dressed was a sensible precaution. Problems arose, however, when the family moved to Australia. In order to encourage him to wear fewer clothes when the weather was hot they provided him with a wristwatch with an integral thermometer, and when the temperature reached a certain level he was told he could strip down to his under-shorts. Because they ensured that these were of the same style as other young men's shorts his appearance in underpants was socially quite acceptable, and Daniel's parents rightly congratulated themselves on their imaginative approach to the problem. Unfortunately, some time later they returned to England around Christmas time. In the middle of a shopping expedition to Harrods, Daniel realised that the temperature had reached the required level, and it was only with extreme difficulty that his parents managed to remove him before he had stripped completely.

Bob was taught by his parents, after some worrying episodes were reported in the local paper, that if a stranger ever spoke to him in the street he was to run straight back to the house. This rule worked relatively well throughout his childhood, but began to backfire when he reached adulthood. If someone innocently stopped to ask him the way he would immediately shriek and take to his heels, much to the astonishment of the innocent questioner.

Nevertheless, despite such drawbacks, rules of some sort are a great deal better than no rules at all. And as time goes on it may be possible to add riders or modifications to the original guidelines to make these more flexible. In Bob's case, as he was a hefty young man over six feet tall, his parents felt there was little risk of his being taken advantage of; moreover, his flight and panic on being asked the simplest question by a stranger made him appear very abnormal. They eventually persuaded him that he should first stop and listen to what he was asked, and if he could answer (he was very knowledgeable about local routes) he should do so and then *walk* on.

In another case, Sarah had caused many problems as she grew older because of her fascination with babies. She would approach babies in their prams and pick them up whenever the opportunity arose. This behaviour was not appreciated by their parents, and as she grew into a young woman there was a real danger of her getting into serious trouble. Her family and the staff at her day centre made an absolute rule that she was not to approach any prams or *ever* touch a baby, and with much vigilance they were able to enforce this. Some time later, Sarah's sisters began to have children of their own, and as it seemed very *inappropriate* to adhere strictly to the rules in their case she was told she could pick up the babies *if* she asked first and as long as someone from the family was there 'in case she needed help'. The rules were further adapted when two staff members from the day centre, of whom Sarah was very fond, also had babies of their own.

On the whole, it seems more successful to begin with a very strict but simple rule, which must be rigidly followed initially and then gradually to relax this as appropriate, rather than to begin with more flexible or complicated guidelines which then have to be made more stringent.

Other 'rules', relating to dress, appearance, how to greet people, contact with strangers and so forth, are also best laid down at an early age. Help may also be required in learning to distinguish between different types of 'stranger'. Thus, while it may be acceptable to talk to or even take sweets from the owner of the local newsagent while out shopping, it is not allowable to accept sweets from a stranger who approaches you on the street. Specific help may also be needed to cope with apparently straightforward activities, such as using a public lavatory. For example, although Matthew's mother had suspected that he was being badly teased at school, it was only when another pupil told her that this was because he always pulled his trousers right down before urinating that she realised why.

Although the value of early guidance or preventative strategies cannot be overstated, the rule 'Better late than never' also applies. People with autism, even those of normal intellectual ability, often remain much more dependent on their families than other young adults, and may accept parental advice long after others would reject it. If this is not the case – and some individuals decide early in their teens that parents should no longer 'interfere' in this way – they may be more receptive to instructions from others. Thus, for example, the 'social stories' technique developed by Carol Gray (1998) can be very successfully adapted to help adults cope in difficult social situations.

Personal hygiene

One area in which many adults who are living independently or in semi-sheltered accommodation may need help is in organising their weekly activities to ensure they manage to cope adequately with tasks such as washing or cleaning. Advice on constructing a daily, weekly or monthly timetable can prove helpful in ensuring that time is effectively and efficiently structured, and experience indicates that few people resent what might otherwise be construed as an intrusion into their lives. Even with such apparently clear-cut tasks, however, it is important to ensure that the individual *fully* understands what is required. Gerald had a fixed routine (largely organised by his mother) for shopping, going to the launderette, bathing, cleaning his flat etc.

She had taken great pains to ensure that everything was fitted in and was therefore most upset to hear that he was having problems at work because of poor personal hygiene. He assured her he did go to the launderette once a fortnight and that he changed his shirts and underclothes on a daily basis as agreed. A visit to his flat, however, revealed that although he *changed* his clothes every day he did not necessarily wash them. If the linen basket were full he would place soiled clothes neatly back in his drawers, and these could well be worn several times before eventually being taken to the launderette. Supplying him with a larger laundry basket, and specifically instructing him to *wash* clothes before rewearing them, effectively overcame this problem.

Although, as noted earlier, the failure to appreciate potentially embarrassing situations can lead to problems, it can also be an asset at other times. Explicit explanations that a behaviour is not acceptable, that clothes are dirty or inappropriate, or even that personal hygiene is inadequate, would be deeply resented by the majority of individuals. But because Gerald, like many other people with autism, showed no embarrassment following the complaints from his manager and was not at all bothered by the involvement of his mother, he was able to return to work without the slightest qualms. Moreover, it is often the case that the person with autism will not appreciate the need to change unless he or she is given such direct feedback and guidance.

Responding to cues from others

As far as social communication is concerned it may well prove impossible to provide someone with autism with a complete understanding of when it is, or is not, appropriate to talk to someone, or whether a particular topic should be discussed or not. Nevertheless, it is usually possible, at the very least, to teach ways of responding to guidance from others. Simply learning not to speak so loudly, so that comments are not broadcast far and wide, can be a great advantage. Similarly, responding to a cue from parents, siblings, teachers or others that discussion of a particular topic should cease forthwith may help to avoid giving offence to others. As a general rule, attempts made *at the time the problem occurs* to explain *why* a behaviour is unacceptable or why a topic is not appropriate for discussion simply tend to exacerbate matters, as the individual with autism is likely to demand reasons for the interruption or vociferously defend his or her right to continue. A clear and unambiguous signal that it is time to stop may help to deal more effectively and immediately with problems of this nature, whilst explanations can be given after the crisis has been resolved.

Appropriate responses to guidelines from others generally need to be established in non-conflictual settings. With time, the behaviours learned in this way can then be generalised to situations in which difficulties actually occur. However, sometimes individuals may be very resistant to 'intrusion' of this kind unless they are fully aware of the possible consequences. John, who was a very able teenager, had an unerring knack of saying just the wrong thing to everyone he met. His mother had tried to teach him to introduce himself appropriately and to make compliments to people he met, or to try to talk about topics in the news, but these frequently misfired. When told that a friend of his mother's had lost a stone in weight, he immediately said it would be a very good thing if she lost another two. To a colleague who called to take his mother to work he suggested it would be a good idea if she became a 'Page Three Girl' because she had such a nice figure, and at social gatherings organised by his left-wing parents he would regale visitors with his very right wing political opinions. Matters finally came to a head when, on a visit to his brother at university in Dublin, he was asked to play the piano in the local pub. He had exceptional musical ability, but unfortunately the first tune he tried to play was 'God Save the Queen'. He could not understand the offence that this obviously caused, and resisted attempts to silence him. Without his brother's intervention he would almost certainly have been physically attacked.

On-the-spot explanations of why such behaviours were unacceptable simply led to further arguments and remonstrations, but away from the situation he was able to accept that he did 'sometimes say the wrong thing'. Because he became quite fearful after the incident in the pub his family managed to persuade him that if he said or did something inappropriate they would say loudly 'Well, I think it's time to go now' and he would then follow them out of the room or building. He would still try to argue with them when he was removed from the situation, but at least this tactic reduced the embarrassment that his behaviour so frequently caused.

Helping more complex social understanding

Formulating rules that are likely to be successful across a range of different situations is difficult enough, even when relatively straightforward social behaviours are involved. Improving more fundamental understanding presents even greater problems. Temple Grandin is reported as trying to deal with the problem by building up a vast library of experiences over the years:

They were like a library of video tapes, which she could play in her mind . . . of how people behaved in different circumstances. She would play these over and over again, and learn, by degrees, to correlate what she saw, so that she could then predict how people in similar circumstances might act. 'It is strictly a logical process', she explained.

(Sacks 1993)

However, much social understanding takes us beyond the realms of logic. For example, although recognition of whether or not someone is a friend comes naturally to most people, few of us could actually define how this understanding comes about. In autism, perceptions of friendship are often based on superficial and possibly misleading cues. The fact that someone speaks to them in a kindly fashion, greets them on a regular basis or even sits next to them at work or in class can quite erroneously be taken as a wish for closer friendship. Alternatively, the individual with autism may take to approaching people directly, and asking them 'Will you be my friend?', a tactic that is almost guaranteed to ensure they will not be.

Some help in dealing with social problems may be obtained from the series Books Beyond Words written for people with learning disabilities by Sheila Hollins and colleagues. These illustrate clearly and explicitly problems of social rejection and can be used to discuss the emotional and practical issues surrounding this. However, teaching someone how to recognize whether or not someone is truly a friend is probably an impossible task. Indeed, many of us will have had experiences of our instincts being wrong and of being let down in the trust we have placed in someone. For most of us, however, persistent errors of this kind are rare in that we are able to learn and profit from earlier mistakes. Often this is not the case for people with autism. Specialised social skills training, as described in a later section, may help to some extent, but this is available only to very few. For others, helping them to recognise explicit signs of rejection or acceptance may be all that is possible, and even this may well require considerable assistance. Giles, for example, was always approaching young female members of staff at his day centre and asking politely if he might sit next to them, a request that they could hardly refuse. It was obvious in his talk with his mother that he believed them to be his 'real friends', unlike the clients at the centre, to whom he considered himself greatly superior. He would become very distressed if a 'friend' subsequently left, or had to deal with him firmly. At the request of his mother the staff discussed the problem and decided, against the better judgement of some of them, that they would have to be more honest in their dealings with him. It was made clear that, although they liked him very much, because they were staff they could not be 'real friends'. Attempts to encourage activities with some of the more able clients at the centre were not at all successful, but developing his role as assistant to those who were more disabled helped to improve his self-esteem and reduced his tendency continually to pursue staff members.

Danny had been in trouble on several occasions for approaching women in his local pub and asking if he could sit next to them, whether or not they were accompanied. His siblings, who were much concerned about the situation, did their best to offer practical guidance. Their first rule was that he should *never* approach a woman who was already sitting next to, or in a group with, other men. The next rule was not to ask if he could sit next to someone – most of the women he asked tended not to give an outright refusal – but to ask instead 'Is someone else going to be sitting here?' (which seemed to give people the excuse to say 'Yes' even if no one actually appeared). *Only* if they said 'No' *and* they moved up to make space for him could he take this as an invitation to sit down. Otherwise, he was to go and find somewhere to sit by himself. On the few occasions when someone actually did move up, he was instructed to ask them one question only (usually something as banal but inoffensive as 'Have you been here before?' or 'Do you come here often?' if he had seen them on previous occasions). If they did not ask him any further questions, he was then told just to sit and read his book or newspaper. His sister and brother kept intermittent checks on his behaviour when they could, and their rules did seem to help to keep him out of further trouble.

Learning to say No

Other social difficulties arise from the fact that, in their desire to make or keep friends, people with autism may try to comply with any request that is made of them. Many find it extremely difficult to refuse requests for help as they believe this will make them appear rude or ungrateful. This desire to please can obviously lead to difficulties, and not necessarily only with strangers. Damien, who had always been very careful with his money and had acquired considerable savings, was approached by his cousin who had recently come to live in the same area. He explained that he needed some cash, and as the banks were closed he asked if Damien would give him money in exchange for a cheque. Damien parted with a hundred pounds, but despite the fact that neither this nor subsequent cheques were ever honoured, his cousin still managed to persuade him to part with similar sums on many occasions. Damien admitted that he knew the money was unlikely to be paid but was too anxious about upsetting a member of the family to refuse.

Helping people to say 'No' politely but effectively, when they are aware that a request can lead them into trouble, is an essential requirement. The experience of more able people with autism suggests that they are usually aware – or at least they eventually become so – that what they are asked to do is unwise or can lead them into trouble. Giving them the opportunity to discuss the problem, helping them to work out what they should or should not do, and providing them with strategies for avoiding or getting out of the situation, can all be beneficial. Because many people seem to find it difficult to say 'No' directly, an alternative way of excusing themselves from the situation may be useful. Jack, who on a number of occasions had been used as a scapegoat for other children's misdemeanours, was encouraged to say 'I'll just check with my mum first' if ever members of the local teenage gang asked him out. If they were up to mischief this response tended to make them depart with speed.

It may also be necessary to enlist the help of other people. Although Damien was encouraged to respond negatively but politely to his cousin's requests for cash, he was not able to tell him that he had no money unless this was actually true. He was finally persuaded to tell his parents about what was happening, and as well as approaching the cousin directly they tried to ensure that Damien did not have enough money available in his current account to make such payments. For a while the problem subsided, but eventually the cousin returned, this time asking for cheques instead of cash, and telling Damien how 'hurt' he had been by his 'betrayal' to his father. Unfortunately, this emotional blackmail resulted in large additional amounts of money being lost until his parents eventually found out what was happening.

Sometimes, too, it may be necessary to take steps to prevent the problem situation from occurring altogether. Robert's mother began to realise that his dinner money was not arriving at school and suspected that this was being used to 'buy' friendship from other people. She arranged with his teacher for the money to be taken in the first lesson each morning rather than at lunch time, and again, for a while, this seemed to work. However, he then began to be waylaid on his way to school and in the end the only solution was for the school to collect the money in advance directly from his parents.

Working with older people with autism, it is clear that almost all experience great difficulties in attempting to be appropriately assertive. Much earlier intervention, when they are children, could perhaps help to reduce later difficulties. Basic strategies such as providing clear guidance on what is right and wrong, when to say 'No' to other children, help to understand that money or goods will not bring them friends, or that saying 'No' will not necessarily make them enemies can all help to reduce the risks of more serious problems in adult life.

Respecting individual difficulties

One way in which more able individuals with autism are able to help themselves is to be explicit with other people about the nature of their social difficulties. Many individuals, for example, are uncomfortable at having to meet direct eye-gaze, dislike physical contact or proximity, or find it difficult to cope with loud noises. If they can be encouraged to explain these problems to those with whom they come into contact, unnecessary conflict can be averted. Judith, a young woman currently studying for a postgraduate degree, finds direct eye contact with others very disturbing but is able now to explain this and to warn people in advance that she would prefer not to look at them. As long as this request is met her interactions with other people go quite smoothly. Veronica, another extremely gifted woman who writes both music and poetry, cannot bear physical contact or being in crowded situations of any sort. However, as long as she is able to make clear beforehand that she cannot tolerate people shaking her hand or touching her in other ways, and as long as she has some predetermined 'escape route' in social gatherings, she is able to tolerate and sometimes even to enjoy these.

This approach clearly contrasts with the methods sometimes used to encourage social interactions, particularly in children with autism. In the past, for example, direct eye contact was often specifically encouraged. However, although behavioural techniques can be used to increase eye contact, such methods can never teach the subtleties of eye-gaze: when it is appropriate to look, when to shift gaze, when to look away. Instead, what tends to be achieved is a fixed and unblinking stare, which is socially much more disconcerting than someone who explains simply that they do not like to make eye contact. Children with other handicaps are usually taught ways of circumventing their difficulties. If a child has physical or sensory impairments they are provided with aids to ameliorate these; they are not forced to try to see or hear without help. In contrast, enormous pressures may sometimes be placed on people with autism to confront their problems directly – pressures that can lead to anxiety, aggression, withdrawal or greater social disruption. Sensitivity to individual needs, and offering ways of avoiding or minimising social pressures, may prove as important for social integration as the teaching of specific skills.

Modifying the demands of the social environment

Whatever strategies are employed to improve social functioning, it is important to recognise that the fundamental deficits are likely to remain throughout life. A focus on changing the expectations or behaviours of others may play as important a role in intervention as concentration on the problems of the person with autism, but this requires considerable flexibility on the part of those other people. Avoiding social situations which, although highly enjoyable for others, may cause distress for people with autism, can be very effective in reducing unnecessary conflict and disruption. However, this may mean a reduction in the variety of activities or outings undertaken, and as such can pose ethical problems for others, especially staff working in residential or other care settings. Similarly, activities involving a high level of participation with others, exposure to crowds or even novel experiences can all place untold stress on someone with autism. Asking carers to allow someone with autism to spend more time alone, to let him or her follow a less intensive programme than other residents, or even to avoid birthday or Christmas celebrations can raise many difficulties and may undermine staff's feelings of competence. The balance between pressure and passivity becomes all-important: not making demands that will result in conflict or distress whilst at the same time attempting to improve the general quality of life. It is essential to offer the person with autism the opportunity to choose between various options. But, in order for that person to be able to make choices he or she must be able fully to understand the options available. If fear, obsessionality, social impairments or communication difficulties interfere with the ability to choose, these problems will need to be addressed directly. Some pressure, too, may also be required in order to persuade the individual with autism to depart from his or her normal routine long enough to experience, albeit briefly, other possibilities. Some sort of 'escape hatch' seems to be essential here, for if the individual has sufficient control over what is happening, if he or she has access to a place of privacy, can escape from social demands if these become overwhelming or can terminate a novel experience if it all becomes too much, then it is much more likely that he or she will be persuaded 'to give it a go'. Over time, exposure to activities that seem to offer some potential for social enjoyment can be gradually increased, whereas activities that invariably precipitate anxiety and distress should be avoided and replaced by more acceptable alternatives.

Learning from mistakes

Because of the pervasiveness of the social problems in autism it is inevitable, whatever help is provided, that difficulties will occur from time to time. However, instead of being discouraged by failure it is important to recognise that errors can in fact be used very productively. Individuals with autism almost always have problems in coping with abstract or hypothetical concepts, and hence attempts to teach rules in isolation are likely to have limited impact. If a problem has arisen this can be used much more effectively as a teaching opportunity: to discuss what may have gone wrong, how cues may have been misinterpreted, or how the situation might be improved in future.

Barry, for example, had attended a number of 'social skills' sessions to help him greet other clients in his day centre more appropriately. When he first began attending the centre he had irritated many people by addressing them, quite deliberately, by the wrong name or title (Mrs Kat, the head of the centre, was always addressed as 'Mr Dog', and clients' names would frequently be distorted in a variety of ways). Attempts to teach him more acceptable forms of address failed entirely, until he was hit by a large and usually docile client whom he had teased for some time. This experience had a much more immediate, and long-lasting impact on his behaviour than had the previous, rather 'academic' strategies used by care staff and made him more responsive to the teaching of alternative responses. Similarly, John, whose unfortunate experience of playing the British national anthem in a republican bar is described above, became much more responsive to his family's suggestions once he was made aware of the potential dangers of his behaviour.

Social skills training

Another approach to improving the social awareness of people with autism is the use of social skills training, Probably because the social impairments in autism are often so different from the social difficulties associated with other disorders, there is little evidence that social skills training in mixed groups is particularly effective. Instead, the groups that seem to have had most effect are those that have focused specifically on the deficits related to autism (Marriage *et al.* 1993, Mesibov

1992, Ozonoff and Miller 1995). However, there are relatively few evaluative studies of the effectiveness of such groups, and the skills taught are not necessarily those most needed in real-life situations. Brown and Odom (1991) noted various problems associated with social skills training programmes, including the often circumscribed nature of the skills taught, limited evaluation, problems of generalisation to and maintenance in real-life settings, and problems in encouraging the use and development of such programmes by care staff, teachers and others. Rogers (1998a) reviews a variety of other programmes (including peer-tutoring, self-management, video modelling, social stories, circle of friends, visual cueing, pivotal response training) to facilitate social interactions in children with autism. Ozonoff *et al.* (2002) also describe different approaches that can be used to improve the 'social world' of children and adolescents with autism and Asperger syndrome. They suggest that the use of 'social scripts' can be particularly helpful, especially for high-functioning children and adolescents. These involve brief written scenarios indicating what the individual might say in order to introduce him/herself, explain their difficulties, or respond to specific questions. Because of the good memories of many people with autism memorising these scripts usually presents little difficulty and if well rehearsed they can be used quite fluently in the appropriate social setting. Krantz and McClannahan (1998) have also demonstrated the value of written scripts or instructions in improving social interaction.

Although few well-documented programmes for adults have been described there is no reason why this approach should not be used successfully with adults as well. Similarly, social stories or being helped to develop a circle of friends could also prove very effective well beyond childhood. Strategies such as those described by Quill (1995a) and Quirk-Hodgson (1995) on solving social problems and developing relationships could also be readily adapted to working with adults.

Mesibov (1992) and Kunce and Mesibov (1998) describe approaches that have been used successfully to increase social competence in high-functioning individuals enrolled in the TEACCH scheme. Their teaching focuses not only on direct social interactions but also on ways of analysing and organising their thinking, understanding the relationships between events and behaviours, learning about perspectives, and developing trust and rapport. Bauminger (2002) evaluated the effectiveness of a cognitive behavioural intervention designed to facilitate social emotional understanding and social interactions, for fifteen high-functioning children and teenagers. At the end of the programme the participants showed more social initiations and made more frequent attempts to share experiences; problem-solving skills and emotional understanding also improved. Class teachers, too, recorded improvements in their social skills. Other programmes have made use of a wide range of different techniques, often involving role-play procedures. Unlike many students, individuals with autism do not seem to be daunted at having to take part in role-play exercises or by appearing on video. Such adjuncts to therapy are valuable in demonstrating and rehearsing the skills required in social settings such as restaurants, pubs, work, shops or parties; in encouraging problem-solving and the development of more appropriate strategies to cope with difficult situations (including assertiveness training); in developing listening, conversational and turn-taking skills; in improving perception of nonverbal cues, such as eye contact, body language, facial expression and tone of voice.

Ways of dealing with situations that are stressful or anxiety-provoking also play an important part in intervention. Although the evaluation of these programmes remains limited, they do indicate that improvements in various areas can be achieved over time. Howlin and Yates (1999) conducted a short-term outcome study of nine men attending a social group for high-functioning adults with autism. There was a particular focus on the use of more appropriate conversational skills, and over the course of one year speech was found to become less repetitive and group members were significantly more likely to attempt to initiate or maintain conversations (e.g. by offering information, asking questions, initiating new topics or developing existing themes). Changes were also reported in social competence more generally. Four individuals left home to live in supported or semi-supported accommodation; two spent some time living abroad and one managed to cope at home by himself when his father moved away. Four managed to find at least part-time employment or embarked on further training schemes (one for a postgraduate qualification). When asked for their own comments on what they had gained from the group, individuals reported improvements in their communication skills, their ability to interpret other people's emotions, their problem-solving and decision-making abilities, and improvement in their ability to relate to people at home and outside. Families also reported improvements in their sons' conversational and social skills, in their self-confidence and general independence, and in their decision-making and problem-solving strategies.

Despite these positive indicators, however, there continued to be difficulties in generalising the skills acquired in the group to settings outside. The individuals attending this group all had good language skills and their intellectual ability was well within the normal range. It was clear that in group discussions and role-play sessions they were able to demonstrate good understanding of social rules and that they also had some perception of other people's feelings and emotions. Nevertheless, once the supports of being in a group were removed and they were left to cope alone with the demands of social interactions, their ability to apply these skills remained limited. For example, in discussion it was evident that group members were fully aware that unsolicited approaches to unknown young women were unlikely to be successful and could well lead to frightening or offending the person approached. However, reports or observations of some individuals in other settings indicated that such behaviours still tended to persist.

Attempts to improve assertiveness skills also seemed to have limited effects. All the group members said they found such interactions very difficult, and they disliked having to try to stand up for themselves, usually for fear of giving offence. For example, Damien, whose cousin had for some time been taking more and more of his money, was helped to recognise that this was both dishonest and manipulative, and that he would never get back the money he was handing out. Strategies were practised that would enable him to say 'No' more effectively, as well as teaching him ways in which he might try to avoid the problem (such as ensuring that he did not have access to large quantities of cash). However, although Damien said that he tried to use these tactics he found it almost impossible to remain firm under pressure and the loss of money continued until his parents actively intervened.

There is also a risk that social skills groups of this kind may run into problems by providing training in certain areas of social inter-action whilst failing to address more fundamental issues. Jerome, who had previously attended another social skills group for people with a mixture of social problems largely unrelated to autism, had been given help and coaching on ways to initiate and maintain conversations with young women. The problem was that Jerome rarely met young women as he lived alone with his family and had few outside activities. His solution for finding the best place to meet as many single women as possible was simple – inside the local ladies' lavatory! When arrested by the police he clearly had no understanding of why his behaviour had got him into trouble, especially as he had been rather proud of himself for solving the problem in this way.

Finally, too, it is crucial that such groups do not appear to promise more than they can actually offer. Teaching young people with autism how to improve their conversational and social skills is no guarantee that they will then be able to find a partner or establish a permanent relationship. From the outset, therefore, it is imperative to make absolutely clear what the group can *and cannot* offer. People with autism suffer constant setbacks and disappointments throughout their lives, and it is all too easy inadvertently to raise false hopes. Clarification, from the outset, of the group aims and limitations is essential if tutors are to avoid the risk of undermining, yet again, their confidence and self-esteem.

Improving the ability to 'understand minds'

Although there have been many investigations of the problems related to 'theory of mind' in both children and adults with autism (Baron-Cohen *et al.* 2002) there have been relatively few attempts to explore whether such deficits can be improved in any way by training.

Those studies that have taken place have concentrated almost exclusively on children and have usually focused on very specific areas, such as understanding false beliefs or distinguishing between appearance and reality (Bowler *et al.* 1993, Ozonoff and Miller 1995, Starr 1993, Swettenham 1995, Swettenham *et al.* 1995) Teaching in these studies has utilised a number of different approaches including computers, actors, behavioural and emotional cues, direct instruction, task repetition and feedback. Almost all the children involved were able to learn to pass the tasks and, in some cases, to maintain the skills over a period of several months. There was little evidence, however, that children were able to generalise what they had learnt to novel tasks or situations.

Research by Hadwin and colleagues (1996) suggests that, at least when working with young children a developmental approach to teaching may be more effective. Using a range of different teaching strategies they were able to demonstrate improvements in the understanding of beliefs and emotions. However, although there was some generalisation to non-taught tasks within the same domain, there was little generalisation to other, non-taught, aspects of theory of mind. Furthermore, few improvements were found in the development of imaginative play activities. Nevertheless, the fact that even a very brief intervention study of this kind was able to make a significant impact on certain aspects of children's learning is promising.

The increasing sophistication of interactive video and DVD programmes also has considerable potential for helping individuals with autism. Baron-Cohen and his colleagues at the University of Cambridge (2002) have recently produced an interactive 'mind-reading' programme that contains over 7000 examples of emotions, using lessons, quizzes, and games to increase understanding. Successful participants can even award themselves a 'certificate of achievement'.

However, the value of these techniques in improving social and emotional understanding in adults has yet to be demonstrated. Recent research at the Yale Child Study Center (Klin *et al.* 2002) suggests that impairments may stem from the earliest years, and may result from the inability of infants with autism to recognise the importance of facial cues (such as eye and mouth movement) in interpreting social situations. Thus, it may well be that in order to achieve long-term success, and improve generalisation to naturalistic situations, therapy may have to begin at a much younger age and focus on a much earlier developmental stage. The need for early intervention is also highlighted by the work of Peterson and Siegal (1995), which suggests that initial impairments in theory of mind may be further exacerbated as time goes on by poor expressive and receptive language abilities, which, in turn, progressively impede individuals' exposure to, and understanding of, mental states as they grow older. Whether or not, therefore, training in adults is likely to have even the limited beneficial results found in studies of children is clearly an urgent topic for future research.

As all the examples cited above indicate, life for many people with autism is frequently lacking in the most basic human comforts, which for the rest of us are so essential for happiness and fulfillment. Social impairments affect relationships within the family, success at work or college and acceptance within residential settings, specialist centres or the wider community. Even the most casual of interactions are likely to be affected, and the chances of enjoying the pleasures that come from close intimate or sexual relationships are severely curtailed. The accounts of more able people with autism make very clear how much some of them, at least, miss the opportunity to be like other people, to have friends, or develop relationships, particularly with the opposite sex. Therese Jolliffe (Jolliffe *et al.* 1992) writes: 'contrary to what people may think, it is possible for an autistic person to feel lonely and to love somebody'.

However, many also recognise the conflicts that a close relationship might entail. Marcia, a young woman in her twenties, described how much she sometimes longed for someone to talk with, but she is perceptive enough to admit to the difficulties that intimacy would involve: 'Half of me would like to have a close friend but the other half knows that it would be too much hassle'. Previous relationships had always ended in acrimony: at school, because she would try to dominate the interaction and exclude all others and later, when she tried sharing a flat, because of her stereotyped and ritualistic activities.

Anne, a young woman described by Margaret Dewey (1991), notes:

> I don't feel as if I have enough friends but I've been feeling a lot
> better recently because of all the things I've been doing. I work
> part time organising the library for the Autistic Society. And I do
> some part-time work with the Developmental Disability group.
> There are some benefits in being alone, too, I can think through
> and be more ready to go out again. I often feel lonely for a man.
> I would really like to have somebody but I'm glad I haven't gotten
> attached yet so I make further progress and be more acceptable.

Other people express the view that they may be better off alone.
Margaret Dewey's son Jack is quoted in the same paper as saying:
'Actually, I don't suffer from loneliness. If I have to relate to people
too much I become nervous and uncomfortable. . . . It is important for
me to please people [but] it is not important that I see them often.'

Still others confess that if it were not for outside social pressures
they might be much more contented with their way of life. Irene, a
woman in her mid-twenties, who has had a number of disastrous
relationships in the past, noted that:

> I don't usually feel lonely, and in some ways I'm better by myself;
> I couldn't cope with the demands of a close relationship. . . . I'd be
> awful. . . . Sometimes I think that if I didn't know about friends,
> or knew other people had them, being alone wouldn't bother me
> at all.

At least such individuals are able to talk about their loneliness and
feelings of exclusion or rejection. Many other people with autism, even
those who may possess relatively good language skills, have far less
ability to express their feelings in this way. Very often, in settings
catering for people with disabilities, clients with autism are often
described as being 'happiest if left alone' or as having 'no desire' for
contact with others. The anecdotal accounts or writings of more able
people, however, suggest that such assumptions (which can, of course,
help to reduce the burden on professional carers and sometimes even
families) may be completely mistaken.

Making use of existing skills

Given the complexity of intimate human relationships, and the pitfalls
they present to even the most socially accomplished of individuals, it is

unrealistic to expect – and certainly dishonest ever to promise – that any form of therapy or training can help to furnish the individual with autism with the skills of empathy, understanding, sensitivity and the countless others that are needed to establish successful relationships. Help can, however, be provided to ensure that as many opportunities as possible exist to increase the opportunities for social contacts, and to ensure that the person with autism is as well equipped as possible in the skills necessary for successful interactions

Even when working in specialist day or residential settings it is crucial to overcome, as far as possible, any behaviours that will make individuals socially unacceptable within their peer group. It is also important to ensure that the person with autism is encouraged and if necessary taught the skills required to interact with other clients. Often, people with autism spend much of their time alone, or in one-to-one interactions with members of staff. For some this may be entirely appropriate, but others may never have learned how to work *with*, rather than simply alongside, others in their daily activities. Very many activities, however, do offer much more scope for sharing, turn-taking and cooperation than is often recognised. Music, cookery, gardening, yoga, art and crafts, as well as more obvious activities such as dancing or games, offer many opportunities for skilled staff to promote inter-actions between clients. Many individuals with autism in institutional or day-care settings are often much more capable in many ways than their peers, and helping them develop a supportive or caretaking role can also foster integration. Jenny, for example, developed consider-able skill in using massage and simple aromatherapy techniques with physically handicapped clients at her day centre, and became a very useful source of additional help to the therapist. Denny is a young man who will spend hours pushing wheelchair users around, as long as he is allowed to follow his own repetitive routes.

Encouraging a wide range of activities, in which social interactions may be further developed, is crucial for individuals of any level of ability. Making use of specific skills or interests in areas such as music, chess, computing, transport, wildlife or environmental issues can also be invaluable in offering individuals the opportunities to mix with other people. Jonas had always had a fascination with railways since a young child and as he grew older accompanied his parents to local groups campaigning for better transport systems. He is now an active lobbyist in the campaign against new motorways, and spends much of his time travelling around the country attending meetings on these issues. Peter, who initially had an obsessional interest in deer and sheep, is now a devoted supporter of the Worldwide Fund for Nature and a tireless fundraiser on their behalf. Anna, whose fascination with stick insects caused many problems at home when she was a child (especially as she always failed to replace the tops of their containers) now has a considerable reputation as an expert in this field, and frequently travels to international conferences. Leslie, a gifted musician, spends several evenings a week playing for local orchestras or choirs, or in residential homes for the elderly and handicapped. Dominic spends almost all his time in activities related to the local church, and weekends and holidays are spent helping individuals with physical disabilities. In the week, he attends foreign language classes so that on the annual trip to Lourdes with the church he will be able to offer better help. All these individuals describe themselves as having many friends, and although the quality of these friendships may be questioned it is clear nevertheless that their time is fully occupied, that they are accepted and appreciated by the groups involved and – most importantly – that they view themselves, with some justification, as popular and valued members of society.

6 Stereotyped, ritualistic and obsessional behaviours

Patterns of stereotyped and ritualistic behaviours in adulthood

A characteristic – but over-simplistic – view of ritualistic behaviours in autism is that of a solitary child lining up rows of bricks or coins, spinning the wheels of toy cars, posting objects down the backs of radiators or chairs, or collecting coins, leaves, pieces of string or plumbing equipment. However, with age, particularly in the case of individuals of higher intellectual ability, the routines, rituals and stereotypes tend to become much more complex. For many individuals, too, they may play a crucial role in keeping fear and anxiety under control. As Therese Jolliffe notes:

> Reality to an autistic person is a confusing, interacting mass of events, people, places, sounds and sights. There seems to be no clear boundaries, order or meaning to anything. A large part of my life is spent trying to work out the pattern behind everything. Set routines, times, particular routes and rituals all help to get order into an unbearably chaotic life. Trying to keep everything the same reduces some of the terrible fear.
>
> (Jolliffe *et al.* 1992)

Environmental and developmental factors also play an important role. The degree to which individuals are able to develop their social, communication and cognitive skills, for example, can have considerable impact on the extent of ritualistic behaviours in later life. The more limited an individual's skills in these areas the greater will be their dependence on ritualistic and stereotyped behaviour patterns. Similarly, the emptier their lives the more such behaviours will predominate (see Turner 1999 for further discussion of the factors associated with repetitive and stereotyped behaviours in autism).

Collecting facts

Instead of large collections of objects, many older people with autism collect information: knowledge about all the different seating systems on British Rail Western Region trains since 1960; the hit songs of particular pop groups or the records published by specific recording companies, rugby scores, the trophies won by Torvill and Dean, Les Dawson, albinoism, sporting events or personalities, astronomy, poisons, quiz shows, pedigrees of Arab stud horses, dimensions of dinosaurs are but a few of the topics about which individuals may possess a wealth of knowledge. A memory for, or fascination with, birth dates or travel routes and timetables is also characteristic. Many more intellectually able people with autism will avidly buy books or magazines related to their special interests, or spend hours in the library reading about them. In contrast to the stereotyped behaviours of childhood, when the obsession itself is a problem (so that families may have the house filled with unlikely objects such as left-foot red wellingtons or blue rubber sink plungers) difficulties in adulthood tend to arise because of the time spent thinking, talking or worrying about these interests, sometimes to the exclusion of other activities.

Damien, for example, was a young man with an obsession with airlines and aeroplanes. Given the registration of a particular plane he could recall with complete accuracy not only where and when it flew but its flight history, the company that owned or leased it and its repair and accident record. The extent of his knowledge was so impressive that as part of a job experience scheme he was given a placement at his nearest airport. His careers adviser had, understandably, thought that his fascination and knowledge of planes would prove a major advantage there, but in fact the opposite proved to be the case. Instead of completing the jobs assigned to him Damien spent the whole day watching or talking about planes and eventually managed to hack into the airport's computer system to gain even more information. Stuart, who had an obsession with the seating systems on British Rail trains, carried around with him albums full of photographs of these. Whenever the opportunity arose he would go through these in detail, and at great length, with anyone who was close at hand.

Generally, the effect of such obsessions is to induce boredom, or at worst irritation in the listener; however, there may be even less desirable effects. Sandy, who had always been interested in warfare, developed a particular interest in the Pol Pot regime of 1970s Cambodia. He would regale anyone he met with the atrocities committed during this period, providing graphic, horrific and unwanted details about the methods of slaughter and the numbers of victims (particularly infants) murdered. His glee in recounting this information and his obvious fascination with violence could make listeners feel most uncomfortable, and there were concerns that he might begin to enact some of his violent fantasies. Obsessional interests can also lead to financial difficulties. Oliver, a young man fascinated by computers, spent all his time and money buying computer magazines and agonising over which model he should buy next, even though he was already seriously in debt.

Involving others

Whilst most obsessional interests will have at least an indirect impact on other people, some may involve others more directly. Owen was a young Welshman whose obsession with rugby had persisted since a child. He knew everything there was to know about teams, players, scores or league tables, and was a devoted attender at his local club. His 'conversations' were dominated by rugby and he would try to involve anyone he met in talk about this. However, he was also very pedantic about the precise terminology used. Players had to be called 'boys' not 'men', jerseys described as 'jumpers', boots as 'footwear', scarves as 'colours' and so forth. If his mother, in her attempts to talk with him, used the 'wrong' word, this could lead to hours of correction and recrimination, often disrupting family activities for the rest of the day.

Sally was a twenty-five-year-old woman fascinated by TV quiz games. Since she was very young her parents had watched these with her as this was one of the few situations when she would enjoy talking to them. Although she became much more sociable as she grew older, she continued to insist that they all watch quiz games together. Twenty years ago, when the obsession first began, there were relatively few quiz games to watch and the habit was not particularly disruptive. As the frequency of these games on TV increased, however, and as her insistence on the family's involvement became more pronounced, the intrusiveness of this obsession became considerable. Even if they went out she would insist on the programmes being recorded on video, and these would then have to be viewed, often until late into the night.

Irene had, over the years, developed various rituals of her own concerning clothes, bedtimes, meals and outings etc. These were generally tolerated by her mother, although they could prove quite disruptive at times. However, major problems arose when her mother remarried and had two more children. Irene dictated their clothing (including insisting that they wore vests in the height of summer, nightdresses not pyjamas at night and woolly hats from November to March), what and when they should eat and what time they went to bed. The children's friends would be sent from the house if they disturbed any of these routines, and conflicts within the household escalated dramatically as the younger children began to resist these restrictions on their lives.

Dislike of change

Although, as they grow older, many people with autism come to accept and even enjoy greater variation in their lives, they may continue to resist changes in specific settings or in certain aspects of their environment; unpredictable changes, in particular, frequently provoke considerable distress. Lise Pyles (2002) recalls 'I once asked John [her son with Asperger syndrome] "What is the definition of hell?" He said without hesitation, "Surprises"'.

David was a forty-year-old man who, after many years of living with his mother, was helped to buy his own apartment. Before leaving he had taken numerous photographs of his previous house and these were displayed throughout his new flat. He also ensured that the layout of his bedroom was as similar as possible to that of his old room. Through the help of his photographs, and with his mother's support, David coped remarkably well with the move. However, unforeseen problems occurred when his mother herself later moved house. David insisted that all the rooms should be arranged exactly as they had been previously, and he became so upset that he had not taken enough photographs of the old house that he wrote to the new owners asking permission to take some more. He was then horrified to discover that they had already begun major alterations to the kitchen, bathroom and garden. He was so distressed at not having enough photographs of the original layout that he spent all his free time searching old photo albums for pictures and cutting them out (ruining his mother's photo collection in the process).

Martin had learned to cope with many changes in his life and after leaving college had succeeded in finding work in a local office. However, at holiday times he still insisted that the family go to exactly the same place, and carry out the same activities, as they had done when he was a child. This was a small, isolated caravan site, not far from their home in the south of England, which in his more disturbed days had been the only place they had been able to risk taking him. The only activity, apart from sitting on the beach, that he would take part in was crazy golf, which they were forced to play for hours on end.

Although the holiday was the highlight of Martin's year, for the rest of the family the mere thought of a whole fortnight there became a nightmare.

Simon, by the time he was in his mid-twenties, was living alone with relatively little support. He had learned to clean and shop for himself and had begun attending day courses at his local college. However, the one area he never changed was his diet. At home he would cook only a certain brand of frozen food and when out ate only chips and cheese-burgers from a particular fast-food chain. Unfortunately, as this was not one of the major chains it severely restricted opportunities to eat out and in turn imposed major limitations on trips or holidays away.

Bonnie was a young woman who, despite having a marked resist-ance to any changes in the home when younger, had learned to cope with alterations over time. However, in her own room everything was kept in strict order, and although she spent much of her time in a residential unit her family were not allowed to move any item, no matter how small, in her absence.

Matthew was an eighteen-year-old who since early childhood had insisted on being washed at the kitchen sink. His self-care skills had developed considerably since he had begun attending a social educa-tion unit, and he was quite able to bath and wash himself. On bath nights (Tuesdays, Thursdays and Saturdays without exception) there were no problems in his using the bathroom. On the other nights, however, he insisted on stripping off completely and washing at the kitchen sink as he had always done. This gave rise to untold embar-rassment if his teenage sister had friends around at the time.

Collecting

The tendency to collect objects of various kinds can persist well into adulthood. Sometimes the focus of interest may remain much the same as in childhood; for others, collections may vary over time or become more sophisticated. Sally, a middle-aged woman with autism and mod-erate learning difficulties, has continued to collect 'diaries' throughout her life. These contain lists of the names and birthdays of everyone with whom she comes into contact, and if the current book is lost or removed (other residents in her group home have learned that this is a very easy way of upsetting her) she becomes very distressed. Sarah, another young woman with learning disabilities, collects small stones wherever she goes, which she keeps in jars all over her room. Stevie, a young man with a degree in electronics, is an avid collector of pop records, of which he now has many thousands. Each of these is catalogued according to its date, publishing company and singer and identified by a complex numbering system. If new editions of any of these records are produced Stevie is unable to rest until he has acquired these, sometimes at considerable expense.

Many families report that the obsession with collecting seems to decline somewhat as individuals grow older, but sometimes the opposite may be the case. Emma, for example, loved collecting notebooks and shiny pieces of paper as a child. In her teens she developed a passion for ballroom dancing and collected any leaflets relevant to this activity. Then, because she worried lest any leaflets became damaged, she began to collect several copies of each. Eventually, she became unable to dispose of pieces of paper at all and as she worked in a printing company would bring home large parcels of waste paper each week. The house and garage became full of boxes of paper, but although she recognised the problems that her collections caused for herself and her family – paradoxically she loved everything around her to be neat and tidy, and this had become increasingly impossible – she could not bear to throw anything away.

Rodney was a middle-aged man who had lived alone since the death of his father. As a young child he had had a fascination with collecting tools and electrical equipment and when older had found work as a porter in the supplies department of a large electrical company. When equipment became obsolete he was often allowed to take this home. The problem was not too bad while his father was alive because he refused to allow new items into the house unless an old item was disposed of first. However, after his death Rodney continued to collect everything he could, until it became almost impossible to enter the house because of the huge piles of equipment stacked everywhere.

Routines

Routine is essential for everyone if they are to organise their lives in an effective way: leaving the house at a certain time, eating at regular intervals, developing regular patterns for washing, dressing, going to work or even pursuing leisure activities can be crucial if life is to run smoothly. It is only when such habits become so fixed that they disrupt other activities, or when a behaviour that was once acceptable becomes inappropriate because of changing circumstances or expectations, that problems occur.

Jim had had a fascination with watching the sun set for many years. At school this had not been a problem, because for most of the year lessons finished well before sunset. When he moved to an adult residential unit, however, and was expected to be engaged in work or other activities, or to catch the coach home later in the day, his insistence on waiting to see the sun set became much more of a problem. Similarly, Bob had been fascinated by the weather since he was tiny and he spent much of his childhood listening to weather forecasts and informing everyone what the next day's weather would be like. As the family lived in Western Australia at the time the predictability of weather conditions was fairly good. Their move to England, however, resulted in enormous disruption when Bob quickly realised that the correlation between the forecast and actual weather conditions was far from perfect.

Marion was a very able young woman whose autism was hardly apparent except to those who knew her well. By her mid-twenties her main rituals were confined to night-time activities which had little impact on other members of her family. Eventually, through her church group, she met a young man to whom she became engaged. Her parents realised that these remaining 'habits' could be a source of considerable difficulty for the marriage. The main problem was that before going to bed she would draw and re-draw the curtains until they were in *exactly* the 'right' position and she also had to pick up every piece of fluff on the floor. Her parents had imposed a time limit on these behaviours in the rest of the house, but in her bedroom at night she would spend hours engaged in these activities. However, it was clear that her fiancé would find such behaviours very difficult to understand or cope with.

Susan was another young woman who had left her family to live in a large residential unit. As a child she had always been given pocket money by her parents, and although she had little interest in the money itself she took great delight in depositing it in her post office account and watching her savings grow. The money was never removed as she was always provided with everything she needed. In her new home she continued, like the other residents, to deposit any money remaining from her benefit payments into an account at the local post office. However, persuading her to *withdraw* this money produced enormous problems. Even taking out enough money to contribute to a birthday card for another resident would require days of wrangling, and she would refuse to go on trips or outings rather than withdraw any of her funds.

Other stereotyped behaviour patterns may present problems in adulthood because behaviours that are acceptable in a child later become entirely inappropriate. Joey, for example, loved to watch the washing spinning around in his mother's machine, and this could keep him still and quiet for hours. The family lived in a small country village, and if his mother's machine were not in action the neighbours were happy to let him watch theirs. In his teens he would wander off to the launderette in the nearby town and happily remain there for an hour or two. When this closed down, Joey was resourceful enough to seek other ways of indulging his passion. He would wander around the neighbourhood looking through kitchen windows, and if he saw a washing machine working would do his best to gain entry. His family only became aware of the problem when he was brought home by the police, having terrified an elderly pensioner who came home to find him sitting in the middle of her kitchen floor.

Stereotyped movements

Stereotyped movements, such as rocking, flicking or flapping are often less in evidence as individuals grow older and if they do occur may be an important indicator of distress or anxiety. Bella was a young woman with moderate learning difficulties who had always flicked and flapped her hands as a young child, but by the time she reached her late teens and was well settled in a local day centre she rarely did so. After a holiday away, however, these behaviours suddenly returned, together with other signs of stress. Having little speech, Bella was unable to explain what had happened, but it was later revealed that a number of clients on the trip had been abused by a worker there. It was never established whether Bella herself had actually been abused, but it was apparent that the distress surrounding these incidents was responsible for the upsurge in stereotyped behaviours.

Precipitating factors are not necessarily as serious as this, of course. A change in routine or an unexpected event which would be of little significance to most people may easily trigger a return to stereotyped motor behaviours in someone with autism. Jeremy was a middle-aged man working in a large office as an accounts clerk. With his formal suit, rolled umbrella and smart attaché case he appeared much the same as all the other commuters at his local railway station. Yet unlike them he could never behave with the same equanimity over cancelled or delayed trains, and it was at these times that he would revert to the rocking, flapping and hand-biting that had been so characteristic in childhood.

Boredom or inadequate stimulation may also be a problem. Individuals who previously showed few signs of motor mannerisms in a structured educational setting may begin to display these behaviours if they are subsequently placed in situations with inadequate stimulation. Raymond, for example, had rarely rocked since being a child, but this behaviour became very pronounced after a few months in a residential unit. On visiting him, his social worker found that he was unable to join in most of the day activities at the unit because of the noise and general overcrowding there, and this was when the stereotypes were most in evidence.

Although problems related to stereotyped behaviours may lessen in adulthood, or be important indicators of other, hidden, anxieties, the main difficulty is that they appear much more out of place as individuals grow older. Whilst flapping and rocking may go almost unnoticed in a very young child, they will rapidly draw attention to an adult with autism, often exacerbating that individual's social difficulties and reducing his or her chances of integration and acceptance.

Anxiety, fears and phobias

Another major problem related to ritualistic and stereotyped behaviours in older people is the high anxiety levels that may result from them, for a variety of different reasons. Fears and fascinations often become inextricably linked, so that children who have an obsession with a particular object at one stage can develop a great fear of it later. Mark's first word was reported to be 'Hoover', and for years his mother would let him play with the vacuum cleaner to calm him down. She even turned it on in order to get him to sleep! However, when she switched from an upright to a cylinder model he became quite distraught, and thereafter the noise of the cleaner would induce such panic that his mother was only able to clean when he was out of the house.

Martin had developed an obsession with video game machines as a young boy and was well known as an expert player at the local games centre. His presence there would attract large numbers of onlookers, keen to see what his scores would be. However, he became increasingly anxious about maintaining his high level of scores, and although he loved playing his fear of 'failing' to meet his onlookers' expectations became so intense that every visit became more and more stressful.

Adam, a young man in his early twenties and of well above average intelligence, had had a fascination with things electrical since he was tiny. By the age of six he would create havoc when his family visited other people's houses by attempting to rewire lamps or other equipment. At the age of seven he wired up the Christmas tree lights to the video recorder to see whether inserting a video tape would make the lights come on! Although, as he grew older, he began to take more heed of his parents' warnings about the potential danger of such beha-viours, he then became obsessional about *never* touching electrical equipment unless it was entirely safe. He would not use any equipment in the kitchen or bathroom because of the proximity to water and was therefore unable to make himself even a cup of tea or piece of toast; bathing was difficult because he refused to have the light on in the bathroom, and he would only use an electric shaver in his bedroom. Eventually he refused to go into the kitchen at all, becoming far more dependent on his mother for cooking and washing than he had ever been when younger.

Robin as a child had developed a very strict sense of 'honesty'. This was so strong that he kept rigidly to every rule he was ever given at school, much to the annoyance of his peer group (continually inform-ing the headmaster of the other children's favourite place for illicit smoking did not enhance his popularity!). When he reached his teens, if he was ever given the wrong change in buses or shops he would always seek to remedy this, even if this involved considerable incon-venience or expense, to return or get back just a few pence. Over time he became more and more anxious that he might inadvertently walk out of a shop without paying for something and be arrested for this, and he would insist on being given receipts for the smallest trans-actions. He then became worried that if the receipt were lost he could still be charged with theft and began to hoard every proof of purchase he could, becoming extremely agitated if any of these were mislaid.

Anita had always been described by her parents as a 'perfectionist' and could not bear anything that was damaged in any way. As a child she would refuse to wear clothes with any marks or faults at all, but as she grew older and acquired a particular fondness for certain garments she became very anxious about what would happen if these wore out. Her solution was to insist on buying at least two or three copies of every garment, so that her wardrobe became full of unworn shoes, trousers, jumpers and T-shirts. The problem then extended to buying food, as she could not bear the thought that she might have bought inferior produce. She would spend hours choosing a lamb chop or pack of bacon, and would often return home with pounds of these items, to ensure she had bought the best in the shop.

Finally, the futility of certain obsessions can be very difficult for families to tolerate. Living in a house filled with collections of stones, shells, pieces of cardboard or sink plungers is hard enough, but it may be even more frustrating when a potentially useful interest develops into a meaningless activity. James's mother was a keen, skilled gardener and she had encouraged him as a child to share her interest in the subject. In his late teens he developed an obsession with daffodils and narcissi and knew everything there was to know about the many different varieties, their flowering habits and so on. He was provided with space in the garden to grow his own and he spent considerable sums of money acquiring rare or new varieties. However, as soon as the bulbs flowered he would dig them up and replace them with others, throwing away even very fine plants. His mother could not bear the wanton destruction of plants in this way but could do little to change this behaviour.

Coping with stereotyped and ritualistic behaviours

Work with children suggests that direct attempts to prevent or prohibit stereotyped or ritualistic behaviours frequently prove counterproductive (Howlin 1998b). Deprived of the opportunity to take part in the few activities that may provide them with enjoyment or relief from stress, individuals may become even more disturbed, agitated and anxious. Even if attempts to stop one form of obsessional behaviour are successful, children may then proceed to develop new rituals or obsessions which can be even more disruptive than the original ones. Similar effects are found with adults. Moreover, as individuals become bigger, stronger and better able to control their environment, attempts to prevent these activities will become ever more difficult. Locking cupboards or doors or trying to place things out of reach are unlikely to hinder a large and determined adult.

A more productive approach is to attempt gradually to modify the behaviour so that it no longer interferes to the same extent with the lives of individuals or their families. A variety of different approaches can be adopted in order to achieve lower levels of disruption, and often a combination of strategies will be required. Determining the best approach will require careful assessment of the problem behaviour and detailed knowledge of the individual involved.

Addressing underlying causes

Stereotyped and ritualistic behaviour in adulthood may persist simply because the individual concerned has always done things in a certain way or has always had an interest in a particular topic. However, as noted above, an upsurge in such activities may well be an indication that someone is particularly anxious or under stress. In such cases, little progress will be made unless the underlying source of stress is identified and, if possible, eliminated.

Sometimes quite simple modifications to the environment can result in a rapid diminution of obsessional behaviours. Sally, who had moved to a residential home, became increasingly ritualistic at mealtimes. She would insist on sitting in a certain place, eating only from particular dishes, and had a variety of motor mannerisms that became more pronounced as the meal progressed. If attempts were made to calm her down she would immediately throw her meal across the room. Staff realised that the behaviours did not occur to the same extent at weekends, when many of the other residents were away. Sally's parents also reported that she generally disliked eating when she was surrounded by too many people or too much noise. Allowing her to sit at a table by herself, well away from the others and in a position that allowed her to leave the room easily if noise levels got too high, soon helped to reduce the problem.

In other cases it may be necessary to modify the expectations or attitudes of other people in order to bring about change. Jonathon was a young man who had recently moved to a residential unit where staff were particularly concerned about his inability to cope with money. Because this restricted his ability to go out alone they decided that teaching him to use money appropriately should have a high priority. What they did not know was that at school Jonathon was almost 'phobic' about maths and had become expert at making himself sick in almost every maths lesson. Shortly after the money coaching was introduced, Jonathon began complaining that 'maths made him sick' and he would repeat this over and over again to anyone he met. It was decided simply to ignore these comments, with the result that Jonathon soon put his words into action, vomiting every time money training was introduced, and rapidly losing weight. When staff sought help to deal with the problem the advice given was to reduce the emphasis on using money, at least in the home, and simply to ensure that Jonathon always had sufficient funds when he went to the shop to buy his favourite magazines and sweets. The vomiting quickly stopped, and although he quite often returned without any change he was unperturbed by this. The staff remained torn between the desire to help Jonathon develop his independence and the need to keep him healthy, and they in turn needed support to accept that few normal adults reach their full potential in all possible fields of competence, and that being able to choose which skills we develop and which we do not is a fundamental human right.

At times, of course, it may not be possible to modify the environment sufficiently to ensure that obsessional behaviours do not occur, and it may be necessary to address underlying anxieties more directly.

Desensitisation techniques

There are many effective cognitive and behavioural strategies that can be used to decrease fears and anxieties. However, many desensitisation programmes rely on the ability of clients to *imagine* themselves in fearful situations, and this clearly poses problems for people with autism. Instead, 'real-life' exposure is usually required.

In the case of Adam, whose obsession with the dangers of electrical equipment resulted in his becoming less and less able to take care of himself, a desensitisation programme was devised to help him overcome his fears. A simple 'hierarchy' of fears was established by getting Adam to indicate, using stick-on faces, how he felt about certain activities involving electrical equipment (see Table 6.1). A chart was pinned on the kitchen wall indicating the task to be worked on each week. In order to reduce his anxiety as far as possible a selection of his favourite tapes was kept in the kitchen to be played whenever he was there. As the tapes were not available elsewhere, this increased his motivation to enter the kitchen. After three months he was able to make toast, put food in the microwave and make toasted sandwiches as long as his mother was close by, but he refused to use a kettle until a circuit-breaker was installed. Once he was assured that this would instantly cut off the flow of electricity if problems arose, he began to make himself hot drinks and to stack the dishwasher. The process up to this stage took six months and Adam continued to be very dependent on his mother's presence. When he began to approach the stage of attempting these tasks without his mother he became increasingly agitated, constantly talking about what would happen if anything went wrong or if the circuit-breaker failed, and he once more began to resist entering the kitchen. It was decided that this level of stress was unacceptable and that it would be better to maintain his current progress rather than push him too far and perhaps cause his behaviour to regress. Although the ultimate goal of the programme was far from being attained, at least some level of independence had been reached, giving Adam a greater sense of self-esteem and allowing his mother some extra freedom.

Graded change

Just as special interests, obsessions and rituals tend to grow gradually, often almost imperceptibly over time, programmes to reduce them work best if carried out in gradual and carefully planned stages. A 'graded change' approach can be particularly useful in helping

Table 6.1 Hierarchy of fears relating to electrical equipment

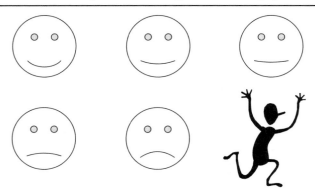

Fear hierarchy	How feeling: IMAGES
	0 Quite happy and relaxed
	1 Not happy, but not upset either
	2 Bit tense; tight feeling in stomach
	3 Very tense and nervous
	4 Very upset and panicky
	5 Want to run away and scream
Fear rating	0 = No anxiety 5 = Panic
1	*(Mother present in kitchen)*
1	Making dry toast
2	Making a toasted sandwich
2	Making a toasted sandwich with tomatoes in
3	Putting dry food (eg cooked rice) in microwave to heat
4	Cooking a prepared meal in the microwave
4	Heating cup of coffee in microwave
4	Putting cup in dishwasher
5	Turning on dishwasher
	Making cup of tea/coffee
4	*(Mother absent)*
4	Making dry toast
4	Making a toasted sandwich
4	Making a toasted sandwich with tomatoes in
4	Putting dry food (eg cooked rice) in microwave to heat
5	Cooking a prepared meal in the microwave
5	Heating cup of coffee in microwave
5	Putting cup in dishwasher
5	Turning on dishwasher
	Making cup of tea/coffee

individuals to cope with environmental changes or alterations in daily routine. David, who became very upset when his mother moved house, tried to insist that she place all her furniture in the same position as in their old home. To begin with, his mother attempted to comply with his wishes despite the inconvenience this caused. However, as time went on David became increasingly resistant to her changing anything. Remembering how difficult it had been to stop his obsessions as a child she decided she must draw. Indeed, drawing, or taking photographs, was exactly what she did. Beginning first in the downstairs kitchen and dining room, where David's 'plans' were particularly inconvenient, she took photographs or made drawings of the layout, explaining to him exactly what she was doing and the changes she planned. As long as he had a pictorial representation of how things had been he agreed to accept some minor alterations. His mother made it clear that she would make no changes without telling him first, and that she would ensure that he had enough photographs or drawings of the original layout. David accepted this, and gradually over a period of several months she was able to organise most of the new house as she wanted. The exception was the spare room, which David used when he visited and which he was allowed to preserve exactly as it had always been.

Encouraging alternative and more acceptable behaviours

Stereotyped and ritualistic behaviours are frequently at their worst when individuals have no access to other, more productive activities with which to fill their time. Attempts to modify rituals or obsessions without replacing them with alternative behaviours are unlikely to prove successful, and without careful planning there is a real risk of even more disruptive behaviours taking their place.

Tessa was a thirty-year-old woman whose fascination with hairdressing had persisted since childhood. If not carefully watched at her day centre for people with intellectual impairments she would frequently cut her own hair, and whenever the opportunity arose she would take aside uncomplaining clients and cut their hair too. If scissors were not available, knives or razor blades removed from the craft room served equally well. It was apparent that this behaviour occurred mainly at lunchtimes, when staff supervision was minimal and when no other activities were timetabled. Once the 'danger periods' had been identified additional help was enlisted to ensure that Tessa was appropriately supervised during the lunch break. A detailed timetable was drawn up, to ensure that the time was filled more constructively and staff managed to obtain some old wigs and wig stands, together with a supply of styling equipment (heated rollers, driers etc.) that could be used by Tessa to indulge her interest without endangering others. At the same time, the whereabouts of potentially vulnerable clients was closely monitored and security in the unit was improved in order to restrict her access to scissors, knives or razor blades. Since staff were aware that Tessa was capable of breaking into drawers or cupboards, or searching through their possessions to look for scissors, they took the additional precaution of routinely asking her, each meal time, whether she had a knife or scissors in her bag or pockets. Tessa would always show them if she had, and this combination of strategies brought the behaviour successfully under control.

Sally was a thirty-five-year-old woman with a severe learning disability who had lived with her parents since leaving school. Because of the inadequacy of local day-care facilities she spent almost all her time at home with her parents, with only occasional input from local services. Whenever she was bored through lack of occupation, or stressed by being pushed into activities that she did not enjoy, Sally would pull or pick her hair until she had become almost bald. The only time she did not hair-pull, apart from when she was asleep, was when she went swimming. Her parents and support workers attempted to try to develop a more appropriate daily programme that was neither over- nor under-stimulating and which involved as many visits as possible to the hydrotherapy pool of a local hospital. Sally loved water, but it was not possible for her to use a public pool as the noise or presence of too many people, and especially children, was very distressing for her. As Sally never tried to pull her hair whilst wearing her bathing hat she was encouraged to wear this for much longer periods each day, a nylon hat replacing the less comfortable rubber one. Over time the combination of the hat with a more constructive daily programme resulted in a marked diminution of the hair-pulling – apart from her fringe, which remained an easy target. Some activities outside the house were then reintroduced, but Sally's appearance was not enhanced by her red- and-black striped swimming cap. Because attempts to remove this resulted in much distress it was covered with a more age-appropriate baseball cap. Eventually, as the seams of the bathing hat began to fall apart, Sally was persuaded to wear just the baseball cap when out, although she still preferred the bathing cap in other circumstances.

Keeping stereotyped behaviours and interests out of sight

In some cases, the main problem with special interests or stereotypes is not so much that they are particularly disruptive in their own right, but that they may bring unwanted attention to the person with autism. Whilst this may not concern the individual concerned, it can cause problems for other family members.

David was a young man who had made good social progress in many ways and who worked in a voluntary capacity at a day centre for people with more severe learning difficulties. He got on well with his two brothers and shared their enjoyment in going to the cinema or the local pub. However, he had a number of facial mannerisms and grimaces that tended to occur if he were not otherwise occupied, and on buses or in queues these were a source of considerable embarrassment to his brothers. Although when he was younger David's parents had taught him to bring his hand mannerisms under control (by developing greater awareness of them and ensuring he always wore trousers with pockets into which he could put his hands), his awareness of his odd facial movements remained much more limited. Eventually his brothers insisted that wherever they went he carry with him a daily newspaper, and if the grimacing began they would make him disappear behind this. If the paper contained something of interest for him, this tended to reduce the amount of grimacing; but even if it did not, at least no one else could see him, which was all that mattered to his brothers!

Alan was an adolescent attending mainstream school where, although rather isolated, he was respected by other pupils because of his academic ability. He had always had a fascination with Sooty and Sweep puppets, but had learned that taking these to school led to teasing or worse and he was content as long as he always had them at home at night. Problems arose when his class went on a geography field trip. His mother was concerned that if other boys found his puppets he would be teased unmercifully; on the other hand, she knew he could not possibly sleep without them. Eventually she sewed them up into a pillowcase, with a gap into which Alan could place his hands, and she hoped that the other boys would not notice. When she discussed the situation with the teacher in charge some time after their return, she was upset to learn that Alan had soon revealed his secret to other children. However, it then transpired that several others had teddy bears, old blankets or other 'comforters' tucked away and Alan's revelation had made it possible for them to talk about their special objects too.

Shaping: contracts and compromises

For anyone, attempting to get rid of a long-standing habit, no matter how undesirable, inconvenient or even health-threatening it may be, is no easy task. For someone with autism, in whom patterns of behaviour are particularly entrenched, the difficulties are even greater.

Often by the time families or individuals seek help, patterns of obsessional behaviour may be so intractable that almost every area of functioning is affected. Attempts to solve many different problems at once usually lead to frustration and failure, and the first important step is to accept that progress will be slow (although it can also be steady) and is generally best achieved by working on one aspect of one problem area at a time. Overambitious attempts to stop behaviours that have had a strong hold for many years will almost certainly prove unsuccessful. Instead, behaviours need to be carefully broken down into their component parts and these then tackled step by step, with the ultimate goal perhaps taking many months or even longer to achieve.

Matthew was an eighteen-year-old whose insistence on washing in the kitchen sink caused his teenage sister such embarrassment that she threatened to leave home. Although he bathed regularly three nights a week, he persisted in stripping and washing at the kitchen sink every other evening. In this case the stages of intervention were as follows. First, the red plastic bowl he used to wash himself in the sink was replaced with a different bowl which he accepted without too much resistance. The original bowl was then transferred to the basin which had been installed some years ago in his bedroom but which he had consistently refused to use. Initially he also refused to use the bowl here, until his mother (knowing that he loved to be able to lock the bathroom door when he went for a bath) offered to let him fit a lock on his bedroom door too. She also supplied him with some favourite towels and soap from the bathroom. When the lock (which could easily be opened from the outside) was fitted he began to wash himself in his bedroom, but only with persistent pressure from his mother, and he continued to try to get to the kitchen sink. However, following an electrical fault all the lights in the kitchen ceased working, and as he hated the dark he became more willing to wash in his room. Rather than have the fault mended his mother left the lights unfixed for several months (at considerable inconvenience to herself) until his new washing patterns were well established.

Because Matthew had very limited speech, his involvement in the planning of this intervention was fairly minimal, although his agreement was sought at every stage. However, with more able individuals it is often helpful to draw up more formal 'contracts' in which the roles of all those concerned are agreed and specified from the outset.

Emma's paper collection had, as noted earlier, grown to such an extent that the garage was full of boxes of theatre, sport and dance programmes, printing leaflets from work (she estimated she had around 18,000 of these) and old school textbooks. Her parents were insistent that something had to go, and Emma herself accepted the need for this. First, a hierarchy of items was drawn up specifying the materials that would be most difficult for her to relinquish and those that would cause least distress. The most disposable were her old school textbooks, the least dispensable her dance programmes. Although she could not bear to throw anything away herself, she agreed to allow her mother to remove the boxes containing school books over a three-month period. The next stage was to work on the theatre and dance programmes. She had many duplicate copies of all of these and after a lengthy discussion agreed that she would throw away any copies in excess of two, thereby reducing the number of boxes by about a third. The next stage involved the removal of all but ten boxes of printed labels that she had got from work. If Emma wished to bring more paper home, this was accepted only if she allowed her mother to remove an equivalent amount. Again, she could not bear the thought of the paper being thrown away but agreed to give them to her mother so that she could use them for notes 'or other purposes'. She stipulated that her mother was not to throw any paper away but that she could take it to the recycling depot as long as she did not tell Emma if and when she had done so. In turn, Emma had to agree not to ask what had happened to the paper (her mother knew this would lead to anxiety and persistent questioning). Future theatre programmes could be collected, but no more than two copies of anything were to be brought home. Each stage of the programme, including planned dates for action, was specified in writing, with both Emma and her mother signing their agreement to the proposed plans. Emma had little difficulty coping with the removal of her school books, but the loss of her precious theatre programmes proved too traumatic and she asked to renegotiate the plan allowing her to keep three of each. Rather than increase her anxiety to a level where she would refuse to cooperate altogether, this was agreed. Eventually the programme resulted in a large quantity of paper being removed from the garage, and thereafter the level was kept fairly stable.

Marion, whose impending marriage was causing her mother such anxiety because of the time she spent, drawing the curtains and picking up fluff before she went to bed, finally agreed that this might irritate her partner. With her parents' help she rather reluctantly attempted to reduce these behaviours. For a few weeks she kept a record of how long it took her to get to bed each night, the average length of time being about two-and-a-half hours. With advice from her psychologist Marion drew up a bedtime schedule on which the time for getting to bed was reduced by five minutes each night. By using this, and with guidance from her parents, she was able to reduce the nightly ritual to about thirty minutes, a time period that it was hoped would be more acceptable to her new spouse. Finally, they invested in a Dyson vacuum cleaner as a wedding present in the hope that this would speed up her carpet cleaning, thereby reducing the time even further.

Anita, whose anxiety about having to wear damaged garments resulted in drawers and wardrobes overflowing with clothes, agreed to attach a 'wear-by date' label on each item purchased. The negotiated expiry period was two years after the original purchase date; thereafter Anita agreed that her mother could take any unworn garments to a local charity shop. On the whole this agreement worked quite well, although occasionally she would buy back certain garments from the charity shop and re-date them, pointing out that this had not been restricted in the terms of the original agreement.

Making rules

Although discussion and compromise are the most desirable ways of effecting change, there may be times when the level of resistance shown is so strong that a firmer approach is required if families or carers are to gain any degree of control. As already noted, attempts to restrict an obsession entirely are rarely successful, but it may be necessary to establish rules about when, where, with whom or how often certain activities can take place. Stuart's preoccupation with photographs of British Rail seating systems, for example, was beginning to discourage people from visiting the house, as he would bombard them with his pictures as soon as they arrived. Finally, in exasperation, his sister demanded, in no uncertain terms, that he must not talk to any of her friends ever again. He was so upset by this that she relented somewhat, promising that he could talk to them on any other topic for five minutes only before they went out. She also promised to look at his pictures with him every Sunday afternoon. She primed her friends to say 'I don't like photos of trains' if he broke the rule, but also encouraged them to talk to him about other topics. This approach proved so successful that the family began gradually to impose further restrictions until the obsession became far less intrusive.

Discouraging stereotyped interests and behaviours by imposing limits on where, when and with whom they can be carried out often proves very effective, and if restrictions are introduced in a planned and gradual way they should not result in too much distress or resistance.

With effective planning, ritualistic behaviours can also be used to reward periods of more productive activity. Caroline, who attended a local day centre, would spend all her time, if left alone, ripping up pieces of paper. Over time, staff dealt successfully with the problem by insisting first that she did not tear paper in the kitchen whilst making or drinking coffee (an activity that was also very important to her). Opportunities for tearing were also reduced by removing paper towels, kitchen rolls or newspapers from the room. Once she had left the kitchen, Caroline was allowed to return to her paper-tearing. Next, tearing was restricted in the dining room and later during musical and craftwork activities, which she also enjoyed. At the same time her involvement in other tasks, such as completing chores, was rewarded by providing her with a small pile of paper to rip up. As the time spent in other activities increased, and as the paper supply grew steadily smaller, her obsession with the activity gradually reduced, until it no longer caused any disruption. However, it could still be used to fill up time if she were not otherwise occupied, or to calm her if she became agitated or distressed.

The same problem was dealt with in a rather different way in the case of Jiro, who returned with his family to live in Japan. There, many day centres for people with learning disabilities produce recycled, handmade writing paper or cards etc. The first stage of this procedure involves tearing up vast amounts of paper into small pieces that can later be pulped by machine. The never-ending task offered Jiro a very important role in his centre.

As noted in the chapter on communication problems, there is one class of ritualistic behaviour that can prove particularly resistant to modification of verbal routines. Whilst it may be relatively easy to restrict the time spent lining up videotapes or to insist that the collection of jam jars be kept in a specified place, placing limitations on verbal behaviours is much more difficult, and the problems of developing *consistent* management strategies should not be underestimated. No matter how hard one tries to resist it is extremely easy to be drawn into ritualistic conversations before even realising it. Particularly if the subject matter is interesting or novel, the individual with autism usually has little problem in finding an audience. Dan, who was fascinated by the subject of albinoism, could readily attract the attention of people who did not know him with his extraordinary knowledge of this subject. Aaron, who spent all his time watching films on or reading about Batman, showed remarkable skill in turning any conversation around to this topic. Repetitive questioning also tends to 'feed' the obsessional interests more generally. Thus, Adam's obsession with electricity and the potential dangers of this was heightened rather than diminished if he were given the opportunity to talk about the subject at any length. Establishing rules early in childhood, or when an obsession first begins to emerge, about *when* a topic can be discussed (e.g. only after a discussion of other topics, or only at bedtimes), *where* discussions take place (only at home), or *with whom* (e.g. with the class teacher, but only at the end of the day's work), is crucial if later difficulties are to be minimised. Attempts to prevent the individual from *ever* talking about his or her special interests, or asking repetitive questions, are likely to result in overwhelming anxiety and agitation. As long as the established rules make it clear that the obsession is allowed at specified times, and as long as carers keep to their side of the agreement too, then a reasonable degree of control is usually possible. However, if complete freedom is allowed in the early years, or if repetitive discussions or questions reach a level where they totally dominate all conversations, intervention in later life becomes far more difficult.

Enlisting the help of others

As is evident from the examples above, reducing ritualistic behaviours to an acceptable level can be a very complex process involving detailed assessments and a variety of different strategies including environmental restructuring. In order for programmes to succeed information, help and support are needed from everyone concerned. Family and carers may also be required to change their behaviours or expectations at least as much as the person with autism. Changing the habits of many years is not easy for anyone, and careful discussion with and agreement from all the relevant parties will be required. Adam's mother had great difficulty in *not helping* him in the kitchen, as she could not bear to witness his distress and anxiety. Over the years she had protected him more and more from the need to use electrical equipment but in doing so had greatly curtailed his self-help skills. Her agreement *not* to offer him support was as difficult to achieve as his agreement to try to use the equipment, and although with time some measure of success was achieved he continued to remain dependent on her presence in order to be able to carry out the necessary tasks.

For older parents, too, the practicalities of offering support can present problems. Although Emma's parents were very willing to help reduce her paper collection, they lived some distance away, and it was not easy for them to visit their daughter on a regular basis to ensure that the terms of the agreement were consistently complied with.

Compromise may well be needed on both sides and it is not always possible to predict, at the start of a planned programme, the degree of stress that may be experienced. However, if anxiety, or distress (on either side) become excessive, intervention will almost certainly fail; hence the need for back-up and professional support, frequent reviews and a rapid renegotiation of plans if problems arise.

Self-control techniques

Because of the strains that an intensive programme can impose on other people, and the problems that can occur if external support is unavailable for some reason, it is also crucial to provide the person with autism with as many ways as possible of controlling their own behaviour.

Sometimes these strategies can be purely practical. Emma, recognising the pain that parting with her paper collection produced, realised that it would be easier for her to *stop* taking papers home rather than then having to throw them away. If offered leaflets or papers on the street she began either to refuse these or to discard them immediately she had read them instead of taking them home. Whilst this strategy did not reduce the amount of paper still left in the garage, it helped to avoid any further worsening of the situation.

Predicting and dealing with change

Although it is often stated that people with autism have extreme difficulties in coping with change, in many cases it is the inability to cope with *unpredictable* change that gives rise to most problems.

Jeremy, whose agitation when the train failed to arrive on time made him appear so odd to other commuters, was helped to deal with his problem in a number of ways. First, he was encouraged to get up fifteen minutes earlier each morning to listen to the travel news on his local radio station; if problems were predicted he would ring up his workplace to let them know that he 'might' be late. He also listened to the weather forecast before going to bed each night, as rain or bad weather were also likely to cause delays. Second, instead of sticking invariably to a single route to work he planned out some possible alternatives that could be used in the case of major disruptions or cancellations. Next, he made sure that his mobile phone was always fully charged in order to be able to contact work if problems arose. Finally, in order to reduce his own agitation he began to listen to his Walkman on the way to work as this helped him to relax. Being able to predict problems, at least to some extent, together with the provision of some simple, practical hints on how to deal with these, greatly improved the journeys to work. Although difficulties were not entirely solved – totally unforeseen delays, for example, continued to cause major disruption – they were significantly reduced.

Bob's distress at the inadequacy of weather forecasts in England was dealt with by his family in the following way. Firstly they agreed that his complaints were not without foundation, and they did not attempt to argue with his frequent suggestions (accompanied by letters to the BBC and the Met Office) that all forecasters should be instantly dismissed. Instead of trying to reassure him that the forecast would probably be correct, they reinforced the idea that it might well be wrong. They encouraged him to keep daily records of the weather conditions that had been predicted and what they had actually been like. As the obsession shifted from distress at inaccurate predictions to a statistical analysis of the inaccuracy of the forecasts much of the disruption that this problem had previously imposed on family life was removed.

Relaxation

Perhaps the major problem associated with stereotyped and ritualistic behaviours is the high level of stress that they can engender. In particular, intense anxiety can occur if the individual is prevented, or has fears of being prevented, from carrying out the activity; because of worries about change, or because of fears of what will happen if the activity is not performed in a certain way. Relaxation techniques, which have proved so effective in dealing with the fears and anxieties of non-autistic people, can readily be adapted to meet the needs of someone with autism. The principle underlying relaxation techniques is that of 'reciprocal inhibition': that is, alternative responses can be elicited in order to reduce, inhibit, or otherwise interfere with the physiological and psychological symptoms of anxiety (Sheldon 1995). Many tapes and books are commercially available to help individuals develop more effective means of relaxation. These involve physical relaxation methods to reduce muscle tension or to improve breathing techniques, as well as psychological methods. The last-named may involve developing powerful visual imagery (e.g. of pleasant and tranquil scenes), which can then be used to disrupt anxiety-provoking thoughts or images; auditory stimulation, involving calming music or other sounds, can be used in a similar way.

For individuals with autism, however, some of the recommended physical muscle relaxation exercises may be too lengthy or complex, or demands on visual imagery and imagination too abstract, for these techniques to be of much practical use (Clements and Zarkowska 2000). Some, even amongst the most able of individuals, complain that the tapes are just boring or meaningless and they have little motivation to persevere with them. However, the basic techniques can be modified to suit people with autism. For example, simple breathing techniques showing individuals how to take four or five deep breaths in a way that decreases rather than increases chest tension (many pull in their stomach muscles when they inhale, which simply increases tension), can be a rapid and effective way of inducing feelings of calmness or relief, and avoids the need for more prolonged relaxation exercises. Instead of trying to promote *mental* visual images – which often proves too abstract a task for people with autism – looking at a photograph, postcard or picture of a pleasant or familiar scene may be much more helpful. The picture needs to be small enough to be carried about easily and may need covering or reinforcing in some way if it is not to fall apart. Alternatively, a series of easily replaceable pictures may be used instead, and postcards can be particularly helpful here. Some people find the 'Magic Eye' postcards (where the apparently abstract foreground of the card needs to be stared at intensely before a 3-D image can be seen) useful sources of distraction. Individually made tapes of music or other relaxing sounds can also be used to promote relaxation.

Whatever exercises or images are found to be helpful, the crucial aspect of relaxation training is that it *must* be carried out at frequent and regular intervals if it is to be of any practical use when anxieties actually arise. Ideally, a daily session should be established, when the individual goes through his or her 'exercises', and as people often find it difficult to set aside special times for these, bath or bed times are often the best periods to choose. Supervision and guidance may be needed at first, but once appropriate techniques are developed individuals should be able to put these into practice themselves, albeit with some reminding, as time goes on.

The main problem then is to ensure that individuals make use of these strategies when anxiety-provoking situations actually occur. For people who have some supervision throughout the day, direct prompts can be given by carers when the first signs of anxiety are recognised. Experience indicates that it is much more effective to intervene immediately the first signs of agitation are apparent rather than to wait until anxiety has reached a higher level. However, for individuals who are living independently or who do not have access to input of this kind, other options will need to be explored. One alternative is to make use of role-play situations that deliberately provoke anxiety or stress and then to encourage the use of relaxation strategies. Perhaps surprisingly, many people with autism seem to respond well to simulation exercises of this kind and have little difficulty in summoning up the appropriate emotional responses. David, for example, had an obsession with 'always being right', and if anyone seemed to be critical of him in any way he would become extremely agitated. Sessions with his psychologist were used to help him cope in situations when someone spoke to him in an angry or annoyed voice or when they had criticised something he had done. As soon as he started to become visibly agitated he would be prompted to practice his deep-breathing and distraction exercises. The psychologist also helped him to recognise his own internal and external symptoms of stress (in his case facial grimacing and a feeling of tightness in his stomach) and to respond more rapidly to these. The programme also involved practical advice about ways of responding to criticism.

Another possible solution for adults living relatively independently is to enlist the help of relevant individuals at work or home. Timothy had a job as a computer programmer, but became very agitated if certain problems over data input arose (usually when he considered that someone else had made a stupid or avoidable error). At such times he would grimace, shout and even throw things: behaviours that were particularly unacceptable if there were visitors in the office. After discussions with his line manager, one of the older secretaries volunteered to take Timothy aside whenever she saw him becoming agitated and would suggest he went outside to the corridor to calm down. Because of her seniority Timothy was willing to accept this guidance and the impact of the problem was greatly reduced.

At the other end of the spectrum, for people of lower intellectual and linguistic ability, self-directed relaxation techniques may be difficult, if not impossible, to implement successfully. Instead, direct help with ways to relax will need to be provided by other people. Massage, aromatherapy, physical exercise, music and dance, and various arts and crafts are all activities that have been reported to be valuable in reducing agitation and distress.

Distracting techniques

A further way of attempting to reduce ritualistic behaviours is to use distracting techniques. Again, these can be of a variety of different kinds and should be adapted to the needs of the individual involved. As with relaxation, the chosen strategies should be employed as soon as the first signs of the obsessional behaviour or the anxieties related to it are noted. Monica was a young woman with severe learning difficulties as well as autism whose main obsession was, 'posting' things (mainly paper items) down the backs of chairs, radiators or cracks in the walls or floors. Several important documents and the occasional twenty-pound note were thought to have disappeared in this way. If she were fully occupied the problem tended to diminish and it arose mainly at times when the unit was poorly staffed. Although the main aim of her care programme was to keep her fully occupied, this was simply not possible throughout the entire day. A large wooden container was constructed, full of holes of different shapes and sizes, and if other activities were not readily available Monica was encouraged to post items into this. Whilst the behaviour was not stopped by this technique, it did at least ensure that the items posted could be easily regained.

John, a young man attending a day centre, had an obsession with coins and would 'collect' these whenever the opportunity arose – a habit that caused considerable resentment amongst some of the other clients. His key worker noted that the 'collecting' tended to occur after John had begun to talk about money and what he would do with this. He found that if he then occupied John in making shopping lists for purchases for the centre, and arranged for a time when he could be taken to the shops, the problems diminished.

Thought-stopping

Another technique, developed from cognitive behavioural work with adults with depressive or obsessive problems, is that of 'thought-stopping'. This, as its name suggests, involves interrupting the train of distressing or intrusive thoughts by introducing conflicting thoughts or self-instruction (Sheldon 1995). Again, however, reliance on internalised verbal techniques of this kind can be difficult for people with autism. Martin, whose anxiety about achieving the highest possible number of points on video games was described earlier, was advised to use thought-stopping techniques to reduce his anxiety. However, telling himself 'I'm the best' if a lower-than-expected score was achieved did not prove helpful, and he even began to argue with his parents and therapist about the 'untruthfulness' of such claims. Instead, it was decided to encourage him to keep a notebook in which to record every score, so that he could then work out his *weekly* average (which was almost certain to be extremely high). Delaying the opportunity for worry, by writing scores down, proved much more effective. Other thought-stopping strategies can also be employed. Jason, who had an obsession that any aeroplane flying overhead might crash, had found aromatherapy helpful in teaching him to relax. His insistence on rushing outside every time he heard a plane proved very disruptive, especially during group activities, and instead he was encouraged to carry a small pad soaked in essential oil that he could smell whenever he heard an aeroplane. Staff reminders to 'have a good sniff' would often distract him long enough for the plane and the anxiety to disappear!

For other people, the use of picture postcards as a distracter, or cards containing a simple written instruction (e.g. 'Relax', 'Don't panic', 'Take a deep breath' or 'Count backwards from ten') may be helpful. Other cues can also be used. Sally, who tended to get very agitated if she were not allowed to line up objects whenever she went somewhere new, was instructed by the staff at her home to 'count to ten' in order to calm her down. As she could only count to ten by looking at her digital watch, and as she insisted on waiting until the seconds were back to zero before doing this, her outbursts could often be delayed long enough for some other distracting techniques to be employed.

Further descriptions of other self-control techniques, which can be adapted for use with individuals of different ability levels can be found in the books of Clements and Zarkowska (2000) and Sheldon (1995). Tryan (1979) also provides a useful review of simple thought-stopping techniques, including non-verbal strategies such as wearing on the wrist a thick elastic band which can be pulled and released if obsessional thoughts begin to intrude.

Improving the general quality of life

Possibly the most crucial element in any intervention programme for stereotyped or ritualistic behaviours is the need to develop and encourage other activities as far as possible. The importance of appropriate stimulation is illustrated in many of the examples above and there is considerable experimental evidence to indicate that such behaviours increase when individuals are inadequately occupied (Chock and Glahn 1983). However, once routines or stereotyped behaviours become established they can prove remarkably resistant to change and hence attempts to expand alternative activities may be strongly resisted. Again, a 'graded change' approach can often prove effective.

Adam, whose obsession with the dangers of electrical equipment was described earlier, spent almost all his time talking about the problems of electricity and its potential perils. In addition to the practical desensitisation programme, attempts were made to increase activities that might distract his thoughts from electrical matters. His other main interest was tennis, but because of his fear of losing he would only play members of his own family (whom he could beat fairly easily). Fortunately, a neighbour discovered that a local residence for people with learning disabilities needed volunteers to coach them in sports such as tennis, and suggested that Adam might give this a try. Since he was almost certain to win every game he was only too happy to spend his spare time at the unit, where his quietness and gentleness were much appreciated by the residents. As he became more involved in his tennis coaching his electrical obsession became less intrusive and his previously overwhelming anxiety about this also seemed to subside.

For individuals of lower ability, attempts to develop alternative activities may also be helpful. Clyde had many problems in settling into a home for people with learning disabilities, and his obsessional behaviours became very difficult to deal with. Before leaving each morning he insisted on lining up all the chairs on the ground floor in straight lines, their backs a few centimetres from the wall. Because of his anxiety that other residents might disrupt the furniture, he refused to leave the house until everyone else had gone, often missing the coach to his day centre because of this, and if anyone remained at home because of illness he would not leave at all. Recognising his need for order, and for greater solitude, staff gave him the responsibility of organising the equipment in the greenhouses and garden sheds. As each item already had a set place, identified by silhouettes or pictures, Clyde did not have the opportunity to impose his own idiosyncratic placement systems and seemed content to replace everything in its allotted position. Few other residents went into the sheds, so that Clyde was generally left alone, and he knew that equipment there was unlikely to be moved. The combination of an ordered environment and greater separation from other residents helped to reduce his other obsessional behaviours to a more manageable level.

Early prevention

The effective modification of stereotyped and ritualistic behaviours in adults with autism will almost always require strategies that are complex and specifically designed to meet individual needs. The more pervasive and entrenched the problems, the more imaginative and resourceful management programmes will need to be. However, there are a few basic rules, which, if followed, could prevent many subsequent problems.

The first is to ensure that, from the child's earliest years, obsessional behaviours are under the control of those caring for the child as opposed to the carers themselves being controlled by the obsessions. Although this may sound far-fetched, there are many examples of families whose lives, over the years, have become dominated in this way. Raymond, now in his fifties, had always shown a marked resistance to change. Even when he was still in his pushchair his sister remembers walks being dominated by his insistence on never taking left-hand turns and his protests if his mother tried to retrace her steps rather than returning by a different route. He was not diagnosed as having autism until he reached his late forties, and although his family had always recognised the fact that he had problems, no explanation and, more importantly, no help for these was ever provided. By the time he was fifty he was living alone with his widowed mother and had absolute power over her, dictating who came to the house, what food they ate, where they shopped, where they went on holiday, and refusing ever to let her throw away anything so that the house was full of old clothes, newspapers and useless equipment. In the end, as his mother's health deteriorated, she was removed by social services for her own protection. Eventually, too, because of his inability to function adequately alone, he required hostel accommodation. Perhaps if the family's need for help had been recognized when he was at an early age and if appropriate advice and support had been offered, the obsessional behaviours would never have been allowed to develop to the level where they virtually destroyed the lives of an elderly woman and her only son.

The second rule, which admittedly requires some ability to see into the future, is not to allow or encourage behaviours in young children that will be unacceptable in later life. All too often special interests or ritualistic behaviours present difficulties as people grow older, not because the intensity or frequency of the behaviours has increased but because other people's attitudes have changed. Behaviours that are acceptable in a little child (such as a fascination with the feel of women's tights, or people's toes) will be viewed very differently when the same individual reaches late adolescence or adulthood.

Joey's obsession with washing machines, for example, had provided his mother with much-needed respite when he was a child. However, by the time he was a large, active teenager he was well able to break into other houses to indulge his obsession, so that a previously innocuous behaviour became a threat to both himself and others. Adam, whose skill in 'mending' electrical equipment was considered a real party trick at the age of seven, by the age of twelve required constant attention and supervision both at and away from home because of the potential danger of this behaviour.

Without help, parents are unlikely to be able to identify potential problems such as these and in order to avoid distressing a young child will very naturally tend to give into routines and rituals, sometimes with disastrous results in the future. It is up to professionals who are knowledgeable about autism, and the pattern that behaviours are likely to take in later life, to advise, to warn, and to develop appropriate strategies for families, schools and others to follow. Coping with a routine of a few weeks' duration may be hard, but it is nothing like so difficult as attempting to eliminate a behaviour that has been well entrenched for many years!

The third point is to remain vigilant and sensitive to the emergence of new or potential problems. Most people with autism will develop new interests, obsessions or rituals over the years. Some of these may be short-lived; others may become very pervasive and disruptive. Knowing when or whether to intervene depends principally on knowledge and understanding of the individual concerned. In some cases it is wisest to pay little attention to new behaviours, in that if ignored they will tend to disappear again fairly rapidly. In contrast, stereotyped behaviours in other individuals quickly become entrenched, and rather than allowing this to happen intervention in the very earliest stages (specifying rules about when, where and with whom) will be crucial if the problems are not to escalate.

A final guideline is to make the best use of any externally imposed changes on the individual's environment or lifestyle. The move from home to a residential setting or from school to college provides many valuable opportunities for change, and even individuals with very fixed routines in one setting may show surprisingly little resistance to modifying these in a totally different environment. However, for such changes to occur it is crucial that steps are taken to ensure that there are no opportunities for the old behaviour patterns to re-establish themselves. If allowed in the new environment the behaviours will be strengthened even further. On the other hand, if different and more appropriate routines are established *from the outset*, major behavioural changes can often be implemented with relatively little difficulty. Sandra, a woman in her twenties, had developed very rigid patterns of behaviour at home with her elderly mother. She would watch television, with the volume on high, until the early hours of the morning; she had lengthy and complex routines for washing and going to bed; and she insisted on her mother cooking meals at exactly the same times each day. Recognising the importance of such routines for Sandra, staff at the home to which she was moving constructed, with her collaboration, detailed timetables specifying the times for each of these activities on a daily basis. The times were changed somewhat from day to day, to avoid over-rigidity, but ensured that TV watching was limited to times that did not disturb others (a mark was also placed on the volume control to indicate acceptable levels of loudness) and that the time involved in dressing and washing was not excessive. Because she was aware, well in advance, of what the routines would be, Sandra accepted the changes with little difficulty.

Recognising the value of obsessional interests

Although ritualistic and stereotyped behaviours or interests may, if not adequately controlled, become the source of considerable disruption, they can play an important role in providing people with autism with comfort, self-occupation or entertainment which, because of their lack of other creative, social or imaginative skills, would be almost impossible to obtain by other means. Special interests or skills can be used to help control fears, for relaxation or as a means of social interaction. Pokemon® or video games have helped many youngsters with autism to relate to their peers. As they grow older the Internet, sports, general knowledge or specific research interests (plants, insects, space, astronomy, the weather) can all offer a gateway to wider social contacts.

The fact that longer-term outcome, too, can be positively affected by the way in which special interests develop was noted long ago by Leo Kanner. In his follow-up of young adults with autism, Kanner found that many of those who had made most progress had done so via their particular interests. Special interests in music, memory or mathematics had, in a significant number of cases, led to the development of valuable work-related skills; others with a fascination for topics such as chess, history, politics or transport succeeded in building a range of social interactions around these.

Asperger, too, reports on cases where early interests led to later success in life. For example, one individual with a childhood fascination with mathematics subsequently became an assistant professor in a university department of astronomy, despite severely impaired social skills, after having proved a mathematical error in Newton's work.

Similarly, in the London-based follow-up of young adults (Howlin *et al.* 2004), several individuals who had done particularly well had made use of their earlier interests. Danny had, ever since he was a small child, been fascinated by angles and directions, and from about the age of three his drawings consisted almost entirely of room plans or the angles made by doors or furniture. By his mid-twenties he was successfully employed in a cartographer's office and despite some problems was a popular member of staff. His popularity was also enhanced by his input to the company's sporting team because of his remarkable skills in orienteering. Maurice, who had been fascinated by collecting scientific facts from an early age, had managed to obtain a master's degree in chemistry and was currently working as a scientific officer for a major chemical company.

From a personal point of view, Temple Grandin (1995) also stresses the value of using obsessional interests:

> Fixations are powerful motivators. It is a mistake to try to stamp out fixations . . . When I was in high school many of my teachers and psychologists wanted me to get rid of my fixation on cattle shutes. . . . I have made a successful career based on my fixation with cattle squeeze shutes. I have designed livestock handling systems for major ranches and meat companies all over the world.

More recently, too, her skills have expanded into developing ways of transporting other animals, and her services are sought from zoos across the world in helping to move particularly valuable or nervous stock.

Even if special interests do not lead to occupational success they can play an important role in developing hobbies or other activities to fill otherwise empty hours. Clara Park (1992), writing of her daughter Jessy, tells of how her unusual artistic skill was put to little use until she discovered that it brought her money, one of the few items in which she did have a particular interest. Although art for art's sake held little meaning for her, art for money's sake did, and by the time she reached twenty painting and drawing had become an important and fulfilling part of her life. Many other people find their obsessional activities a source of comfort if they are anxious or tired or have to cope with novel or stressful experiences. Others use their obsessions in order to relax. Jonah, who works as an accounts clerk in a busy company, spends an hour or so at the end of each day at his local railway station collecting train numbers. Caroline, who was always fearful of the dark when younger, now reports that it is much easier for her to sleep if she has managed to watch the moon in the sky for half an hour or so on clear nights.

Obsessional interests can also offer support at times of severe stress or loss. Dennis, who worked for his father in their small family shop, was the victim of a vicious attack in which both he and his parents were shot and wounded. Although unable and unwilling to talk about his suffering or fears after this incident, his obsession with collecting and drawing a particular make of old-fashioned radio clearly gave him some relief. Over time his desire to talk about his interests overrode his avoidance of social contacts, and eventually it became possible for him to make some use of professional counselling.

Sometimes, too, obsessions may serve to reduce anxiety as well as proving productive in other ways. Temple Grandin first constructed a 'squeeze machine' to reduce her own anxiety and obsessional fears, and this later became the basis for her later, highly successful, cattle-restraining devices.

Finally, particularly for less able individuals with autism whose range of interests and abilities may be very restricted, the opportunity to indulge in stereotyped activities can be an important means of increasing other skills. David Premack, in the 1950s, was one of the first psychologists to show that the use of ritualistic, repetitive or other apparently meaningless activities as a reward for more appropriate behaviours may be a very effective strategy in increasing behavioural repertoires. Since then many other studies have shown how stereotypic, obsessional or attachment behaviours can be used to increase more constructive activities in people with autism (Wolery *et al.* 1985, Sugai and White 1986). Whilst such strategies do not aim to eliminate obsessional or ritualistic behaviour, they can be highly effective in reinforcing and encouraging short periods of alternative behaviours, with the result that the obsessions themselves gradually diminish in frequency or intensity.

As the examples above illustrate, dealing with stereotyped behaviours, rituals and routines is by no means an easy task, and successful interventions will require time, patience and often the implementation of several different strategies in tandem. The principal guidelines for success, however, are: early intervention; a graded approach to the introduction of change; the provision of a more appropriate or stimulating environment in order to encourage other activities; and the establishment of basic rules about where, when, with whom or for how long ritualistic or obsessional behaviours may take place. The aim should generally be not to remove the obsession entirely but to ensure that the behaviour no longer intrudes in a distressing or unacceptable way into the life of the person with autism or that of his or her family or carers. Once an acceptable level of control is reached, stereotyped behaviours or interests may actually have many beneficial effects. Indeed, Lise Pyles (2002) the mother of a boy with Asperger syndrome, suggests that special interests are often portrayed more negatively than necessary, and quotes another mother as saying 'Since I have yet to see an obsession or interest that hasn't helped (my daughter) in some way (though that may not be immediately clear), my tendency is to encourage them . . . as much as possible'.

7 Secondary education

A recent report by the National Autistic Society has estimated that in the United Kingdom one in every 152 children has a formal diagnosis of an autistic-spectrum disorder (Barnard *et al.* 2002). This is higher than most previously published figures, and indeed estimates of the prevalence of autism have been steadily revised upwards over recent years (see Fombonne 1999, 2003). Whilst these figures seem to reflect a heightened awareness of autistic-spectrum disorders among professionals and the public rather than a true increase in incidence (Wing and Potter 2002), they clearly have major practical implications for educational services.

Currently, there is a variety of different educational options for pupils with autism. Placements may include specialist autistic schools or units such as those run or accredited by the National Autistic Society in the United Kingdom (see National Autistic Society Publications 2003) or schools for children with moderate or severe intellectual impairments, emotional and behavioural problems, or communication disorders. Within the mainstream sector, pupils with autism may be placed in a regular classroom – with or without additional support – or spend all or part of the school day in a separate unit on the same site. Each of these options has certain merits, but there are also potential disadvantages (see Howlin 1998b). Arguments for and against inclusive education are as rife in the field of autism as for any other disability (Burack *et al.* 1997, Mesibov 1990, Simpson and Myles 1993) although evidence in favour of either specialist or mainstream schooling remains equivocal. Reviews of research in this area indicate that both mainstream and segregated education have benefits and drawbacks, and outcome can vary according to the type of setting, the needs of individual children and the severity of their difficulties (Howlin 2002a). Thus whilst some studies conclude that academic and social attainments are enhanced by inclusion, these have tended to be conducted in highly specialised, experimental classroom settings (Harris *et al.* 1991, Hoyson *et al.* 1984). Other research suggests that mainstreaming does not necessarily improve social, cognitive or language skills (Burack *et al.* 1997, Harris *et al.* 1990, Sigafoos *et al.* 1994b). The appropriateness of different educational provision is also likely to vary during the course of an individual's school life. Thus, whilst specialist (and hence largely segregated) provision may be entirely appropriate for autistic children with additional severe learning and behavioural difficulties, it is unlikely to benefit more able children with autism, especially as they reach secondary school age when access to the normal school curriculum is essential for their future academic and employment prospects. The crucial issue for them is not *whether* integrated or segregated education is best, but how the mainstream can be appropriately adapted to meet their social, emotional *and* educational needs.

Research into effective school environments has consistently indicated that both typically developing children and those with special needs do best in settings that are well structured, offer appropriately individualised programmes, emphasise 'on-task' activities, and have goals that are clear to both teachers and children and that can be modified according to children's needs and abilities (Rutter 1983). Very similar factors appear to be important in educational programmes for children with autism. Over thirty years ago, Rutter and Bartak (1973) demonstrated the benefits of a structured teaching programme, with a direct focus on educational goals, in improving both academic and social competence in pupils with autism. The highly structured teaching approaches that form the basis of the TEACCH programmes of Schopler and his colleagues (Schopler and Mesibov 1995, Schopler 1997) have since been widely adopted, and appear to be highly effective in reducing behavioural difficulties and enhancing learning skills. Koegel and Koegel (1995) also illustrate how traditional behavioural techniques can be successfully adapted for use in more naturalistic school settings. Other strategies that can be incorporated into mainstream settings include the use of peer tutoring (Kamps *et al.* 1994, Strain *et al.* 1996); cooperative learning groups (Dugan *et al.* 1995); 'circle of friends' (Newton *et al.* 1996) and 'social stories' (Gray 1995), although evaluative studies of these approaches is limited (see also Schreibman 2000).

A number of general texts for teachers in mainstream schools on how to meet the needs of children with autistic spectrum disorders have recently been published. Cumine and her colleagues (1998, 2000) provide practical suggestions for teaching children with autism and Asperger syndrome, and Jordan and Jones (1999) describe ways in which the teaching procedures can be made more 'autism-friendly' and hence more effective. However, it is clear that effective teaching requires adequate support. The development of successful teaching programmes also requires detailed individual assessments, specially adapted teaching techniques, environmental restructuring, and often considerable attitude change (see Quill 1995a).

Research evidence suggests that, with adequate support structures in place, inclusive placements for young children with autism can be effective (Howlin 2002a), and there is a number of studies indicating that input from normal peers can have very beneficial impact on play and social interactions (see Rogers 1998a for review). However, even with this younger age group, interactions between children with autism and their peers need to be carefully structured and reinforced by teaching staff; the type of play equipment used and the general structure of the classroom are also important, otherwise the enthusiasm of the typically developing children tends to be short-lived (Lord 1984). Full integration for older, secondary school children is more difficult to achieve, and research suggests that the risk of rejection rises steadily with age. It is evident, too, that support systems for pupils with autism and their teachers in mainstream schooling are far from adequate. The recent National Autistic Society survey (Barnard *et al.* 2002) found that almost half the respondent schools considered that neither pupils with autism nor their teachers were getting the assistance they needed; 72 per cent were dissatisfied with the extent of staff training in autism, and only 22 per cent of teachers had received some autism-specific training. There were particular concerns about provision, support and training in secondary schools, where rates of autism-related exclusions were particularly high. Moreover, at secondary school stage the range of alternative placement options tends to diminish. For example, whilst there are many primary classes or units for pupils with communication difficulties – which can sometimes offer a very appropriate educational environment for higher-functioning children with autism – few such units exist at secondary level.

In mainstream settings, discrimination by peers and teachers alike tends to increase for a number of reasons. First, because of a lack of support, coupled with increasing pressures to perform well in academic 'league tables' or similar forms of assessment, many schools have become more reluctant to accept pupils who are likely to have a negative impact on their ratings. If a pupil shows very disruptive behaviour, this, too, can be detrimental to the work of other children.

Second, in adolescence the need to conform and to be accepted by peers becomes of paramount importance. Deviations from the 'norm' are far less likely to be tolerated, and those individuals who do not fit in become increasingly marginalised. Recalling her adolescence, Clare Sainsbury (2000) writes:

> When I got to secondary school. . . . I was just continually aware that no one liked me, that whenever we were told to pair up, in lessons for example, I was always the one left over. Even if there were even numbers in the class, the teacher would have to order someone else to form a pair with me.

Third, the structure of secondary schools is very different from that of primary schools and poses far more problems for pupils with autism. In primary school, children often remain with the same peer group for six years or more. Lessons are conducted in the same classroom, with the same teacher for almost every subject, and many children remain with the same teacher for two years or longer. Schools tend to be relatively small in size, so that teachers become familiar with all the children and their parents. Staff will usually learn to tolerate 'unusual' behaviours (such as making loud comments in assembly or correcting the teacher in the classroom) once they understand that this is done not out of malice or rudeness but because of a lack of social understanding. Classmates, too, often become used to, and accept, the child's 'odd ways'; indeed, these may prove a welcome distraction from the usual tedium of lessons. In such environments it is also possible (although by no means always easy) to keep a watch on bullying or teasing and for staff to agree on consistent approaches to education and management.

In contrast, secondary schools are large, sometimes on split sites; although there may be some familiar children from primary school, most will be unknown to the individual; lessons, classrooms and teachers change at hourly intervals; most teachers will never get to know the children well, or understand the problems associated with an unusual and specific disability such as autism. Thus, collaboration between teachers in establishing an appropriate educational programme for a pupil with special needs can prove very difficult. Because of the numbers and ages of the other pupils it is impossible for teachers to exert the same amount of control over bullying or teasing. Furthermore, the very uneven profile of skills and difficulties shown by the child with autism can prove very disconcerting for teachers, possibly even undermining their own self-esteem. If the child with autism has the reputation of being, say, an excellent French scholar or one of the best mathematicians in the school, why is it that he or she cannot ever bring the correct books into lessons or even learn to tie shoelaces properly? If an individual has an excellent spoken vocabulary, it can be very difficult to accept that *comprehension* of language may be much less well developed, or that problems in cooperation are due to the pupil's failure to understand rather than disobedience. Instead of these problems being accepted as fundamental deficits over which the child has little control, teachers may understandably interpret the student's difficulties as being due to deliberate non-compliance. As one individual in Claire Sainsbury's book (2000) comments: 'As far as my teachers were concerned, I was bright but perverse and lazy. . . . My great mistake was in not being mentally retarded.'

Gunilla Gerland (1997) also remembers how:

> My very uneven achievements in school seemed to provoke them. I got top marks in Swedish English French and Art. I often had to correct my teachers of Swedish because I knew all the alternative spellings a word could have and I always adhered to the spelling which I considered most correct . . . but then, in Geography I might be completely absent, not answering when spoken to and getting few of the answers correct in tests. . . . My behaviour drove the teachers demented.

However, it is not only pupils' uneven learning profiles that give rise to difficulties. Giles was a thirteen-year-old of high intelligence whose autism appeared relatively mild. Unfortunately his social difficulties had already led to his exclusion from one secondary school on the grounds of 'gross rudeness to teachers', and he had been removed from another after his parents found out that he was kept in the school building every break and lunch time because teachers were afraid of physical bullying by the other boys. Not wanting to have their son 'labelled', they rapidly transferred him to another school without informing staff of his problems. In the first week he marched up to the headmaster in the middle of assembly and commented loudly – and publicly – on the redness and spottiness of his face!

Fred also ran into problems over his tendency to correct other people's mistakes and his insistence on keeping firmly to rules. His memory and general knowledge skills were excellent, and he would continually correct teachers over minor errors of fact or dates. This clearly did not enhance his popularity, and although his peer group were kept entertained by his arguments with teachers they in turn were alienated by his constantly admonishing them and informing their teachers if they broke any rules. On one occasion he was badly attacked in the playground after he had openly informed the head teacher about certain pupils' smoking habits. He had no awareness of why his honesty had caused such problems, insisting that he was 'only doing his best to help the school'.

Damien was another child whose generally high intellectual ability tended to disguise marked deficits in specific areas. In particular, his understanding of language was extremely literal and in junior school he had frequently been in trouble because of this. When told to paint a flower vase in the art lesson, he had done just that – and broken it in the process! When told to take off his clothes for gym lessons, he would remove every item unless specifically told what to leave on. He was even accused of ruining the school photograph because, having been told by the photographer to 'look up', he stared so intensely towards the sky that all the other children followed suit. In secondary school he ran into major problems with his maths teacher in the first week. The children had been told to go out into the playground and measure the area of tarmac – a task that Damien totally refused to do. The head teacher was asked to intervene, but Damien remained so adamant that his parents were requested to take him home for a few days 'until he changed his mind'. Eventually his mother managed to elicit the reason for his rather uncharacteristic stubbornness. He explained that he could not possibly calculate the *area* of tarmac since tarmac, being three-dimensional, could only be measured by its *volume*.

In secondary school, too, there may be much greater reluctance among staff to accept novel or unconventional approaches to dealing with problems. Thomas had made good progress at primary school, where his teachers had shown considerable inventiveness in using his obsession with Dr Who as an incentive for working on every subject from art to maths to geography. At secondary school, however, such flexibility proved much harder to achieve. His teachers had been informed that allowing him to draw a picture of Dr Who at the end of each piece of work would almost certainly ensure his cooperation, but he was frequently banned from or even punished for doing this because 'it spoiled the appearance of his work'. Deprived of his primary motivation, he became increasingly anxious and non-compliant, refusing to complete work assignments and eventually refusing to go to school at all.

Stevie was a child with autism and mild learning disabilities who had just been accepted by his local secondary school, with support from staff in the special needs unit there. One of his main problems was his inability to find his way in unfamiliar places, and if he got lost or confused he would throw quite alarming tantrums. His mother asked that he be given some additional guidance, before the school opened in September, which would enable him to familiarise himself with the layout. She also asked for extra help in the first term to ensure that he was able to find his way from one lesson to another without difficulty. Although the head of the special needs unit was sympathetic to her requests, the head of the school was adamant that no student could enter the school during the holidays, and additional funding for a school 'guide' was refused on the grounds that the special needs unit was already well staffed. In the first week of school, Stevie became so distressed and violent that he was threatened with exclusion.

Peter was well known at his junior school for avoiding work of any sort unless he was firmly pressured into doing it. His class teacher monitored each page of work carefully and there were strict limits on the amount of time he was allowed to complete each page. His parents cooperated in this programme, and each evening they received a note from his teacher informing them of the amount of homework to be completed. When he transferred to secondary school, his statement of special educational needs made clear his problems and the recommended strategies for dealing with these. Unfortunately, few of the teachers at his new school had the time or inclination to either monitor his work or enlist the help of his parents in the same way, with the result that his output declined rapidly and dramatically.

Stuart had a tendency to throw all his books and even strip off his clothes when upset, and although pupils and teachers at his primary school had learned to ignore such outbursts, it was clear that they could not be tolerated in secondary school. One of the main reasons identified for his becoming disturbed was a lack of structure and predictability. If he knew where he was going, where he could sit and what books he would need, such problems were much less likely to occur. In the early months at the school a special needs teacher was allotted to try to help him get to the appropriate classroom on time, and she also attempted to ensure that he had the right books and equipment. However, to avoid his being singled out as having problems she tried to avoid going into the classroom as Stuart was quite capable of dealing with the academic requirements of lessons. Unfortunately he was unable to cope with the mad rush towards tables as the children entered the classrooms for each lesson, and he was frequently left distressed and bewildered and still looking for somewhere to sit long after the other pupils had settled down. His mother suggested that this problem could be readily overcome if Stuart were allowed to have a fixed place to sit in every lesson, preferably at the back of the class where he would be less of a distraction to other children. She even offered to buy some tables and chairs for his personal use if necessary. Some teachers were happy to implement her suggestions, and Stuart's behaviour in these classes improved rapidly. Others announced that they were not willing to change their teaching practices for anyone, with the result that his behaviour in these settings was generally appalling, and highly disruptive for the other children.

These examples are by no means isolated ones, and, as Clare Sainsbury's book of anecdotes graphically illustrates, far too many individuals with autism have vivid memories of the difficulties they encountered from both teachers and pupils in mainstream settings. Many children experience multiple changes of school, with their first 'expulsions' sometimes occurring in pre-school or nursery! Others describe an almost total lack of understanding of their educational, social or behavioural needs. Occasionally the situation can be transformed by a sympathetic teacher:

> The god-send person was my fifth grade teacher. . . . She took me to the side and worked with me. She took the time to teach me some social skills. I went from making straight F's to straight A's. (Later) she requested an IQ test, which took me out of special ed and placed me in the gifted and talented program. This small act made it possible for me to have a wide range of freedom for the rest of my school years.
>
> (Carol, quoted in Sainsbury 2000)

However, such opportunities seem to be due more often to chance than to appropriate educational planning, and all too many pupils with autism in mainstream school struggle through miserably: unsupported, misunderstood and often mistreated.

Therese Jolliffe writes:

> I hated school . . . the children cannot tell anybody they are suffering and if you do end up with A levels it does not really make people want you, so it seems you cannot use qualifications to obtain, let alone keep, a job. Although ordinary schooling enabled me to leave school with . . . a few A levels and then to obtain a degree, it was not worth all the misery I suffered. . . . The teachers pretended to be understanding but they were not. I was frightened of the girls and boys and everything there. . . . I was kicked, hit, pushed over and made fun of by the other children.

When I attended a place for autistic people life was a little more bearable and there was certainly less despair. . . . Parents of autistic children should never think of sending their children to ordinary schools because the suffering will far outweigh any of the benefits achieved.

(Jolliffe *et al.* 1992)

This, of course, places many parents in an insoluble dilemma. All too often they are aware that the school will not be able to cater for their child's social and emotional needs, and they are terrified of the stress that this will almost certainly cause. On the other hand, if children of average academic ability are denied access to the normal curriculum, their chances of making progress in later life will be significantly reduced. Therese Jolliffe herself, for example, went on to gain a Ph.D. in psychology, and it is almost certain she would not have been able to achieve this had she been educated exclusively within the special needs sector. Despite the fact that special schools are expected to incorporate the 'normal curriculum' into their teaching, the extent to which this can be done is obviously limited. Few schools for children with autism, learning or communication difficulties, or emotional and behavioural problems are able to offer their pupils an appropriate level of teaching in maths, physics, computing, ancient Greek or cell biology, although these are subjects in which intellectually able children with autism may excel.

Among the follow-up studies reviewed in Chapter 2, only around 20 per cent of participants had been educated largely in mainstream schools, and around half had spent most of their school lives in specialist autistic provision. Although the proportions attending mainstream school were somewhat higher in the more recent studies and/or those involving individuals of higher IQ, integration still tended to be the exception rather than the rule. In the London-based study of sixty-eight relatively able young people (all with a childhood IQ of at least 50, Howlin *et al.* 2004) only 15 per cent had been educated predominantly in mainstream schools. Almost half (43 per cent of the total group) had spent most of their school years in specialist autistic provision; 13 per cent had attended schools for children with more general learning disabilities, and around one-quarter had spent the majority of their time in a variety of other educational settings such as hospital schools, schools for pupils with emotional and behavioural problems, language units, home tuition etc. For most, school placements were relatively stable, with fewer than three changes of school during either primary or senior school. However, the majority (78 per cent) left school without any formal qualifications, and amongst those who did obtain academic qualifications most were at GCSE level; only two had obtained A levels. Even basic academic skills were disappointingly low. Over one-third of the group was unable to score at all on tests of spelling or reading accuracy or comprehension and the average age equivalents of those able to score on these tests were only around nine to eleven years.

Clearly, much needs to be done to improve current provision in order to ensure that children with autism have access to educational environments capable of meeting their academic needs while at the same time catering adequately for their social, communication and behavioural difficulties. Unless their very specific patterns of skills and deficits are adequately understood, children with autism may become extremely isolated, lonely and rejected, and hence adequate training and support for the regular classroom teachers is essential (Jordan and Jones 1999).

Educating teachers about autism

Although, as noted above, there is no good evidence to suggest that there has been an increase in the numbers of children born with autism (Wing and Potter 2002), it is clear that over recent years recognition and diagnosis of children with autistic spectrum disorders has grown steadily. The incidence is now estimated to be around three to six per 1,000 (Fombonne 2003, Wing and Potter 2002, Gillberg 1984) (i.e. around ten times the rate reported in earlier, but more restricted epidemiological studies, Lotter 1966) and thus it is almost inevitable that *most* teachers will encounter several children with autism in the course of their careers. Despite this, a recent study showed that one third of local educational authorities were unable to supply figures concerning the numbers of children with autistic-spectrum disorders in their primary schools and those that did tended to produce much lower figures that would be expected on the basis of epidemiological data (Evans *et al.* 2001). As in the NAS survey cited earlier, this study also expressed concerns about the lack of training for teachers of children with autism and related disorders. Even educational psychologists, unless they are working primarily with children with special needs, are unlikely to have detailed knowledge about the condition. Much more effective dissemination of information about the autistic spectrum and strategies for intervention is clearly crucial. Successful teaching models do exist, but these require flexibility and support from educational authorities if they are to become more widely adopted. For example,

Hesmondhalgh and Breakey (2001) describe the development of an integrated resource centre at a high-achieving secondary school in the north of England. This now provides placements for twenty-four pupils with autistic-spectrum disorders who participate in the regular school curriculum whilst also learning a range of additional life skills, from road safety and the use of public transport to understanding and coping with social and sexual relationships.

Since the introduction of the 1981 Education Act many courses for trainee teachers have introduced modules related to children with special needs, but time constraints mean that the time that can be allotted to any specific condition, such as autism, is very limited. Thus continuing professional development courses clearly have a crucial role to play. In the United Kingdom the National Autistic Society and the TEACCH organisation run frequent teaching courses for teachers. Newly introduced programmes, including distance-learning courses, can also offer additional academic qualifications. Birmingham University, for example, offers a number of qualifications specifically in autism (Advanced Certificate, B.Phil. and M.Ed. in education) for professionals working with older autistic children and adults. In Scotland, Strathclyde University offers a postgraduate diploma for teachers involved with pupils with autism, in both specialist and mainstream settings.

Specialist training is vital in helping teachers to identify and understand pupils with autism. Identification in secondary mainstream schools can be particularly difficult, because most pupils who have managed to stay in 'normal' provision up to this stage will show milder or more subtle handicaps than those who are diagnosed earlier. Although such pupils will almost certainly have been singled out as having behavioural or emotional difficulties in the past, unless the nature of their problems has been recognised they tend to be labelled as showing 'disruptive behaviours' or as being 'emotionally disturbed'. One particular problem, for example, is the apparent rudeness of a child with autism. Constantly being corrected in class, having one's physical imperfections highlighted or being faced with direct refusals to cooperate are not easy things for any teacher to deal with. However, the knowledge that a child is acting in this way not out of deliberate malice but out of a failure to understand the impact of his or her behaviours on others can help to make the situation a little more tolerable.

Other difficulties may arise from children's social impairments or from their ritualistic tendencies. In many circumstances intervention tends to concentrate on the outward manifestations of problem behaviours, or on presumed difficulties within the family, rather than addressing the underlying basis of the child's disorder. However, if the fundamental disorder is correctly diagnosed and accepted, this will have major implications for intervention and can also have a marked impact on teachers' willingness and ability to cope.

The failure to recognise autism can also present problems for staff and pupils in non-mainstream settings. Oliver was an eleven-year-old boy with Down syndrome who had recently moved to a secondary school for pupils with learning difficulties. In his previous school, also for pupils with special needs, teachers had found him extremely difficult to cope with because of his 'stubbornness', his 'lack of cooperation' and his 'failure to join in with other children'. For many years his parents had felt that his progress was very different from that of other children with Down syndrome, and in desperation they finally sought a further diagnostic assessment. This revealed that he was clearly autistic in addition to having Down syndrome – a diagnosis that led to a much better understanding of his difficulties both at home and at school.

Approaches to teaching

The mere understanding that a child has autism does not, of course, lead to the disappearance of problem behaviours. Changes in approaches to management will also be required, and there are now a large number of books and pamphlets available that may be of help. *The Current Issues in Autism* series of books edited by Schopler and Mesibov (1992, 1983, 1986) contain many valuable accounts of teaching techniques, and textbooks such as those of Quill (1995a), Jordan and Powell (1995), and Powell and Jordan (1997) provide a wealth of information on both well-established and more innovative teaching strategies. Helpful guidelines for teachers working with children with autism and Asperger syndrome, which are closely based on evaluations of good classroom practice, have also been produced by Cumine *et al.* (1998, 2000), Hesmondhalgh and Breakey (2001), Jordan and Jones (1999), and some education authorities (e.g. Leicestershire County Council and Fosse Health Trust 1998). Wendy Lawson's recent book *Understanding and Working with the Spectrum of Autism* (2002) also offers invaluable advice to teachers on ways of understanding and helping with the difficulties experienced by pupils with autism. The recent journal *Good Autism Practice* is a further important source of practical information for teachers. However, if there is one book that should be made compulsory reading for all teachers, it is probably

Clare Sainsbury's *Martian in the Playground*. This contains an account of her experiences and those of twenty-five other individuals with Asperger syndrome during their school years. Their recollections are often deeply disturbing, and it is all too apparent that the lack of understanding and support for pupils with this condition can have a major impact, not only during their time at school, but often for many years subsequently.

Literature of this kind provides a wealth of practical ideas that can be implemented in a variety of educational settings. There are, however, a few fundamental principles that should be kept in mind at all times.

The need for structure

Classroom organisation

Since the work of Rutter and Bartak many years ago, numerous studies have stressed the importance of structure in teaching children with autism (Howlin and Rutter 1987, Short 1984, Jordan and Powell 1995). The TEACCH programme, developed by Schopler, Mesibov and colleagues, illustrates how highly structured teaching programmes can have a very positive impact on both the behaviour and the learning abilities of pupils with autism. The whole TEACCH framework, including the physical design of the classroom, is designed to provide the students with visual cues to aid understanding. Work areas are clearly differentiated from play or leisure areas; individual teaching areas may be distinguished from group areas; there may be a clearly delineated 'time out' area in which to be quiet or establish self-control. Partitions are used to indicate the types of work activities to be carried out in particular places, and even the positions of chairs and tables may be indicated by the use of sticky tape on the floor. Work materials indicate the tasks to be carried out; their position indicates in what order tasks should be completed, and different coloured containers indicate where finished work should be placed. Although specialist 'packages' of this kind may need to be modified to suit pupils in mainstream provision, many elements of the TEACCH approach are relevant to almost any setting. For example, simply altering the position of a student's desk or table can have a major impact on performance. As noted earlier, providing a child with a desk and some basic writing materials in a quieter area towards the back of the room can reduce disruption within the class, and increase on-task behaviour. Close proximity to other people can be a source of anxiety for many students with autism, and allowing them rather more desk space can have a significant impact on work output. Another account in Clare Sainsbury's book describes how one pupil was always made to sit at the front of the class, next to the teacher's desk, because of her disruptive behaviour. This made her even more of a target for teasing by other children, and did not improve either her work or her behaviour. However, when a new teacher took over 'I was allowed to sit along the wall of the classroom at the very back but it was not quite in the corner of the room. I was able to see everyone without them seeing me or staring at me.'

Many components of the TEACCH approach are valuable for almost all students with autism, no matter how able they are. Small signs or pictures placed inside a rucksack, for example, can help to ensure that books/computers/gym kit etc are packed in an accessible way. In science or technology lessons, visual 'jigs' can help to indicate how to lay out materials, the order of the procedures to be followed, and where to put away equipment at the end of the lesson (this latter strategy should help with all students). Many individuals with autism have specific problems with route-finding (Clare Sainsbury was still unable to find her way around school after five years), but this can easily be helped by providing a simple map and showing the student how this should be followed. However, it is also vital to ensure that the visual cues are fully explained. One contributor to Clare's book noted that he spent a whole year in high school before he realised that any room number beginning with three was on the third floor. Furthermore, only as an adult did it dawn on him that the picture placed over his coat hook in kindergarten had been meant to indicate where to hang his coat. Instead he had always found his way to the right hook by 'some sort of special navigation', and he had developed a routine of walking at a certain angle towards the pegs in order to end up in front of the correct hook!

Timetable organisation

Problems in school are usually most in evidence if the daily timetable is poorly organised. If difficulties are to be minimised the programme for the entire school day should be clearly specified, so that the tasks required for any time period are made absolutely explicit. Thus, in addition to the regular school timetable the student with autism may need to be provided with an extra, personalised timetable indicating the materials or books required for each lesson and the amount of work (number of written pages/problems to be solved etc.) to be produced during each lesson. The timetable can be in the form of a personal diary or stuck on the inside of the pupil's desk or locker. For children who lose everything that is given to them, a security belt, with a discreet inside pocket, can hold small plastic-covered cards with the daily timetable pinned inside. In the case of pupils whose main difficulty is maintaining a satisfactory level of work output, picture cues can be used to indicate the number of tasks to be completed within a set time. For example, 'tear-off' clock faces indicating the passage of each quarter of an hour can help students keep track of the amount of work completed in a specified period of time and is far more effective than asking them simply to 'keep an eye on the time'.

Because of their dependence on structure, major problems can arise for children with autism outside lesson times. Although breaks from lessons are designed to provide normal children with the opportunities they need to relax and to interact with their peers, for a child with autism such periods can be extremely stressful. Children who are able to behave quite acceptably when involved in guided and structured activities frequently appear much more 'odd' or unusual at times of free play. Stereotyped and ritualistic behaviours may become more apparent and exposure to teasing or bullying is much more of a risk, especially because staff supervision at such times is greatly reduced.

If, as is often the case, it is simply not possible to offer greater structure or supervision in the playground, avoiding the problem by allowing children *not to go out to play* may be the best solution. Break times, after all, are intended to offer children relief from the pressures of the classroom; they are not designed to increase stress, although this is just what they may do for children with autism. Carol was a fourteen-year-old girl in a school for pupils with mild learning difficulties. Although able to cope in lessons, at play times her inability to join in with the other girls, and her tendency to rock and flap her arms, led to teasing and mockery. The anxieties associated with break times became so great that she began to complain of sickness and headaches each morning, showing increasing reluctance to leave the house. After discussions between her teachers and her parents it was agreed that she would be allowed to remain in the classroom during break as long as she completed certain chores. Far from resenting this, Carol was delighted at the opportunity to be able to keep the room tidier, and she was soon able to remain in the classroom without supervision. In similar cases, the situation has been greatly improved by allowing children to spend the time in the school library or computer room or even to go home for lunch.

School meals can be another major source of difficulty, and it is clear from personal accounts that having to tolerate the noise and smells of meal times in a crowded school canteen can be almost akin to torture for individuals with autism. Being forced into close proximity with other students, or made to eat food of particular textures or mixed altogether on the plate (many individuals cannot bear separate items of food touching each other) can be extremely stressful. Clare Sainsbury recalls that she 'nearly vomited on a regular basis'. Even understanding the rules that apply when queuing for food can be a major challenge. Again, Clare writes:

> The potential for making mistakes (and the anxiety caused by the fear of making mistakes) is enormous. One of my most vivid memories of secondary school is being hauled out of the lunch queue by one of the dinner ladies shouting angrily, and made to stand to one side; she refused to tell me why. Only after I had burst into tears was I allowed back . . . nobody ever explained what I had done wrong . . . and to this day I still have no idea.

A quiet corner in which to eat, being allowed to eat slightly earlier or later than other pupils, or being permitted to bring sandwiches are among the simple solutions that can transform a 'nightmare' into a perfectly tolerable activity. If the principal problem is not knowing what to do, then the basic rules can be explained simply – and discreetly – beforehand.

Games and PE lessons are also frequent causes of stress for pupils with autism, who may lack the motor coordination, the ability to follow rapid instructions or unwritten rules and the social reciprocity required in order to contribute to these activities in any useful way. Of the twenty-five individuals interviewed for Clare Sainsbury's book none could see the point of insisting that pupils with Asperger syndrome should take part in sports against their will, and terms such as 'nightmare', 'torture', 'punishment', 'trauma', 'stress', 'failure', 'humiliation', 'hate', 'fear' and 'nemesis' abound. Competitive cooperative sports are a particular problem and are probably best avoided altogether, both for the sake of the person with autism and the rest of the class. However, physical health can be improved by encouraging activities that improve body awareness and coordination. Yoga, swimming, golf, walking or gymnastics, if sensitively taught, may later become enjoyable leisure skills and a means of relaxation. Some individuals become adept at sports such as badminton, billiards or bowls, whilst others with a good visual memory and sense of direction can prove very competent in activities such as orienteering.

The organisation of teaching materials

No matter how good the overall organisation of the school day, children with autism will generally require direct supervision and monitoring of their work if standards are to be maintained. Many, even amongst the most able, have problems regulating their own progress or even continuing to work unless they are continually supervised. Constant attention to the work output of one child is rarely feasible, even in specialist provision where staff ratios are relatively high. Within lesson times, therefore, it may be necessary to attend to the design of work materials order to ensure that tasks are satisfactorily completed. For tasks involving a variety of different materials, such as cooking, it may be preferable to present the student with a row of trays or boxes containing small quantities of the necessary ingredients rather than expecting them to select and measure from a large array. Once the first ingredient has been weighed or measured, it should be returned to a specified 'finished' position before the pupil moves to the next stage. If the amount of material to be worked with is limited, the task requirements clearly indicated (by pictures or written lists etc.), and completion marked by the return of equipment to a specific setting, the activity is more likely to be completed without the need for constant prompting. Breaking down a longer task into smaller stages also provides the student with more frequent opportunities for reinforcement. In addition, having a visible finishing position helps the teacher to monitor progress from a distance.

Academic tasks can be broken down in a similar way. Henry, a fifteen-year-old in mainstream school, had experienced problems when it came to completing coursework for his GCSE examinations. While the rest of the class could be left unsupervised to get on with their project work, Henry was unable to cope without continual guidance. His geography teacher provided him with a timer and placed 'Post-it' labels at intervals in his workbook, specifying the work to be done within the time set. At first the timer was set for quite brief intervals, the amount of work to be completed being relatively small, and each time the timer went off the teacher was reminded to check. As the term progressed, work assignments were made longer and the intervals between checks increased, until Henry was capable of working consistently for periods of up to thirty minutes at a time. A few other teachers then followed suit, and his independent work improved considerably. Later, his parents provided him with a wristwatch timer so that his need for this additional help became rather less conspicuous.

Comparable procedures worked well for Sally, a thirteen-year-old in a school for children with learning disabilities. Because of her very demanding behaviour she was provided with one-to-one help for part of each day. However, she would still not work without constant reassurance. Sally had an obsession with 'Happy Eater faces' and the classroom assistant fortunately managed to obtain a large quantity of these before the restaurant chain providing them closed down. She also stuck a small 'Post-it' label at the end of every work item. When this was completed, Sally would take the label to her teacher and be rewarded with a 'happy face' sticker. Initially labels were placed in her workbook after each work item, then after two items, and then three and so on, gradually increasing the time and the amount of work to be completed before Sally received her reward and reassurance that she had done well. By the end of a term Sally was able to complete a whole page of work at a time before requesting further help.

Homework assignments can be another major problem. Even if pupils with autism manage to take the right books home, they are very likely to forget what needs to be done by the time they get there. In many cases, unless the help of parents is enlisted, work tends to be left undone or the wrong exercises are attempted. From Roger's first days at secondary school his parents and teachers worked together to overcome this difficulty. In his junior school they had found a 'school-home' book, which travelled between them on a daily basis, invaluable for dealing with problems, and his new form teacher agreed to continue with this. In the first term, with the cooperation of other teachers, homework instructions were written in the book each night as were details of the books to be taken home. Before Roger left school each evening his form teacher checked that he had the necessary books and his parents ensured that homework was completed before he went to bed each night. Obviously this arrangement imposed extra work on school staff, so the next stage was to encourage Roger to write down homework instructions for himself. The books used for each subject did not alter much over the term, so a general instruction sheet indicating the books needed for each subject was inserted in his 'school-home' book. Every evening before leaving school he ticked off the books that he needed as he packed them. The book list was replaced weekly by his form teacher, but otherwise, by the beginning of the second term, Roger needed little additional help to monitor homework assignments.

Using computers

The allure of computers for children with autism has often been noted, but although there are some reports of the use of computers to enhance communication or teach basic academic skills such as reading (Tjus *et al.* 1998), their use as a general classroom aid has yet to be fully exploited. Hardy *et al.* (2002) have developed a guidebook for teachers which describes the many benefits of computers for children with autism. In essence, computer programmes succeed because they are predictable and controllable; tasks have clear beginnings and endings; choices and options are clearly presented; feedback is rapid so that mistakes can be easily identified and rectified. They are also, in themselves, highly rewarding for many children. Specialist software packages are available to address syndrome specific difficulties such as emotional understanding (e.g. Baron-Cohen *et al.* 2002); visual cues can be rapidly produced in conjunction with digital cameras, and there are also various programmes available to develop reading, writing and number skills; to improve use and understanding of spoken language; and to enhance communication by alternative means such as pictures and symbols. Voice recognition software also has a potentially important role to play, both in helping students whose written skills are poor because of coordination difficulties and in providing individualised and direct feedback to pupils who have difficulty following instructions in group settings. Properly used, computers can also help to increase social interactions. Keyboards, switching mechanisms and mice can now be easily adapted for use with almost any pupil, and there is even software that taps into children's obsessional interests, such as, for example, www.thomasthetankengine.com. Hardy *et al.* (2002) describe how students' potential computing skills can be assessed and utilised, and they present numerous examples of situations in which computers can enhance learning across many different domains.

Learning the rules

Most children at school develop some sort of sixth sense for understanding what is appropriate and what is not; which games/clothes/pop stars are 'in' and which are 'out' at any time. How they do so is poorly understood – the important thing is they do it so easily and so well. For autistic children, who have difficulty understanding or following explicit social rules, making sense of these unwritten and often apparently inexplicable ones is virtually impossible. Matthew, now twenty-five, describes his experiences of the first years at secondary school (having previously attended a very small and sheltered primary school) as being like 'those of someone from outer space'. He generally had no idea what was going on, and having finally recognised that a particular 'craze' or sporting activity was in vogue he would belatedly equip himself with the necessary equipment only to find that it was no longer in fashion. He also failed to follow the other children in other, more important, ways. For example, in his first term in particular, he suffered extreme teasing from other pupils. Eventually his mother found out that this was because when he used the urinal he would pull his pants and trousers down completely instead of just undoing his zip.

Other children get into trouble because, in their desperation to make friends, they will do whatever anyone asks of them – and are unable to recognise the difference between children laughing at and laughing *with* them. Tales abound of children, especially in mainstream school, getting into serious trouble for following the instructions of their peers: to call a teacher by an insulting nickname, to remove their clothes in the middle of assembly, or even, in one case, to defecate in the school piano (immediately admitting to this when confronted). (For many other examples, see Sainsbury 2000).

The factors governing successful social engagement are so complex that even normal children are unlikely to understand them fully, although they will recognise immediately any minor infringements of the rules (Wolfberg 1995). For the autistic child, however, the most ordinary of social behaviours can cause problems. Darren began to get into trouble at school for laughing every time the teacher spoke. The problem was that, having recognised that the teacher was pleased if the other pupils laughed at her jokes, he would then guffaw loudly at *everything* she said. He was unable to work out when to laugh and when not to, and so, to be on the safe side, pretended to be amused by everything.

Because of the complexity of even apparently simple social interactions it is impossible to provide any child with a full understanding of why and how they should behave. Nevertheless, there are some fundamental rules that can help to enhance acceptability in school. Dressing appropriately (which may mean parents keeping a careful look-out for the latest fashions); never removing clothes in public; urinating only in private; never doing things that are known to be 'naughty' or 'silly', however many children ask you to; not correcting teachers, however wrong they may be; not informing teachers about the activities of other children without discussing this first with parents; not commenting on people's physical characteristics.

These are all simple guidelines that can make the difference between tolerance and rejection. Learning to wait and watch what other children do can also help. Temple Grandin (1995) notes that although she always had problems understanding social interactions, she would store up memories of how other people had acted and then, when similar situations arose, replay the scenes in her imagination like 'tapes in a video' as a guide to what (or what not) to do. At a simpler level, Darren's inappropriate laughter was modified by instructing him not to laugh *unless other children did so first*. Although his laughter remained somewhat exaggerated, this advice did help to reduce the disruption he caused in class.

As noted in the chapter on social behaviour, there is often little to be gained by offering detailed explanations of why certain behaviours are unacceptable. This may have no impact on the behaviour, and can lead to prolonged and futile arguments. At least in the initial stages of dealing with a problem it is often preferable to lay down a simple rule and insist that this is kept. Explanations can be given later, when the behaviour is well under control. Difficulties then arise, of course, because almost no social rules are invariable. Because of Michael's propensity to remove his clothes in primary school his parents and teachers had enforced the rule that no clothes could be removed unless his parents or a teacher from his school gave permission. This worked well, even in senior school, until he broke his leg racing at another school. The sports master there immediately took him to hospital, but neither he nor the doctor in the emergency clinic quite fitted the rule's specifications and he refused to undress until someone from his own school, several miles away, was sent for.

Similarly, staff at Billy's school had become concerned after a number of students had been approached by a man outside the grounds who was offering them trips in his car. Billy's vulnerability, together with his love of cars, clearly made him a potential victim and so the head teacher gave him a long talk on how he must not talk to strangers, and how he must never go in a car unless it was driven by a relative, a close family friend, or someone connected with the school. A few weeks later, when the school bus failed to arrive, his mother called a taxi to take him instead. Billy, sticking steadfastly to his teacher's warning, became very agitated and refused to board it. His parents had to work extremely hard to convince him that taxis were acceptable even though the head had not originally mentioned these.

Despite such potential problems, it is generally better to have even inadequate rules than none at all. Schools can also help by providing additional guidance for pupils whose understanding of social relationships and how to deal with them is often very limited. Hesmondhalgh and Breakey (2001), for example, describe how, within their specialist resource centre, they were able to adapt the mainstream curriculum to help students with autistic-spectrum disorders discuss their problems related to social and sexual understanding, and how strategies were developed to avoid or minimise difficulties in these areas.

Dealing with change

Despite their dependence on routine, children with autism are required to learn to tolerate many changes throughout their years at school. Very often it is not so much change itself that causes difficulties but the *unpredictability* of that change. Adequate preparation is therefore crucial, though not always easy. Even very able pupils with autism may continue to have problems with abstract or hypothetical concepts, and verbal explanations about what may be about to happen are frequently misunderstood. By the time they reach secondary school most normal children have no problems coping with daily variation in the timetable. For children with autism, this variability can be a nightmare. Having a timetable (in a folder or diary) that they can carry around with them, with instructions about *where* lessons will be held and what books or equipment will be needed, can be of considerable help. A simple chart displayed at home can also be a useful reminder of what equipment they need to take to school on a particular day. However, visual reminders alone will not always suffice. Joe, who had just started secondary school, had charts and timetables displayed all over the place, but he still managed to turn up late for most lessons and without the necessary materials. Only when his parents made up checklists that he was required to tick off at appropriate intervals did the situation improve. Initially the checklists were very simple and were merely used to ensure that he took (and brought back home) his games equipment on Thursdays. Gradually they became more sophisticated, covering every day of the week, and over time this strategy helped to improve his organisational skills considerably. A similar system worked less well for Fred, another twelve-year-old in mainstream school, because he constantly lost any pieces of paper given to him. Laminated pieces of strong card indicating the lessons and books needed for each day were firmly attached to his rucksack, and this helped to improve things to some extent, although he also lost his rucksack at frequent intervals.

Visual materials can also assist less able children to cope with alterations in routine. Fran was a fourteen-year-old in an autistic unit who was always extremely upset by changes in staffing. The situation became so bad that if any of the staff's cars were missing from the car park when she arrived at school she would scream and protest loudly, even if the staff member were actually there. Fran's class teacher collected photographs of all the staff in the school, and each day she was encouraged to stick up on a board the pictures of those who were 'in'; underneath went the photos of staff who were 'off'. This activity seemed to deflect her agitation over absences, and when it was known in advance that someone would be away, their pictures were placed in the appropriate section before Fran went home for the evening, thereby giving her plenty of warning for the next day.

Peel-on/peel-off pictures can also be used to indicate changes to the regular timetable. For example, if swimming or riding or outings tend to take place at different times of the week or term, photos or drawings of these activities can be used to replace pictures of other, regular activities. 'Picture calendars' (or normal calendars for more able pupils) are invaluable for preparing for major disruptions to the school routine such as holidays or trips away, and the complexity of these can easily be modified to suit the ability of the children involved.

The need for additional cues or special aids

An important factor, incorporated in many of the programmes outlined above, is the need to make use of alternative, often visual, cues when teaching children with autism. Even the most able are likely to have problems in dealing with complex or abstract information and additional aids to comprehension can make a considerable difference. This is particularly true when it comes to teaching *sequences* of activities. Although children may pick up isolated aspects of the task, they are unlikely to grasp all the stages required. Activities such as cooking or preparing drinks can be easily broken down into their component parts, and these simply illustrated, in the manner indicated in Figure 7.1.

With an appropriate level of prompting, many children should be able to complete tasks of this nature, even if they have difficulties with verbal instructions. Photographs of the *actual* materials to be used or the people involved may be required for less able children, but for others pictures, sketches, symbols or written instructions may be sufficient. By adapting the system to the individual child a whole range of activities, from putting away equipment to completing a physics experiment, can be made much easier. Donna Williams (1992) and Temple Grandin (1995), for example, both note that they were unable to cope with maths problems unless every step was first written down.

At an even simpler level, visual cues can help children to dress appropriately, or to keep better track of their belongings. A coloured label discreetly sewn inside *the front of* T-shirts or jumpers can help to

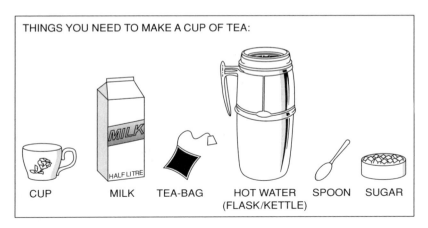

THINGS YOU NEED TO MAKE A CUP OF TEA:

| CUP | MILK | TEA-BAG | HOT WATER (FLASK/KETTLE) | SPOON | SUGAR |

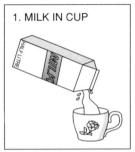

1. MILK IN CUP

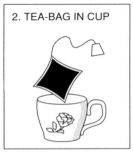

2. TEA-BAG IN CUP

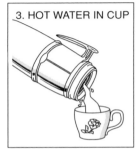

3. HOT WATER IN CUP

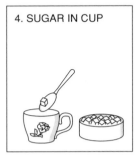

4. SUGAR IN CUP

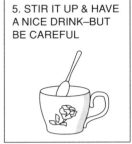

5. STIR IT UP & HAVE A NICE DRINK–BUT BE CAREFUL

Figure 7.1 Stages in preparing a cup of tea (NB: A flask is often safer to use than a kettle; putting milk in first can increase safety; if necessary, liquid can be pre-measured to avoid spills). Items in the 'menu' may be ticked off as completed; alternatively, they may be in the form of stick-on labels that can removed after each step.

indicate which way round clothes should go; a red mark inside right shoes and a yellow (lemon) mark in the left shoe can avoid considerable discomfort; a bright identifying mark on bags, sportswear or other belongings can also help reduce losses. Sally's obsession with 'Happy Eater faces' was used to encourage her to take greater care of her books, bags and clothes, which she was continually losing. Her mother stuck or sewed 'Happy Eater faces' (black outlines drawn on yellow felt) on all her school belongings. These helped to motivate Sally to collect her things before leaving school, and, equally importantly, ensured that her belongings were readily identifiable by all the staff.

Visual cues can assist in many other ways. By having work materials set out in a set sequence, or identified by particular colours, pupils can be helped to complete tasks with less direct help from adults. A filing tray placed to the left of the desk when the child begins work in the morning might, for example, contain three different-coloured files (e.g. blue, red and yellow) each containing a different activity. When the task in the blue file is completed the pupil can be taught to replace this in a specified place (perhaps a tray indicated by a blue sticker), the red file can then go in the tray with a red sticker, and so on. In this way it is clear to the student how many tasks need to be completed, and what should be done when they are finished; the teacher too has clear and easily visible information about the rate of progress. (Many other examples of strategies of this kind are to be found in the TEACCH programmes and Jordan and Powell 1995).

Visual 'jigs' of the sort used in industrial settings to indicate the correct placements of objects can also be helpful. Placing a knife, fork and plate on a plastic mat that has the items already drawn on makes setting a place at a table much easier, and if mats are laid out for everyone a whole table can be set with only minimal prompting. Such cues can also be helpful in ensuring that equipment is put away properly, or even in helping with activities such as dressing. Richard, an adolescent with many physical problems in addition to his autism, was supplied with special orthopaedic shoes to wear at school. Because he had great difficulty putting these on the correct feet, even with colour cues, his teacher drew the outline of each shoe, correctly positioned, on a mat by her desk. Each morning Richard matched his shoes to the outline and then simply stepped into them.

Thought also needs to be given to the materials used when teaching new tasks or activities. A flask with a press-button top is much safer for making tea than a kettle for someone who has little understanding of danger (or a tendency to throw things). Velcro fastenings or self-tie laces, which automatically wind together, make putting on shoes a great deal easier. Food that can be heated in a microwave rather than laboriously prepared by hand can motivate even the most reluctant students to try their hand at making a meal.

Finally, the setting in which learning is to take place needs to be given due consideration. Most people find concentration difficult if surrounded by crowds or other distractions, but autistic children are often expected to learn in noisy, open-plan environments. As indicated earlier, Stuart's difficulties in settling in the classroom were greatly helped if he was allowed to have his own table at the back of the room. Other, more active, pupils may find it easier to remain still if they are seated in the corner of a room, with their back to the wall and a table in front of them, so that it is less easy for them simply to get up and walk away. Movable screens can also help provide some degree of privacy, or freedom from distraction, when children are engaged in specific teaching tasks. These can also serve as a visual cue for 'on-task' activities, whilst being easily removable at other times.

Protection from bullying

Unfortunately, teasing or bullying by other pupils is a significant risk for children with autism, particularly in mainstream schools. Problems may occur for a variety of different reasons. First, pupils with autism may require extra attention from teachers, thereby limiting the amount of time available to other students and causing resentment or jealousy. Second, certain characteristics such as ritualistic behaviours, the need for constant reassurance and in particular repetitive questioning can become extremely irritating for classmates as well as teachers. Inappropriate attempts to socialise, or lack of awareness of social rules or personal space can also antagonise others. Even the characteristic honesty of many people with autism can be a problem, since openly informing school staff about the misdemeanours committed by other pupils is not a good way to gain popularity. In addition, because of their social naivety, often coupled with a desire to be accepted by other pupils, children with autism can be very 'easy prey'. Clare Sainsbury found that teasing and bullying were almost invariably part of the school experience of the individuals she interviewed, and physical and sexual violence were not uncommon. One man, for example, remembered: 'I got hanged (with wire) and other kinds of what the staff called mild teasing. . . . Someone ejaculated over my trousers in front of the whole class . . . no one helped me. . . . It was torture and abuse.' Bullying can also be much more subtle; Imogen, for example, was the butt of other girls' jokes, because of her 'weird' clothes and hairstyles, and they would deliberately suggest she wear even more bizarre garments, which then produced further amusement. A group of girls also pretended to be her 'best friends' and at weekends would make arrangements for them all to meet up at a particular venue in the evening. Imogen would spend the whole day preparing for the occasion, but when she turned up the others were never to be found. Clare Sainsbury notes that many children also quickly realise that they can terrify their classmate with autism without having to lay a finger on them, by exploiting their gullibility and literal-mindedness or making fun of their obsessions. The inability of children with autism to stand up for themselves and the ease with which they can be reduced to tears of rage or frustration by others make them 'perfect victims'. Often they are unclear if they are being bullied, or if what is happening is their own fault, and lack of support from teachers further exacerbates the problem. 'Severe beatings and abuse were pointedly ignored by school staff. . . . They turned a blind eye. . . . Teachers insulted me and said it was my fault for behaving like a prat.' Unfortunately teachers, too, may be responsible for bullying. Tony, who has a mannerism of shaking his head when anxious, remembers that his teachers always referred to him as 'Noddy'. Clare Sainsbury even cites the example of a boy who was locked in the nurse's room each day for several hours, and verbal abuse by teachers was reported by many of her informants. Numerous other examples, of more subtle mistreatment, are also described in her book. When one individual was asked 'What would you like teachers of kids with Asperger's to know?', he replied 'That they have the capacity to damage a kid for life'!

If integration is to mean anything, such experiences must be prevented. However, this will only happen if teachers themselves fully understand the nature of the difficulties shown by children with autistic-spectrum disorders; if they are prepared to be vigilant against bullying, both overt and covert, and to offer their pupils the protection they need; and if they are willing also to address the behaviours that can lead to bullying and to assist their pupils with autism to develop more effective social strategies, or avoid behaviours that give rise to difficulties.

Using additional resources

Although none of the procedures described above are particularly complex or time-consuming, for teachers who are already hard pressed, implementing even very simple additional programmes can prove difficult. Again, a few basic guidelines can help.

First, make optimum use of additional professional help whenever possible. Psychologists, psychiatrists, paediatricians, social workers or other professionals with knowledge and experience of working with autistic children may all be able to provide guidelines for action, or suggestions about strategies, even if they have no instant solutions to problems.

Second, for those not working in specialist autistic provision, calling on the help of those who do can prove very illuminating. There is now a range of teaching programmes that have been specifically developed to meet the needs of children with autism. Many specialist schools and other services also exist. The NAS list of accredited or affiliated schools, for example (NAS 2001) includes around 400 different establishments, and there are over 130 centres listed on the NAS list for adults and adolescents. Visiting specialist autistic provision, or having the staff come to visit or advise can be better than reading a hundred books (though, hopefully, these too will offer some guidance). For teachers already working in special schools, talking to staff from other schools may provide ideas about alternative strategies for dealing with behaviour problems or developing learning skills. The National Autistic Society also provides training, in a variety of different forms, from on-site training to off-site courses, for those working with children with autism.

Third, consider the use of other pupils as possible sources of help. After Stevie's special needs teacher (his route finding difficulties are described earlier) had her request for additional support refused, she enlisted the help of one of the sixth-form students to help him find his way around school. This pupil was hoping to get a place on a psychology course, and because her timetable was often free at the start of the day she was keen to use this opportunity to help a pupil with special needs. As noted earlier, several programmes in the United States have utilised peers as therapists with younger children, and there is no reason why, with adequate structure, teacher support and appropriate reinforcements, these strategies should not be adapted for use with older students, too. In their book on fostering inclusion, Hesmondhalgh and Breakey (2001) also describe the role of 'typical' students in ensuring the success of special programmes.

Fourth, make use of other people's ideas or strategies. There have been many different programmes published for teachers of young autistic children, and although a 'package approach' to education is not necessarily appropriate, modified versions of these can often be a useful adjunct to regular teaching procedures. Strategies developed by Wolfberg (1999) for increasing group play, by Sherratt (2002) and Thorp *et al.* (1995) for play and drama skills, by Gray (1998) for improving social understanding, and by Dalrymple (1995) on environmental methods for developing flexibility and independence, although all focusing on younger children, can be readily modified to suit older children in a variety of school settings. Kunce and Mesibov (1998) provide examples of how the educational environment may be adapted to meet the needs of higher functioning pupils with autism and Asperger syndrome, and Bauminger (2002) describes the successful use of cognitive-behavioural strategies for increasing social initiations and interactions with typically developing peers. As already noted, books such as those by Cumine *et al.* (1998), Hesmondhalgh and Breakey (2001), Jordan and Jones (1999) and Schopler *et al.* (1998) are also valuable resources within the classroom.

Fifth, take note of any advice or information that parents can offer. However expert the teacher, they will know their own child better than anyone else and are also likely to have evolved effective strategies for dealing with or avoiding problems. The example given above of Stuart, who had problems finding where to sit in the classroom, indicates how the advice of his mother worked extremely well, at least for those teachers who were willing to listen.

Finally, if problems are to be minimised it is important that staff agree on the ways to approach problems and that they work together to deal with these. Consistency in management is of crucial importance and disagreements between staff will jeopardise even the best-constructed intervention programmes. Agreement among staff can, however, be difficult to establish in a large school where teachers may have very different educational views or backgrounds. David, a fifteen-year-old starting a new secondary school, had a tendency to throw his bag and belongings across the floor if upset or confused. The head of special needs at his school discussed this with the other staff, and, on the advice of David's previous school, suggested that the best approach was to take little notice other than quietly and firmly asking him to pick everything up and continue on his way. Whilst some teachers were able to accept this approach, others insisted on taking a more punitive approach. The resulting variability in teachers' responses led to a rapid escalation in the behaviour and even after several (often ill-tempered) staff meetings it proved very difficult to reach a compromise. Eventually, with the support of the school's educational psychologist, those who did not agree with the approach were persuaded, for a limited period at least, to ignore the throwing and call on the help of another member of staff to deal with it. Thereafter the problem steadily declined, although if throwing does occur this still tends to be in the presence of staff members who are most likely to react.

Adopting a flexible approach to teaching

Few of the suggestions made in this chapter are particularly complex or difficult to implement, but they do require greater flexibility on the part of all concerned than is usually the case at secondary school level. This need for flexibility can also extend to many other aspects of teaching, including the organisation of individual timetables. Few autistic children, even those of above average intellectual ability, will be able to cope with all the subjects in the curriculum. As already mentioned, sporting activities, with all their demands on social and physical competence, can be a particular source of stress. In such cases, allowing the pupil to avoid activities that are beyond their competence can significantly reduce unnecessary confrontation. After all, few schools would insist on children in wheelchairs joining in sports activities unless they wanted to, yet group games may be just as impossible for a child with autism. Graham, now in his twenties, remembers other children in the school fighting over him at Wednesday afternoon games sessions because *no one* wanted to have him in their team! Little is to be gained by further alienating children from their peers in this way, and it does nothing to enhance self-esteem. Allowing the child to spend time in another activity, or even to join in lessons with another class will be much more productive.

Avoiding core curriculum subjects may be more of a problem, but if a child has a particular difficulty in certain topics then the relevant teachers should be made aware of this and helped to modify their teaching and expectations accordingly. Daniel, a fourteen-year-old in secondary school, developed a surprising talent for French and German and had an excellent vocabulary in both these languages. His ability to cope with English lessons, however, was well below that of other pupils. His English teacher was unable to understand this discrepancy and viewed it as a deliberate lack of cooperation on Daniel's part. When it was made clear that Daniel's success in French and German was largely dependent on his excellent rote memory, whilst success in English depended on very different skills, his teacher was able to take a rather more sympathetic attitude. He also reduced the demands made on Daniel in lessons and agreed to modify homework assignments in order to help him succeed more frequently rather than constantly failing.

Flexibility is also important when it comes to developing existing abilities to the highest possible level. If these are in French or German, as above, then the way ahead is fairly clear. Sometimes, however, the skills of someone with autism may have less obvious implications for educational progress. Nevertheless, it is generally much more productive to concentrate on areas of competence rather than deficit. Gemma was a young teenager in a school for children with mild learning disabilities. Although she was intellectually more able than many of the other pupils, her social skills were very impaired. Attempts to increase her social competence had produced little improvement, but she did excel in one particular area – computer games. Although games were prohibited in the classroom, they were deliberately encouraged in other situations because staff recognised that her expertise brought her considerable admiration and attention from other pupils.

Sometimes special abilities may be more circumscribed: for example, a child may only draw high-rise buildings or may read at an adult level of accuracy but without comprehension. Teachers may argue, with some justification, that such skills are of little value in themselves and may even try to discourage them. Nevertheless, because they are of such inherent interest to students with autism they can be very potent in motivating them to complete a range of other activities. Dan had an obsession with albinoism, and as long as he was allowed to write a paragraph about this topic at the end of his work (no matter how incongruous this was) his written exercises gradually improved. By the time he reached the third year of secondary school the 'albino notes' had become restricted to three or four sentences only and had to be written on a separate sheet of paper so that their intrusion into his regular work was minimal.

For other children who may, for example, be fascinated by numbers without being able to use them in a practical way or able to read without understanding, the challenge to the teacher is to make these activities more meaningful, rather than discouraging them. David had somehow taught himself to read, probably by watching adverts on television, and spent all his free time reading the TV pages of newspapers, most of which he did not understand apart from the names of his favourite programmes. In school, his teacher provided him with sheets of written instructions to follow (involving a variety of social and practical activities), and these had to be completed before he was allowed access to the newspapers. Learning to follow the instructions gradually improved his reading comprehension, and made good use of a previously purposeless activity. With appropriate guidance from teachers many children with autism can be helped to use their skills to foster social interactions or to increase their acceptance within the class. Allowing a student who is good at spelling or arithmetic to help other less able pupils can greatly enhance self-esteem, whilst someone with a particular skill in drawing, or an extensive knowledge of specific topics, may be a useful contributor to class projects.

Flexibility of provision

Finally, flexibility of provision is also crucial for the appropriate educational placement of children with autism. This applies both to the range of provision on offer and to the ease with which children are able to move from one type of school to another. For some children, early access to specialist provision may be needed to help deal with the behavioural or obsessional problems associated with autism, but transfer to mainstream provision may later be necessary on academic grounds. Other pupils may be able to cope with mainstream school in the primary years but then require more specialist intervention at the secondary-school stage. The transition from one setting to another requires time, patience and careful planning if it is to succeed.

Kelly, aged thirteen, had always attended a school for children with autism, but her teachers felt that they were failing to meet all her social and academic needs. Because most of the other pupils were boys she had no female peer group with whom to interact, and she was also academically more able than most of the other students. It was arranged for her to spend some sessions in the local girls' school where she began attending music and home economics classes with an aide from her own school. Later she was introduced into gym and arts classes, and despite being unable to cope with more academic subjects by the end of a year she was able to attend the school unaccompanied and clearly profited socially from her time there.

Dominic had attended mainstream school up to the age of twelve, but because of his continuing social and behavioural problems it was agreed that he would not be able to cope at the local secondary school. Instead he transferred to a specialist unit for high-functioning children with autism in the grounds of a mainstream school, spending part of his day there and attending some lessons in the main school. Gradually his time in mainstream was increased, and by Year 12, with the continuing guidance of staff from the unit, he was able to take several GCSE examinations.

In contrast, Ben, who had attended specialist autistic provision when younger, gained a place at a boys' public school when he was thirteen. Although the school was very academically orientated, its small classes, vigilant attitude to bullying and focus on individual skills rather than weaknesses made it ideal for him. He excelled at maths and Greek, and the school's willingness to seek outside advice when needed resulted in the placement being very successful. His tendency towards out-spokenness and a critical attitude to what he was taught were accepted by most of his teachers, whilst his occasionally outrageous remarks in the middle of assembly rather endeared him to other pupils!

The small size and greater structure offered by private schools may in some cases make them much more appropriate placements than larger state schools. Most parents, of course, are not able to afford this option, but occasionally local authorities can be persuaded to pay the fees if it can be demonstrated that no suitable alternative exists.

Generally, it is essential to be aware that the educational needs of a child with autism can fluctuate widely over time and hence these need to be closely monitored. Academic progress at some stages may be much greater than expected; conversely, behavioural, emotional or social difficulties (or changes within the school) may result in disruption to a previously satisfactory placement. Provision may need to be reviewed, and possibly changed, much more often than is the case for other children. A placement that seems appropriate at five years of age may be quite wrong by twelve, and careful and regular monitoring of the success of placements, for both teachers and other pupils as well as for the child with autism, is essential.

Summary: Meeting the needs of pupils with autistic spectrum disorders

Because of the many difficulties faced by secondary school pupils with autism and related disorders the National Autistic Society in the United Kingdom has recently published a number of general guidelines for schools (Powell 2002). The twenty recommendations are designed to make life easier for both teachers and children, and to reduce the current very high rates of exclusion that these pupils experience (estimated as one in four, Barnard *et al.* 2000). The guidelines focus on the need for education authorities to develop clear policies for students with autistic-spectrum disorders, and to provide appropriate support in the following areas:

> Identification of all pupils with autistic-spectrum disorders, whether or not they have behavioural difficulties or statements of special educational needs (SENs);
> Outreach services for mainstream schools;
> Training and practical advice for *all* staff (from governors to playground supervisors) to encourage 'whole-school awareness and strategies' for pupils with autistic-spectrum disorders;

Implementation of environmental modifications to meet the needs of these students;

Collaboration between special educational needs coordinators (SENCOs) and students' families, teachers, and any other relevant external agencies and support groups;

The development of individual education plans (IEPs) covering issues such as general learning skills, developing linguistic and social competence; consistency of teaching staff and assignment of a 'named person' to deal with personal difficulties; modification of exam procedures; protection from bullying, and clear strategies to ensure home-school communication;

Careful preparation for work placements;

Development of links with local universities.

Implementation of such guidelines – and much wider recognition generally – within educational services, of the needs of people with autistic-spectrum disorders could help to make the school years a happier time for many pupils, and avoid the high levels of school failure which in turn will affect the whole of their adult lives.

8   Further educational provision

Access to college life for people with autism

Until relatively recently few students with autism were provided with the opportunity to take part in further educational activities of any kind. Many children went immediately from autistic schooling into residential provision, often spending their entire lives with other people with autism. Whilst such a lifestyle ensures consistency and familiarity, it is a long way from the concepts of integration or 'normalisation' espoused in other areas of education or daily living. In their recent follow-up study of sixty-eight relatively high-functioning young adults with autism, Howlin *et al.* (2004) found that very few had received any form of further education. Fifty-three (78 per cent) had received no education after the age of sixteen, and only five had gone on to college or university. On leaving school most went straight into specialist residential autistic provision. A similar picture emerges from the review of other follow-up studies (see Table 8.1). Only 11 per cent of participants in these studies had received a college education, and only 10 per cent had obtained a degree or professional diploma. The real difficulties, however, can often be traced back to much earlier in school life. Many children attend specialist schools which are unable to develop their particular skills and interests to a level that allows later entry to college. Others, attending mainstream schools, may be provided with so little support that access to the full curriculum is effectively denied them, thereby limiting the opportunity to move on to further education.

In the wake of the movement towards integrated schooling there have been increasing pressures for people with special needs to gain better access to further education. Support services are relatively well established in the United States, and although provision in Britain is less advanced there is now an obligation on colleges in England and Wales

Table 8.1. Reported educational histories in follow-up studies of adults with autism*

Study (N)	Year	Age (years)	IQ	Years in school	% in mainstream school	% attending college/university	% with degree or diploma
Mittler et al. (26)	1966	7–27	24–111		22		
Lockyer and Rutter (38)	1970	16+	x=62	33% no school	2		
Kanner (96)	1973	22–29			3	9	7
DeMyer et al. (120)	1973	X=12		68%<5 years	8		
Lotter (29)	1974b	16–18	55–90	55%<5 years	0		
Rumsey et al. (14)	1985	18–39	55–129		57	14	14
Szatmari et al. (16)	1989b	17–34	68–110	All>5 years	50	50	43
Chung et al. (66)	1990	>12	24%≥70	12% no school	21		
Kobayashi et al. (201)	1992	18–33	23%≥70		27	2	
Venter et al. (22)	1992	18+	x=90		52	7	4
Tuffreau et al. (49)	1995	12+	89%◊50		0	0	0
Ballaban Gil et al. (45)	1996	18+	31%◊70		1		
Larsen and Mouridsen (18)	1997	32–43	78%◊50		44	0	0
Mawhood et al. (19)	2000	21–26	70–117	All>10 years	10	22	11
Howlin et al. (68)	2004	21+	51–137	All>10 years	15	7	4

* Includes only follow-up studies in which specific data on schooling and/or further education are available. Blank cells indicate no relevant information available.

to 'have regard for students with learning difficulties or disabilities' (Further and Higher Education Act 1992). All young people are entitled to full-time education up to the age of eighteen and this change in the legislation has led to a steady growth in colleges, or special college courses, for people with learning disabilities, together with a rapid expansion of 'learning support units' in mainstream colleges. The development of courses leading to a wide range of vocational qualifications has also helped to ensure that a much higher proportion of students with special needs have access to courses that suit both their interests and their ability. For example, the system of NVQs (National Vocational Qualifications or SVQs (Scottish Vocational Qualifications) means that there are now many more training courses available on a part- or full-time basis. There are several levels of competence within the NVQ framework, from very basic work-related activities that are routine and predictable (Level 1) to much higher levels (Levels 5 or 6) that may be equivalent to degree status or higher and which require complex knowledge and considerable individual autonomy and responsibility. The more basic levels are often very suitable for people with autism, although some individuals may well be able to progress to higher levels. The City and Guilds system also offers qualifications with a more practical emphasis than those offered by most regular degree or diploma courses.

In principle, this expansion in training should be greatly to the benefit of people with autism, who, for a variety of reasons – academic, social or behavioural – may have been unable to obtain formal qualifications at school. However, as is the case with schooling, the curriculum for students with more general 'special needs' is often not designed to meet the specific needs of those with autism; nor do tutors on such courses necessarily have any specialist knowledge about the condition.

The uneven developmental profile of students with autism, and the problems this poses for teaching, have already been discussed at some length in the previous chapter. Such problems tend to persist into tertiary education. Most special needs courses are designed to meet the requirements of students who are 'slow learners'. That is, they have no specific deficits in any one area and, although development generally is delayed, their social, communication and academic skills will, on the whole, be at a similar level. This is rarely the case for students with autism, who, almost by definition, will be impaired in certain areas – especially those related to communication and social understanding – but may have much higher levels of academic competence. Other courses may cater for the needs of students with specific learning difficulties, such as dyslexia, but while often being academically more appropriate for people with autism these are still unable to cater for their social and emotional needs.

All too frequently, students with autism who manage to find a place at college either become bored at the low level of teaching or frustrated by their lack of ability to cope with the more abstract components of the course. Harry, for example, was an eighteen-year-old with a passionate interest in all things mechanical. He could mend most electrical equipment with ease, but although his general intellectual ability was in the normal range he had no formal school qualifications and poor literacy skills. On the recommendation of a special careers adviser he enrolled in an electrical course at the learning support unit of his local college. He was outraged to find that the main purpose of this course was to teach students how to *use* a toaster or washing machine, not how to repair or build them – and he soon left in exasperation.

Rather different problems were experienced by Patrick, who was accepted on a mechanical engineering course for mainstream students, with support from 'special needs' staff. Following some early difficulties, it was decided to modify his course so that there was less emphasis on the academic and written aspects and greater focus on his practical abilities. However, because his practical skills were so good many tutors were unable to appreciate the depth of his problems in other areas and consistently expected him to achieve at a higher level than was possible. Thus, despite the support that was offered, Patrick became increasingly anxious and depressed over his inability to cope, his tutors became more and more frustrated, and his constant requests for explanations in class steadily alienated his fellow students. Matters came to a head when a group of students confronted him outside college and threatened to 'kill him' if he did not keep quiet in class. Terrified by their threats, Patrick refused to return and thereafter remained at home unoccupied and miserable.

Not all attempts at integration, of course, fail so disastrously, but success can require considerable preparation. Ben, who had transferred from an autistic school to a boys' public school at the age of thirteen, had succeeded well academically and was preparing to go to university to study mathematics. His teachers recognised that his poor social skills would be likely to cause difficulties and were concerned to find him a place at a college that could offer him a high degree of support. As Ben's mathematical expertise was also somewhat specialised the maths syllabus on offer was carefully examined until a particular university was identified that seemed to meet all his requirements. Ben was successful in gaining a place, and throughout his course a special tutor was assigned to monitor his progress. If difficulties arose, help was also sought from Ben's psychologist, and eventually he obtained a second-class degree in maths and computing.

Other individuals find that after the difficulties they experienced at school – in having to cope both with a wide variety of topics and less than sympathetic classmates and teachers – college life may actually be a pleasant change. Indeed, unconventional dress or behaviour may convey certain social advantages, and even being viewed as 'nerdy' or a 'computer freak' is not necessarily a drawback. Ivor, for example, had always been badly teased at school because of his failure to take part in 'laddish' activities, his lack of fashion sense and his almost obsessional interest in biology. He managed to obtain a university place, and although his social life was rather limited he did develop one or two relationships with like-minded students. With help from two particular tutors he achieved a moderately good degree, but by this time his particular expertise in cell biology had been recognised and he was accepted as a Ph.D. student. Left to pursue the one topic that had fascinated him for years, he blossomed academically, and also began to make much closer relationships amongst other people working in the same field.

Unfortunately, for many college students the support systems on which they depended at school disappear once they enter university. Although Equal Opportunities legislation means that colleges are obliged to offer some assistance to students with special needs, this often tends to focus more on physical or sensory impairments, or on specific disabilities such as dyslexia, rather than a pervasive, developmental condition such as autism.

Personal accounts

The lack of support experienced by many mainstream students with autism is vividly illustrated in personal accounts by past, or current university students such as those published by Dawn Prince-Hughes (2002). Research based on a questionnaire survey of students is also reported by Powell (2002). A particularly informative source of personal experiences, which should be read by all teachers in further education, is the Internet site 'University Students with Autism and Asperger Syndrome' (www.users.dircon.co.uk 2003). This contains advice, based on personal experience of how to cope with the curriculum generally, and exams more specifically. The following are a few of the practical recommendations suggested:

- You will be expected to structure your own time and plan your work to meet long-term deadlines. It can be very hard to judge on your own if you are doing too little work, or too much, especially if you tend towards either disorganisation or perfectionism, and so it is important to make sure you get adequate feedback from tutors.
- If functioning in group situations is a problem, then seminars and discussion groups can be difficult. If you are still deciding which universities to apply to, find out what their main teaching methods are: one-to-one tutorials, seminars, lectures, lab work, or computers. For some people, one-to-one teaching can be better adapted to their needs, while others might find it too intense. If you think you might be unable to cope with a campus environment, investigate those offering distance learning or online tutoring.
- Find out about any resources your university has for blind, deaf or learning disabled students, such as books on tape, or transcripts of lectures. Software designed to adapt computers for people with disabilities can also be useful for autistic students with visual or coordination problems.
- Videotape lectures and/or ask for copies of overheads and diagrams – many people with Asperger syndrome cannot read what is on the board, take notes and listen all at the same time.
- Get an advanced copy of the syllabus (or a rough draft) before term begins in order to prepare for some of the change in routine, and to arrange for adaptations to materials.
- Arrange for a distraction-free environment for study and for taking exams – crowded lecture halls can be stressful for students who have problems with physical proximity – turn up early enough to get an aisle seat, request to be allowed to sit apart (or even in a separate room) for exams.
- Request twice the allotted test-taking time – particularly important for multiple choice exams.
- Determine where your exam is to take place and familiarise yourself with it. Be sure to arrive well in time so you will not panic if anything delays your journey.
- Seek whatever accommodations you feel appropriate (separate room, computer, amanuensis or whatever) Do not be afraid of what other students might think or how professors will react; these are your right and may make the difference between success and failure.
- Prioritise anything else that is going on in your life so it will not compete with your time for preparing for and revising for exams and otherwise stress you out.

Many other hints for college survival (including some very helpful email sites dealing with topics as varied as anxiety, socialising, celibacy, sexual identity, rape, exercise and drug-taking) are offered. Advice on securing appropriate accommodation, and finding one's way around college, both metaphorically and literally, is also provided. A further important issue that is discussed is whether to divulge to college staff or other students the fact that one has autism or Asperger syndrome. In helping students make this decision the following points are highlighted:

- Most universities now make adequate provisions for people with physical disabilities, but few have even *heard* of HFA/AS, let alone considered the possibility that it might affect any of their students. Many people still assume that if you can talk, let alone go to university, you can not *really* be autistic. If you have any special needs, or just want university staff to be aware of areas in which you may function differently, you may have to educate them yourself.
- Some people choose not to tell (especially if they are concerned about privacy or think staff may be unsympathetic or even hostile) but it does make things harder if any autism-related problems do arise.
- If you do choose to tell, it is best not to leave it until a crisis; this makes it more likely that ignorant people will assume that it is just an excuse. It is easier to get any unexpected special needs met if people have been informed of your disability well in advance.
- Remember that you do not have to choose between 'telling everyone' and 'telling no one'. You can choose to tell a few people you trust, and ask them to keep it strictly confidential.
- The most useful thing you can have is an official medical letter stating your diagnosis and giving a brief explanation of the ways it is likely to affect you (keep a copy with you at all times). If you can anticipate in advance any special requirements, ask your clinician to specify them in the letter.
- The second most useful thing you can have is a short paper explaining HFA/AS with particular reference to people of university age (although the contributor to this website adds 'I'm still working on finding this one. . . .')

Particularly informative in the website are the autobiographical accounts of individual students. These include undergraduates and postgraduates enrolled in courses ranging through maths, physics and computer sciences to media studies and history. On the whole, few report major difficulties with the academic demands of university life.

However, organisational problems related to work assignments and exams often resulted in grades being much lower than expected. Difficulties in socialising with other students, and especially problems in sharing accommodation, were a frequent cause of distress. Lack of understanding from staff, teasing and bullying by other students, inability to ask for help or to make important decisions, feelings of failure and incompetence are all cited as significant precipitants of anxiety and depression. Nevertheless, most accounts are characterised by a determination to 'beat the system', and many offer practical tips for doing so.

Although websites of this kind are, without doubt, of enormous value, it is disturbing that, sixty years after autism was first recognised, professional support and understanding remain so limited. The inflexibility of the educational system, and the reluctance to modify this to suit students with autism is of particular concern, especially when very minor modifications (such as allowing students who dislike close physical contact to have an aisle seat during exams) can make such a major difference. Without help, only the most determined and intellectually able students with autism are likely to survive three to four years of university life relatively unscathed *and* with a degree befitting their level of intelligence.

Specialist support schemes

Over recent years, a number of schemes have been developed to help people with autism acquire the necessary skills to enter and cope with college. Some also offer training for college staff who may be involved with students with autism. In America, the support offered by the TEACCH organisation in North Carolina has enabled many students to benefit from further education courses. On a much smaller scale, INTERACT (Graham 1999) in England offers teaching in social, communication and problem-solving skills for individuals wishing to enter college. Some on-site support is also provided in colleges to enable students to follow vocational training courses and ongoing assistance, and advice can be provided to students and college staff, as necessary. The LEAP scheme, run in the United Kingdom under the auspices of the National Autistic Society, is also designed to help students acquire the skills needed to enter college. The focus is on individuals who still need help to develop communication, social, creative and leisure skills as well as to improve self-care and independence. Students may attend the LEAP unit full time, or spend part of their time in special education centres or similar units.

Another example of a specialist scheme is the partnership between the integrated resource centre at King Egbert's School in Sheffield and the five separate units that comprise Sheffield College. The scheme assists students in completing application forms, attending interviews, choosing appropriate courses, and developing strategies for enhancing learning and minimising problems. The essential components of the programme include good communication between college staff, the resource centre and students' families; adequate information for and preparation of college staff concerning the needs of people with autism; explicit timetables and work programmes; clear rules governing social behaviour and standards of work; continuous monitoring and feedback on performance, and the development of social and independence skills. The impact of the physical environment is also recognised, and areas of potential difficulties (having to negotiate around the college site, passing through large noisy crowds of students, even coping with faulty vending machines) are all modified as far as possible. If situations cannot be changed (e.g. crowds of students smoking around main entrances) the individual with autism is helped to find alternative routes or encouraged to seek help from college staff (e.g. when vending machines refuse to accept coins). Although this particular scheme is only able to assist relatively small numbers of students at any one time, it provides a liaison model that could be developed among many other schools and colleges.

Somewhat similar programmes have been developed in Nottingham, where the Highfield House project was set up in order to integrate 16–20-year-old students with autism into the learning support unit of the nearby college of further education. Support for students attending the college is provided by staff in the residential unit, and the programme incorporates training days for the college staff. Oakfield House, a special unit in Birmingham, also assists students with autism in local colleges. Each student has a key worker at college, and training is provided to improve the college staff's knowledge of and ability to deal with the problems associated with autism (see Morgan 1996, for further details of these schemes). Another important initiative, based at Birmingham University, is the distance-learning course in autism for staff working in further education settings, which is designed to improve understanding and management skills.

There are a number of other groups around the United Kingdom that assist higher functioning students with autistic spectrum disorders to access tertiary education. These include the Farleigh Education group in Somerset; the Northumberland-based 'European Services for People with Autism' (EPSA), which offers a range of further education provision, and the Nautical College in Glasgow, which has input from the Scottish Autistic Society. Such centres are also an invaluable source of advice for staff working with students with autism in other, non-specialist placements.

Colleges or special courses for students with learning disabilities may be of help to people with autism who have difficulties coping with the social and academic demands of a regular course and can prove a helpful stepping stone towards eventual mainstream placements. Susanna, for example, had previously failed to complete a word-processing course at her local college because of her fears of having to cope with large numbers of unfamiliar students and lecturers. A year on a special residential course for students with disabilities, where staff had had training in autistic-spectrum disorders, gave her the courage to try again – this time, successfully.

Sometimes, however, it can be difficult to enlist appropriate support even within specialist provision. Annabel was a twenty-one-year-old woman in a residential home for people with autism. Although at first she had settled well, she soon became bored with the limited daytime programme that the unit was able to offer. The manager applied on her behalf for a place on a special needs course at the nearby college, but because the home had a reputation for taking on 'challenging' clients college staff were very reluctant to accept her. However, after the college principal finally agreed to accept Annabel for a trial period of three half-days per week, on condition that the home arranged for her transport and a staff member remained with her at all times. Despite such inauspicious beginnings Annabel thrived; she did well on the practical courses and clearly enjoyed being with more sociable, non-autistic students. Soon the only time that supervision was needed was at break or meal times, mainly because of her outbursts if anyone sneezed or coughed. Eventually a member of the college staff who had developed a good relationship with her offered to accompany her at such times or to arrange for someone else to do so, so that the presence of staff from the home was no longer required.

More information about colleges or training courses for students with special needs, many of which are appropriate for people with autism, can be obtained from a number of different sources. In the United Kingdom, these include the directories published by NATSPEC (Association of National Special Colleges); COPE (*Compendium of Post-16 Education and Training in Residential Establishments for Young People with Special Needs*), 2000, MENCAP (*Directory of Specially Designed Courses in Further Education for People with a Learning*

Disability) 1990b, or the Disability Information Service (*Opportunities Related to Training, Education and Employment Provision for Disabled People*). The Learning and Skills Council also produces a booklet on further education for young people with learning difficulties and/or disabilities, and the Department for Education website provides information on post-16 education and training courses (*www.dfes.gov.uk*).

Changing attitudes

Although attitudes to students with special needs are gradually changing, barriers to integration still persist. Inclusion remains particularly difficult to achieve for students who show severely challenging behaviours, but problems also arise for those who are relatively mildly affected. As in schools, difficulties can occur because of a lack of understanding, misinterpretation of behaviour and inflexibility, either on the part of staff or other students or within the organisational structure.

Even staff who are used to teaching students with special needs may still have difficulties coping with the communication and social impairments that are characteristic of autism. The majority of students in special colleges, for example, are unlikely to possess the very specialised knowledge or interests or memory skills that are typically found within the autistic spectrum. They are unlikely to correct lecturers' factual knowledge or to complain about the way in which the course is being run. Many students with autistic-spectrum disorders, however, show no reticence in giving voice to their complaints, nor do they necessarily learn to express these in a diplomatic fashion. Brian caused total chaos in classes during his first term at college by continually commenting on the tutors' handwriting. He was particularly concerned if they did not dot the letter 'i', and lectures were constantly disrupted because of this. Raymond announced that he would not attend classes taught by anyone who was black or female. Such behaviours, understandably, can result in students being viewed as rude or as 'troublemakers'. Rather than recognising their need for *more* help, lecturers whose competence is called into question in this way are likely to become markedly less sympathetic and may even call for the exclusion of such students from their classes.

Rejection may even occur before the student even gets to college. Louis had a first degree in engineering and subsequently applied for and was accepted for a master's degree at another university. His psychologist and careers officer, who had remained involved since he left school, were aware that he might have problems on a course that depended largely on project work requiring considerable self-discipline and strict adherence to deadlines. Because the university had a special needs department the psychologist, with Louis' permission, contacted them to explain the potential problems and to discuss possible ways of dealing with these. Two days later the psychologist received a letter stating that 'in view of the problems, and limited staff resources, it would be advisable for the candidate to withdraw from the course'!

Other students, too, may need to be given advice or practical support in order to help them understand the problems and needs of someone with autism. Even at college, problems of teasing, bullying, provocation or rejection can occur. Ben, who was completing a degree in mathematics, was deliberately put forward by other students as a candidate for the president of the union because his outrageous speeches were a continuing source of amusement to them and they knew that he was certain to make a complete fool of himself.

Jason, who attended a special college course, was also quickly identified as an 'easy target' by other students. He was desperate to find a girlfriend and, recognising this, other students would deliberately lead him into compromising situations (for example, suggesting that he follow women into their changing rooms or toilets) where he was almost certain to be rebuffed.

Other students with autism may be taunted for their 'stupidity' if they are unable to cope with more complex or academic components of the course. They may also, as in the case of Patrick described earlier, be the source of considerable irritation and disruption to other students because of their constant requests for help, explanation or reassurance.

Ways of coping

Despite the potential problems of coping with college life, whether this be in a mainstream or specialist setting, success at this stage is crucial if the individual with autism is to have any real chance of living and working independently. As with schooling, there are some general procedures that can help to circumvent or minimise difficulties and the NAS provides a helpful leaflet for staff working particularly with higher-functioning students with autistic-spectrum disorders (www.nas.org.uk). Other organisations that may be able to offer advice for people with autism, their families, or teachers, are the Further Education Funding Council (for information about obtaining funding, especially post-nineteen years); SKILL, the National Bureau for Students with Disabilities, and ACE (Advisory Centre for Education).

The first step, however is to ensure that the transition process is adequately planned and managed.

Transition from school to college

The move from the relatively supportive environments of home and school to the adult world of college or university is a time of potential upheaval and stress for most young people. Although for many students the wider social environment and the removal of parental restraints will actively foster personal development and greater maturity, for those with autism these factors may significantly interfere with their ability to make progress.

Transitional programmes from school to college are generally better established in the United States than in many other countries. Over fifteen years ago, for example, Wehman and his colleagues (1988) described in detail the facilities and programmes that had been used to help individuals with disabilities make the transition from school, stressing the importance of long-term planning and the roles that both teachers and parents can play in preparing students for this significant stage of their lives. Recently, the National Autistic Society has published a set of guidelines designed to improve the transition process in the United Kingdom (Powell 2002). It is recommended that all local authorities should have a planning group for autism and Asperger syndrome and that this should include all professionals relevant at the transitional stage from school (i.e. representatives from local colleges and universities; senior educational psychologist and senior SENCO from the local secondary school network; Connexions personal adviser for complex needs in mainstream schools, and a social services representative). This group should be responsible for mapping out links between schools and colleges and agreeing a support pathway for transition. This planning should start with identification of pupils with autistic-spectrum disorders and the development of close liaison between educational and social services *from the age of fourteen*. The student should then be assigned a personal adviser, and families and the young people themselves should be involved at all stages of the planning process. Among the practical strategies recommended are:

- A *comprehensive* assessment of needs and agreed plans for meeting these needs and monitoring progress.
- The student's personal adviser should be responsible for getting to know the student and, on the basis of that knowledge, for developing appropriate plans for future college placement.

- There should be opportunities to visit suitable colleges/universities with support, and link courses should be considered to 'test out' the appropriateness of potential placements.
- The student's ability to meet course requirements (with regard to academic ability; learning styles, social competence, self-organisation, independence, etc.) should be assessed and any difficulties addressed.
- Once a college place has been decided upon, there should be a clear plan of the help needed to meet learning and support needs (personal, tutorial, learning support, counselling, extra financial provision etc.).
- The personal adviser should oversee the process of application to and entry into college, and should inform college staff of all the student's potential needs. Schools should provide all relevant information (IEPs, statements etc.) to college or university staff.

Maintaining links with and support from schools

One particularly crucial link in the chain of support is the knowledge and guidance of staff in secondary schools. Whether education has been in a mainstream or segregated setting, information from staff who are familiar with the individual's strengths and weakness can be vital for the success of later placements.

Many schools for children with special needs do their best to actively prepare pupils for college life. They may also have close links with local colleges, so that staff at the different establishments are well known to each other. A planned and gradual introduction to college life during the final years at school is often the most successful form of preparation for both students and college staff. With a gradual and flexible approach to college entry potential problems can be identified at an early stage, and staff at the parent school can help to advise on strategies to deal with these. School staff may also be aware of difficulties that may interfere with an individual student's future progress at college. Jeremy's school, for example, recognised that he would not be able to cope alone at times when there were no formal lectures. He was fascinated by electrical equipment, and if not otherwise occupied would be likely to roam the campus looking for things he could take apart. During his final year at school a teacher was allotted to accompany him to classes at the local college twice a week. As time went on he was able to remain in class without extra support, and efforts were then devoted to finding ways of occupying him during 'free time'. His teacher identified a number of possible activities including visits to the library, some sessions in the gym, trips to the canteen and a walk around the grounds, all of which could be used to fill this time. Because Jeremy enjoyed having a set timetable to follow the college staff, in collaboration with his teachers, constructed a very detailed weekly timetable for him. No free periods were indicated on this at all; instead, each day was filled with specific activities, many of which – such as a tour around the grounds – Jeremy was soon able to accomplish alone (or with only minimal supervision). In this way he was able to enter college successfully and with relatively little extra input from college staff.

Collaboration with parents

Parents' own knowledge of their children is also likely to be an essential ingredient in determining the success of further educational programmes. Unfortunately, since one of the major goals of post-school education is to foster students' independence the need to liaise with families can sometimes be difficult for staff to accept. However, failure to take account of information from such a vital source can prove disastrous. Johnny had attended a school for children with mild learning difficulties throughout his secondary school years and had done surprisingly well there. He himself was of above average intelligence but his social and communication skills were such that he functioned much better with students of lesser ability. His parents had requested a place, for a one-year preparatory period, in the learning support unit of the local college as they were certain that Johnny would not cope, at least initially, without this help. Because of his relatively high intellectual level and his impressive ability to talk about subjects that were of particular interest to him, the admissions tutor felt that his parents were being 'overprotective' and considered that it was time Johnny 'stood on his own two feet'. As his parents predicted, the contrast between the protective environment of school and the unstructured world of college proved too much for him to cope with unsupported, and by the end of the first term Johnny's anxiety and agitation reached such a level that he had to abandon his studies.

In another case the parents of Jan, a young woman who had previously attended a special school, requested help with transport to college. They felt she would be able to cope at college when she arrived but doubted her ability to get there alone. However, the local authority argued that she did not need special transport, that the college was not far away, she had no physical difficulties, and she was intellectually able to cope with the journey. Despite the fact that a coach stopped at the end of the road to pick up a more severely disabled student, Jan was not allowed to travel on this. She became so anxious at the thought of having to walk to college alone, even though she knew the route perfectly well, that she got up earlier and earlier each day in order to make preparations for the journey. Eventually she would hardly go to bed at all, and her parents became so concerned for her welfare that they increasingly gave in to her demands to remain at home.

Many parents of children with autism will admit to being 'overprotective' but feel that they have little choice in the matter. Their concerns are not just for the possible physical danger to their sons or daughters but relate to the emotional trauma – and the widespread effects of this – which can result from inappropriate expectations or the failure to meet the young person's needs. Clearly, parents and children do need to move apart as time goes on, but few students with autism will have acquired the social competence or the level of independence required to survive when they first enter college. To expect them to be able to cope without support from their families is to deprive them of a vital back-up system and college staff of a valuable source of information.

Links with social service provision

For some students it may not be possible to arrange access to college courses immediately after they leave school. They may need the opportunity to settle first into some other form of day care or residential provision, and only after this has been successfully achieved can plans for their further education be made.

Joe, who was not diagnosed as having autism until his late teens, had been excluded from the local school for children with learning difficulties because of his behavioural problems. He was transferred to boarding provision, but was clearly very unhappy there and made several unsuccessful attempts to run away. Finally his parents took him away from school altogether, and he remained at home, looking after himself during the day from the age of fifteen to nineteen. Local social services became involved after he was attacked by a group of youngsters in a nearby park. Despite his reluctance to leave home his social worker made a determined attempt to get him into college. The principal agreed to a programme of gradual introduction, with Joe at first just attending art classes, where he was allowed to indulge his obsession of painting the designs from 1960s record covers. His social worker accompanied him initially, but as time went on and more classes were introduced she gradually faded from the scene, though remaining available for the staff to seek advice from as necessary.

Many social education centres (also known as adult training centres) that offer daytime provision for people with learning disabilities also cater for clients with autistic-spectrum disorders. Frequently, however, the programme within these centres is too unstructured, the environment too noisy and crowded, and activities too reliant on social interactions between clients to be suitable for someone with autism. The opportunity to attend part-time courses at local colleges can therefore be of enormous benefit, although this may well require additional support. Tessa, aged thirty-five, attended a day centre, and her previously aggressive behaviours (mainly due to a very unsatisfactory residential placement) had improved to such an extent when she moved to a new residential home that it was felt she could begin to attend a special computer course at the local college. Unfortunately, when informed of her past difficulties, the college was very reluctant to accept her. Considerable negotiation was required, and initially she was accepted only if accompanied by staff from the day centre. Gradually it became possible, by ensuring a high degree of structure within the sessions, for her to remain in computer classes with only minimal extra support.

Input from other professional sources

During their childhood many individuals with autism will have had contact with a wide range of professionals. Psychologists may have been involved in assessment or intervention programmes; language therapists may have advised on ways of developing communication skills; occupational or physiotherapists may have provided help with motor or self-help skills; psychiatric help may have been sought for emotional or behavioural problems. Many of these professionals may be able to provide valuable advice: on the most appropriate type of courses to follow; on situations that are likely to exacerbate problems or techniques to minimise these; or on ways of developing students' skills in different areas. Unfortunately, just as many students reach college age access to children's services ceases so that there is little opportunity for these professionals to offer continuing support. College staff, too, may be reluctant to seek advice from those formerly involved in a *child's* care, believing this to be inappropriate for someone on the threshold of adulthood.

Failure to make use of the knowledge and expertise of those who have known the individual for many years is clearly wasteful, and if proper planning for college life is to take place these resources should be utilised as much as possible. Recognition of the very different strands of information and advice that different professionals are able to offer and a willingness to employ these in a constructive way can help to optimise progress and prevent many avoidable problems.

Professional help may also prove useful if unexpected problems arise. The efforts made to ensure that Ben succeeded with his maths course at university are described earlier in this chapter. On the whole the support offered by his tutors proved very successful, but occasionally even their resources were strained. Just before his final exams, for example, Ben announced that conventional notions of algebra were quite unsatisfactory and hence he had developed a system of his own. His tutor was rightly concerned that he might fail badly if he went ahead with this, and the psychologist who had been involved with Ben and his family for many years advised that gentle dissuasion was unlikely to work. Instead, Ben was firmly instructed that he could not work on his own system until after the exams had been completed. If he did well in these the maths department would then consider his proposals, but until then there was to be no more discussion of the issue. Such advice is hardly in keeping with the desire to foster independent thought in students, but from past experience it was clear that if allowed to follow his own ideas as he wished Ben would have become entirely obsessed with them and his output would have been totally unproductive.

Joe, who was helped into college through the support of his social worker, also needed further help when it became apparent that other students there were deliberately provoking him. Groups of young women would approach and ask if he wanted to be their boyfriend or to kiss them. As soon as he tried to take up their offers they would scream and rush away, instantly attracting the attention of everyone around. Formal complaints about 'sexual harassment' were made to the college, although Joe's social worker was convinced that these incidents had been deliberately provoked. She ascertained from Joe that the incidents occurred mainly at the bus stop on the way to or from college. Although college staff confronted the female students concerned, this had little effect. Instead, arrangements were made for Joe to be escorted to and from college by either his social worker or a member of his family. Meanwhile Joe began to attend some social skills sessions to teach him more appropriate ways of responding in such situations; he was also encouraged to inform his social worker whenever the problem arose. Although the problems continued to re-emerge from time to time, the frequency became much less.

The need for structure and consistency

Many problems for students attending college, or for those involved in their care, arise from the behavioural, social or communication difficulties described in earlier chapters. Possible ways of dealing with such problems have already been described in some detail. However, the crucial factor that must be incorporated into college life, whatever the individual student's level of functioning, is the dual combination of structure and consistency. As stressed throughout this volume, it is under conditions of structure and predictability that people with autism function at their best. If they are unsure what should be done, if the situation is unpredictable or if rules vary from time to time, place to place or individual to individual, then progress will be slow and inappropriate behaviours difficult to change.

Supervisory structure

In most schools the management structure is relatively easy to understand, even by children with severe learning difficulties. In college settings, this hierarchy is often less clear. Even in learning support units the student may have to deal with a range of different tutors; contact with personal supervisors may be limited, and if things do begin to go wrong it can be some time before problems are recognised or appropriate strategies implemented. Unless a student's disabilities are very marked or his or her behaviour very disturbed, staffing levels often mean that it is impossible to provide all the help needed, even when that student is recognised as requiring additional support. The lack of any systematic monitoring system or the presence of a key worker to turn to at times of stress can quickly tip the balance between success and failure. It is crucial, therefore, that in planning entry to college, at whatever level, specific agreements be made concerning *who* will be responsible for monitoring progress or ensuring that work assignments are completed satisfactorily; *what strategies* will be implemented if problems occur, and *where* the student should turn to for support. Ideally, for less able students the number of people involved should be as few as possible, although those in mainstream settings will clearly have to cope with a larger number. Annabel, whose gradual introduction to college was described earlier, soon became well known and accepted there. However, not everyone was aware of what to do if problems occurred, in particular if she became very upset when someone either sneezed or coughed loudly. Like all the students of her age Annabel had an identity badge, but under her name was also written the name of her department and the internal phone number of a key worker to contact. As the latter could change from day to day different badges were supplied on different days of the week. Although her identity label was slightly different from the other students', the variation was sufficiently great to single her out as being 'different' and indeed would only be noticed by anyone who needed to approach closely.

As is the case for establishing acceptable patterns of behaviour generally, it is essential that staff collaborate in developing rules and that they cooperate in the procedures to be followed if problems occur. Without consistency, even the most sophisticated strategies will be of little use. However, it is important not to underestimate the difficulties of achieving this: hence the need for an agreed and well-established structure that is clear and acceptable to everyone concerned.

Structuring work tasks and timetables

At whatever level the student with autism is functioning, whether it be completing a doctorate or learning basic daily living skills, the task structure and requirements must be clearly specified. The value of the TEACCH approach for less able students, and the need for a high level of cues and checks, has already been noted in the chapter on secondary education, and these are all procedures that can be readily incorporated into adult teaching programmes. For more able students this level of guidance will be neither appropriate nor practical, but structure is nevertheless crucial. Students must know *where* they should be, *what* they should be doing at all times, and *to whom* they should turn if problems occur.

Even leisure activities or obsessional behaviours may need to become part of the daily timetable. Gary was a young man who had just begun to attend a social education centre after leaving school. He was delighted to find that he was allowed free access to the kitchen and dishwasher, and that he could fill and empty this as often as he wished – an activity that previously had always been strictly controlled. This behaviour soon escalated to the level where he was doing almost nothing else. Other students began to be resentful of the fact that he took no part in daily activities, and also because he refused to allow them in the kitchen whenever he was there as he did not wish them to disrupt his stacking of places and so on. If attempts were made to stop this, he would become resentful and aggressive. In order to reduce the problem a picture timetable using PECS symbols was drawn up for him, as shown in Figure 8.1. There was little attempt initially to make any

dishwasher	dishwasher	relaxation
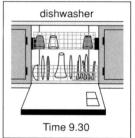	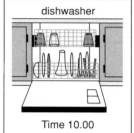	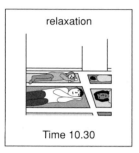
Time 9.30	Time 10.00	Time 10.30

dishwasher	music class	lunch
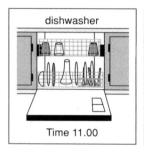	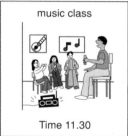	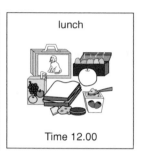
Time 11.00	Time 11.30	Time 12.00

dishwasher	video	trampoline
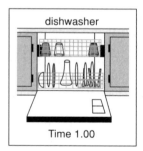	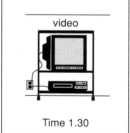	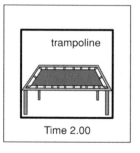
Time 1.00	Time 1.30	Time 2.00

dishwasher	apparatus	home
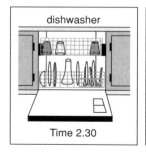	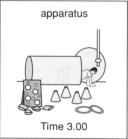	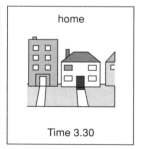
Time 2.30	Time 3.00	Time 3.30

Figure 8.1 Gary's timetable

major changes to Gary's day. He would already take part – if somewhat reluctantly – in relaxation and music or physical education classes, and he loved watching videos. The main alteration in his programme was that these activities, along with his 'dishwasher' sessions, were specifically timetabled, as were the staff who were to be involved. Gary had always had picture timetables at school and seemed happy to have his daily programme laid out in this way. It was made clear that the timetable would be changed as time went on, and gradually more and more activities replaced the dishwasher stacking. The time allotted for each session in the kitchen was also reduced until he was following as full a timetable as most of the other students in the centre and time spent in the kitchen was kept to a minimum.

Students of higher ability levels will usually be accustomed to following a set timetable, but they may need additional help when they are required to complete longer work assignments, and again the timing of these will need to be precisely specified. For many students with autism, being given a piece of work to complete by the end of term is a recipe for disaster. A few may get into a panic and try to complete the project immediately, thus giving the work insufficient attention and preparation; many, however, will find themselves at the end of the year having produced nothing at all. Tutors need to be prepared to break down the task into more manageable units, which then have to be completed within a clearly specified period; they may also need to take on the responsibility for checking progress at each stage.

If necessary, too, the help of other family members may need to be elicited. Dominic was a skilled photographer trying to obtain an A level in photography at a local college. For his coursework he had to prepare a portfolio of photographs, and whenever asked by his tutor how he was getting on would assure him that everything was 'fine'. Just before the final deadline his tutor, who had not seen any photographs at all, telephoned his mother to check what was happening. It then became apparent that *nothing* had been prepared. After a frantic weekend, and considerable expense to get the photos processed by an express service, he did manage to produce some work, but this was of a much lower standard than he was capable of and resulted in his A level results being considerably poorer than they might have been.

Even attendance at college may require careful monitoring. By the time most students enter further education it is generally considered that they should be responsible for their own behaviour and that if they fail to attend lectures then that is their concern. However, for someone with autism this freedom may be entirely inappropriate. Without any clear rules for attendance they may begin to attend very erratically or even, over time, cease to go to college altogether, drifting gradually back into a life of ritual, obsession and solitariness. Self-regulation is unlikely to occur, and if the student is to profit from the educational facilities on offer the requirement for regular, punctual and daily attendance should be made explicit.

Finally, it is essential that tutors are absolutely honest to students about their capabilities, and that they do not allow them to continue on a course that is inappropriate or unlikely to meet their needs. Gareth had enrolled for a wide and disparate range of modules at college in London. It was clear to his family and to his psychologist, who had carried out detailed assessments of his ability, that the work generally was far beyond his capabilities. Moreover, the mix of subjects chosen would be of little use when it came to finding a job. Year after year he failed most topics, just managing to scrape through a few others. It was evident from his feedback forms that lecturers found his inability to cope very frustrating and that other college students were also irritated by his constant demands on staff time. Nevertheless, as he was paying his own fees in full no one asked him to leave, and attempts by his psychologist to meet college staff were unsuccessful. His mother and psychologist both tried to persuade him to take a more appropriate course, but the situation was not helped when he began attending an assertiveness-training group. There he was advised that he must manage his own life and not be dictated to by his family. He became progressively more resistant to accepting help, ceased to visit his mother and terminated counselling sessions with the psychologist. Contact was only resumed again after he was admitted to psychiatric hospital suffering from severe stress and depression.

Flexibility of teaching programmes

The other crucial component of a successful educational programme, again at any level, is the need for a flexible approach to the provision of training. Apparently minor modifications to the environment, curriculum or teaching materials can have a significant impact. During exams, for example, having extra time, being allowed to use a computer, sitting in a separate room or at a distance from other students, even simply being allowed to sit on the end of the aisle, can make the difference between a good pass or total failure. In coursework, explicit instructions on how to complete assignments can greatly affect the standard produced. Allowing students who have problems taking notes to record lectures using audio or video tapes can also improve output.

Computer-assisted learning programmes can be extremely successful, but because of poor organisational skills many students with autism will require explicit guidance on how to make best use of these. Attention to sensory problems can also pay dividends. Some students with autism, for example, report that they find it difficult to cope with the glare from white paper, and using grey or other coloured sheets can make a huge difference. For students who are hypersensitive to noise, access to a quiet room can significantly improve the quality of their work. Other students have found that a 'noise buster' device, which filters out background sounds electronically whilst leaving voices and other foreground noises clear, extremely helpful. (Information from www.nctgroupinc.com).

Since change is particularly difficult for many students with autism to cope with, flexibility is also required in the transitional stage from school to college. As noted earlier, few students with autism are able to cope with this without help, and a much longer introductory period may be required than is the case for other students. An extended preparatory stage may also be needed by college staff if they are to develop effective ways of managing problems and encouraging learning. Gradual introductions, over a period of a year or two (or even more), may be necessary if the transition is to be accomplished without difficulty; college staff may need to be prepared to accept the presence of a support teacher, at least initially, and ideally will need to undertake some additional training themselves. Initial reductions in the amount of work required, especially in the early stages of a course, can also be beneficial. Many students with autism find the demands of a full day's teaching programme excessive, or they may have difficulties coping with the range of subjects offered to other students. It may be more productive to allow such students to attend on a *planned, part-time* basis initially rather than expect them to succeed in classes where they are overstressed. Similarly, more able students may find they cope better with modular courses that allow them to build up to degree level gradually rather than attempt to fit everything into a more rigid three- to four-year course.

Warren's behaviour had become progressively more disruptive after leaving school, and as college attendance was clearly out of the question he began attending a social education centre. However, the daily programme there was not adequate to meet his needs and he quickly became bored and frustrated. Negotiations with a local college resulted in his being allowed to attend specified classes there, and gradually, as he settled in, the time was expanded. He is still not able to attend for the whole day, but the flexibility of the arrangement between the centre and college has ensured that his week is well structured without imposing excessive social or cognitive demands.

At the other end of the spectrum was Martin, who had obtained good A level results but then suffered a 'breakdown' in his first term at university, mainly because of his social and obsessional problems. He attempted a simple clerical job, but again was unable to cope. Eventually he left work, and with the help of a very sensitive social worker began to learn basic daily living skills and to overcome some of his obsessions. After a couple of years he was confident enough to do some voluntary work at the local MENCAP centre; this in turn gave him the confidence to take up an Open University course, concentrating on modules in computing, and he has now enrolled for a full-time university degree.

Flexibility is also required in attitudes to funding further education as well as to teaching. Currently, funding in the United Kingdom is generally available only for courses leading to a 'recognised qualification'. For individuals with autism, especially those with additional learning difficulties, such qualifications may be inappropriate, at least initially. One way around this restriction is to seek funding to enable students to develop independent living or communication skills which will then enable them to enrol in an accredited course. Students can be helped to draw up an independent living plan with individually specified goals, but these goals must be met if funding is to continue. This has led to concerns that objectives could be set to very low levels in order to avoid any risk of failure (and hence withdrawal of funding) with the result that the student's capabilities are not fully stretched.

There are also problems in funding when part-time placements in different settings are required. For example, a student may need to remain on roll at a secondary school whilst spending more and more time at college; or there may be a need to combine funding for attendance at a day centre with funding for college attendance. Many authorities do manage to overcome such financial complexities, but if resources – or motivation – are low, the resulting bureaucracy can seem insurmountable. Moreover, if funding is not forthcoming this can involve parents, teachers, tutors or care staff in unnecessary battles to achieve a settled and appropriate educational environment for the individual concerned.

Even with adequate funding, achieving the appropriate environment for individuals with autism in further education is likely to present many challenges. Almost anyone involved in providing services for adults with autism will probably need to be involved in the teaching of basic life skills, no matter what professional role they usually occupy. The problem is that such teaching is unlikely to be optimally effective unless it is conducted in the context where those skills are actually needed. Herein lies the 'Catch-22': in that people with autism may be unable to enter further education if they lack the necessary social, communication, practical or cognitive skills. However, very often these skills cannot be learned in isolation and will need to be taught in the context of the educational setting.

Summary: Meeting the needs of students with autistic-spectrum disorders

Further educational opportunities for individuals with autism have improved immeasurably over recent years and soon tertiary education may be expected to be the norm rather than the exception. A wide range of potential provision is available, but in order to gain access to and profit from this the special needs of students with autism must be fully recognised. Guidelines designed to improve the current situation for both students and staff have recently been published by the National Autistic Society in the United Kingdom (Powell 2002). The principal recommendations are for:

- Training to improve awareness of autistic-spectrum disorders among-teaching and other staff (e.g. welfare officers, student union officers etc.) and the development of a 'good practice guide' /training package for staff.
- Liaison between local colleges to develop good practice and share information on how best to support these students.
- Provision of effective pastoral and social support networks for students (including a named staff member to help with personal issues or deal with social difficulties, befriender schemes, etc.).
- Identification of and training for a member of staff who can provide advice concerning autism and offer support to tutors if required.
- Flexible approaches to teaching, exams and the physical environment (e.g. allowing students to tape lectures, provision of quiet areas for relaxation).
- The development of information packages for people with autistic-spectrum disorders and their families.
- A coherent protocol for entry into college (including enrolment procedures, induction and orientation courses, funding for additional support; contact with parents).

- A coherent protocol for leaving college (including realistic plans for the transition to work).
- For students who may not currently be able to cope with mainstream placements, the development of 'open learning' or outreach courses.

And – if everything works? Wendy Lawson tells of her success in finally obtaining her certificate in education. Scouring the lists for her marks, she remembers:

> I thought I would explode with the tension . . . suddenly my friend found my name. I was jubilant. The tears rolled down my face at the relief and realisation of what it meant to have secured a place at university. 'What an achievement!' I shouted. Now I was free. I felt the sky was the limit and I would fly forever, I could be anyone, go anywhere, and the world would not look down its nose at me any longer. . . . I was not dumb.

9 Coping with and finding employment

For individuals with any form of disability the chances of finding or keeping employment in the open work market are greatly reduced. It is estimated, for example, that even individuals with mild intellectual disabilities have unemployment rates as high as 60–70 per cent. Although specialist vocational training programmes do exist, most tend to be pitched at a very low level and many potential trainees fail to gain access to courses that adequately meet their needs (Harrison 1996). Moreover, even for those who manage to find work, job status and stability are typically low (Zetlin and Murtaugh 1990), and work experience is frequently very negative (Szivos 1990).

Table 9.1 summarises the employment rates reported by the follow-up studies reviewed in Chapter 2. Although, over the years, there appears to have been some increase in the proportion of individuals with autism finding work, the numbers are still relatively low, with the average proportion in work according to studies post-1980 being only around 20 per cent. In some studies no individuals were employed, and even amongst those with a focus on higher functioning employment rates were rarely above 30 per cent; the highest proportion reported in work was 47 per cent (Szatmari *et al.* 1989a). The majority of placements that were found were menial and poorly paid, in positions such as kitchen hands, unskilled factory workers, or backroom supermarket staff. In addition, jobs had often been procured through the efforts or personal contacts of families rather than through the normal channels (Howlin *et al.* 2004). Employment stability, too, was poor, with many individuals experiencing lengthy periods without paid work. In the group studied by Howlin and colleagues (2004), for example, the average IQ in adulthood was 75, with one-third having performance IQs of 80 or above. Although around 20 per cent had obtained formal qualifications (several had degrees or diplomas), only eight were working independently, one was a self-employed fabric

Table 9.1 Reported employment outcomes in follow-up studies of adults with autism*

Study (Total N)	Year	Age (years)	IQ	N in work	Type of jobs highest	lowest level
Mittler et al. (26)	1966	7–27	24–111	None		
Lockyer and Rutter (38)	1970	16+	x=62	3	No information	Factory work
Kanner (96)	1973	22–29		9	Military, bank, clerk, chemist, accountant	Store hand; kitchen work
Lotter (29)	1974b	16–18	55–90	1	No information	
Rumsey et al. (14)	1985	18–39	55–129	4	Librarian, cab driver, data input	Janitor; most sheltered workshops
Szatmari et al. (16)	1989b	17–34	68–110	7	Librarian, teacher, salesman	Factory; workshop
Kobayashi et al. (201)	1992	18–33	23%>70	41	Bus conductor, mechanic, cook	Industrial work
Venter et al. (22)	1992	18+	x=90	6	Bartender	All but one low level
von Knorring and Hägglöf (38)	1993	10–29		2	No information	
Tuffreau et al. (49)	1995	12+	89%>50	None		
Ballaban-Gill et al. (45)	1996	18+	31%>70	5		All 'menial'
Larsen and Mouridsen (18)	1997	32–43	78%>50	4	Driver, office boy, gardener	Sheltered factory work
Mawhood et al. (19)	2000	21–26	70–117	5	Lab Technician	Voluntary, sheltered work
Stein (28)	2001	21–36	30–94	None		
Howlin et al. (68)	2004	21+	51–137	24	Scientific officer, computing, accounts, cartographer, office and electronic work	Washing up, supermarket, gravedigger, charcoal burner, factory jobs

* Includes adult outcome studies in which specific data on employment are reported

printer, twelve worked on a supported/sheltered or voluntary basis, two for the family business and one in a shop run by his residential centre. One other man, previously employed in a factory, had been unemployed for some years. Even amongst those in higher level jobs involving computing or accountancy, the level at which they functioned was often lower than their educational attainments would have predicted. Only three or four individuals (a cartographer, a scientific analyst for an oil company and two computer programmers) were employed at a level fully appropriate to their qualifications. Those who were not employed attended general work/leisure programmes within their day or residential units. If anything, employment prospects tended to worsen with age, and in a subsequent follow-up of the same group some time after the initial data had been collected Hutton (1998) found no increase in the numbers in independent work and three previously employed individuals were no longer working.

There are clearly significant financial and social implications related to such low employment rates. The costs of adequately educating individuals with special needs, whether in integrated or special schooling, are substantial. Failure to transfer the skills acquired through education to the workplace is a clear waste of resources. Continuing and unnecessary reliance on state benefits is also extremely expensive, as are the indirect costs of treating emotional and psychiatric disorders related to long-term unemployment (Mawhood and Howlin 1999).

Problems within the workplace

Inability to communicate effectively or to understand instructions are amongst the most obvious problems faced by someone with autism, but other cognitive, social and behavioural difficulties may all have a significant impact on the ability to cope with work. Here, for example, is a graphic illustration from Donna Williams (1992) on the pitfalls of starting a new job.

> I was to begin on the easiest of machines; the button-holer. . . .
> I worked hard and I worked fast. Soon the box of fur coats began to fill up, and the boss passed by, impressed with the speed of my work. He decided to check on the quality.
> A horrified look grew upon his face, and he began to shout . . .
> 'What have you done?' he screamed over and over. 'Button-holes in the sleeves, button-holes in the collar, button-holes in the back panel. Get the hell out of here.'
> 'Can I have my money?' I asked shyly.

'No!' he screamed. 'Do you know what you've done? You've cost me thousands of dollars in damage. Get the hell out of here before I kick you out.'

I hadn't realized that button-holes were meant to go anywhere in particular.

Wendy Lawson (1998) also remembers her job as a nursing assistant on a children's ward. She rather liked it, especially on night duty when 'I heated up any leftovers from the children's supper in the sterilizer, along with the metal kidney bowls, and enjoyed a meal during my dinner break'. She was also undismayed by tasks such as washing dead bodies. Although she kept the job for two years she became progressively more aware of her inability to cope with change or complicated procedures. Eventually, after she had forgotten to return an elderly patient's false teeth and taken them home with her instead, her nursing career came to an abrupt end.

As the above anecdotes illustrate, failure to understand the basic requirements of the job can lead to major problems, even dismissal. Further examples, all taken from clinical practice, are noted below and demonstrate how the problems associated with autism can affect the ability to cope with work in many different ways.

Communication difficulties

The inability to communicate negatively affects many aspects of work. Ned, employed as a computer analyst by a major engineering company, was excellent at identifying the bugs in other people's computer programs. However, he was quite unable to explain to his colleagues in a coherent way what the errors were, why things had gone wrong or how the situation could be corrected. Requests to keep written notes were of no help, since no one could understand these either. Whereas his analytical skills could have made him a great asset in any team-based work, his problems in reciprocal communication meant that he was only able to function in a solitary, and hence far less effective, capacity.

Failure to appreciate social 'rules'

Stuart, who was on a work experience scheme, constantly made remarks about the sex or colour of people working next to him. Although he had no intention of being offensive, his comments were most distasteful to other staff. Adrian 'drove people mad' by standing too close, touching them, or asking personal questions, whilst Gerald's poor personal hygiene led to other staff in his office demanding that he be given a room to work in by himself.

Inability to work independently

Although people with autism may be able to work well if closely supervised, lack of self-initiative or inability to monitor their own progress can cause considerable difficulties. Randell, a computer programmer, had many problems at work because he would only complete assignments satisfactorily if *every* stage of the task were specified. Without explicit instructions he would do nothing, even if the job were well within his capability. Sean, another young man with considerable skill in computing, was employed to enter data for a large shipping company. Although his work was very precise when supervised, if unmonitored he became very slow and careless, making no attempt to check on the accuracy of his work.

Inappropriate work patterns

Rodney, who was responsible for the mail in a small local firm, decided that since all their work was so important everything had to be sent first class. He paid no heed to instructions to the contrary and, unless closely monitored, would waste large amounts of money in this way.

Leslie worked in an office sorting files, and as he appeared to be able to do the filing systematically and without difficulty the initial supervision was rapidly faded out. Each evening files were neatly put away, but it was only when he was on leave some weeks later that it was realised that he had developed a totally idiosyncratic filing system that no one else could understand.

David, who also worked for a small company, was very sensitive to noise around him, and because he could not concentrate on his work if other people were chatting he was allowed to listen to his personal stereo when the office became very busy. As time went on he spent less and less of the day working and more and more time listening to his music. When his manager finally insisted he stop using his stereo he became very upset and was quite unable to understand why.

Obsessional behaviours and resistance to change in routine

Margaret, although a competent typist, insisted on having her work checked at the end of each page of typing. If a letter ran on to two pages, even by a few lines, she was unable to proceed until the first page was checked. This behaviour understandably became very irksome for her line manager. Simon, generally a gentle and quiet worker in a library, became very upset if the work routine was disrupted in any way. His insistence that union meetings were held at lunch times or after work rather than in working hours did not endear him to his colleagues, and when he tried to insist that even birthday or Christmas celebrations should be held outside working hours they became most annoyed. Graham, working in a voluntary capacity in a hospital, also became upset over small changes. One day, without warning, he threw his coffee over the woman who brought around the drinks trolley because she had put the milk into a different container.

Other behavioural difficulties

Other difficulties may also interfere indirectly with work. Anthony, who eventually managed to find employment after a period of several years, had developed the habit, whilst unemployed, of going to bed extremely late each night (partly because of his many night-time rituals). When he started the new job he made no attempt to change his sleeping habits, with the result that he was usually late and always tired, often falling asleep at work. Jim had an obsession with watching the sun set from a nearby railway bridge. As the year progressed he began to make excuses to leave work earlier and earlier, becoming very disruptive when he was requested to stay until leaving time.

Coping with promotion

Although, perhaps, this is not a common problem for people with autism, promotion itself can give rise to unforeseen difficulties for those who manage to succeed well in work. Julian was employed as a research worker in a university science department where his attention to detail and painstaking experimental work were much appreciated. Eventually he was promoted to the post of senior lecturer, which required his attendance at meetings and some administrative work. Having worked in a very isolated way for many years, he was quite unable to cope with these demands. Louis had gradually, if slowly, moved up the managerial ladder at work, and was expected to spend more and more time in meetings. However, he had always found group discussions very difficult to follow, and he also became very agitated if schedules were not precisely followed. A change to the order of the agenda or a meeting running over time caused him enormous stress, and he would rush out of the meeting, even if it were his turn to present. Richard, who had a clerical job in a civil service department, was put forward for promotion long after his contemporaries. This involved taking on a supervisory role with junior staff, but his poor social and management skills resulted in complaints from all concerned.

Mistreatment by others

Because of their difficulties in social interaction and their failure to understand the behaviour of others, people with autism may be very vulnerable to teasing or bullying. Paradoxically, these problems are often greatest for individuals whose impairments are least severe. If someone has a very obvious impairment it is much easier for outsiders to recognise and – one hopes – to show greater sympathy towards the person because of this.

Clare, aged twenty-three, suffered from autism and also a marked speech defect. She had a job stacking shelves in the local supermarket where all the staff were aware of her disabilities. Moreover, because of her obvious communication problems they tended to leave her to herself, which was just the situation in which she worked best. In contrast, Jeremy, who was of a similar intellectual level to Clare but with *superficially* good language skills, had a much more miserable time. Despite working in a south London warehouse he had a very 'upper-class' way of speaking and a very sophisticated vocabulary. Although his manager was sympathetic and supportive, whenever he was away several junior staff took delight in teasing and bullying Jeremy. Eventually he hit out at one of his attackers, who of course denied having ever provoked him in any way, and because he was unable to explain the reason for his actions he was dismissed. Jo, a cleaner in a jewellery shop, was so appreciated for his honesty that his employers would sometimes leave him to lock up the night safe. A new nightwatchman was quick to recognise Jo's vulnerability, and offered to 'look after the keys' for him. Jo willingly handed these over, and when the robbery was discovered the next day he was actually charged with being an accomplice. Although this charge was dropped, his employers reluctantly decided that they could no longer employ him because of his inability to judge other people's motives.

Strategies for intervention in the workplace

Supported employment schemes

The effectiveness of the supported employment model for individuals with intellectual disabilities is now well established (Kilsby and Beyer 1996, Hughes-Brown and Rusch 1996, McCaughrin *et al*. 1993, Pozner and Hammond 1993, Stevens and Martin 1999). Over the past two decades, the numbers of such schemes has grown enormously, particularly in the United States, and evaluative studies suggest they result in higher work levels and increased social interaction with non-disabled workers (Kilsby and Beyer 1996). Crucially, too, these schemes appear to lead to higher levels of job retention and job satisfaction for individuals with learning disabilities (Moon *et al*. 1990), and generally result in a better quality of life and improved economic benefits than do more traditional sheltered workshops (McCaughrin *et al*. 1993). Supported employment offers assistance *in the regular workplace* for individuals who for a variety of reasons are unable to compete in the open job market. Once an appropriate placement has been found (often through collaboration between specialist employment agencies and voluntary support groups, such as MIND or MENCAP) a job coach is employed to work alongside the client in order to ensure that *all* the components of the job (including the social and personal aspects) can be carried out satisfactorily. The amount of support required depends on the skills and abilities of the individual employee. Although initial costs can be high, if the wages earned and the cost of unemployment benefits are taken into account the financial outlay can usually be recouped over a five-to-seven-year-period.

Supported employment schemes for people with special needs in the United Kingdom are far more limited, than in the United States, and funding has been described as 'sporadic . . . piecemeal and fragile', with many projects relying on temporary financial support from social services or charitable organisations, rather than the Department for Works and Pensions (Pozner and Hammond 1993, Wertheimer 1992). Most initiatives have been developed for individuals with mild to moderate learning difficulties, and the jobs involved have largely been routine, low-level, unskilled and low-paid. Moreover, even in the United States it is only relatively recently that such schemes have been extended to meet the specific needs of clients with autism. Smith and her colleagues (1995) describe a wide variety of successful job placements in their Maryland support scheme. These included manufacturing jobs, such as simple assembly type work (twenty-five clients); backroom retail work (forty-four clients); printing and mailing jobs (thirty-one); food services (twenty-three); warehouse work (twenty); recycling and delivery (twelve); and jobs with government organisations, mainly janitors, and office clerks (fifteen). The programme is remarkable, not only for the large number of clients finding work, but also because of its success in placing individuals with very limited language, low intellectual ability and challenging behaviour, as well as those who were more able. In another US-based programme, Keel *et al.* (1997), evaluating job outcomes in over a hundred TEACCH clients, found that almost all were in work of some kind. Sixty-nine were in individual placements, twenty worked in 'enclaves' (i.e. small groups with a job coach in one setting); seven of the least able clients worked in 'mobile crews' providing house cleaning services. Jobs were mostly in the food-service field, but around a quarter involved clerical or technical posts.

Although often highly successful, the focus of such schemes has tended to be on relatively low-level jobs, and few programmes have been specifically designed to meet the needs of more intellectually able adults with autism, despite their considerable potential. Nevertheless, specialist support for this particular group can prove highly effective. In collaboration with the NAS, Howlin and Peacock (1994) developed the first supported employment scheme, Prospects, specifically for individuals with autism in the United Kingdom. The focus was on skilled, well-paid employment for higher-functioning individuals, and jobs were sought with major international companies involved in banking, transport, telecommunications and food retail. Unlike many supported employment schemes, which rely on temporary funding, often from social services, financial support for job coaches and preparation for work was obtained from the Department for Work and Pensions, making use of monies available for *existing* Access to Work schemes. There was also an emphasis on close liaison with other disability employment services. The staff employed by Prospects are highly trained in working with people with autistic-spectrum disorders, and hence the focus of training has been less on job-related skills (the individuals concerned already possess a relatively high level of competence in these areas) and more on ways of improving the social and emotional deficits which so often prove to be the main barrier to successful employment for people with autism.

The first evaluation of this scheme was conducted with thirty high-functioning individuals with autistic-spectrum disorders living in London (Mawhood and Howlin 1999). All had a formal diagnosis of autism or Asperger syndrome, a Wechsler IQ score of 70 or above, and had been actively seeking work for some time. Twenty per cent had university degrees and two-thirds other academic or vocational qualifications. Their work outcomes were compared to those of a non-supported, matched comparison group. During the course of a two-year pilot programme over two-thirds of the supported group obtained paid employment, compared to only one-quarter of the control group. Moreover, in the supported group the majority of jobs was clerical or administrative in nature whilst only one individual in the comparison

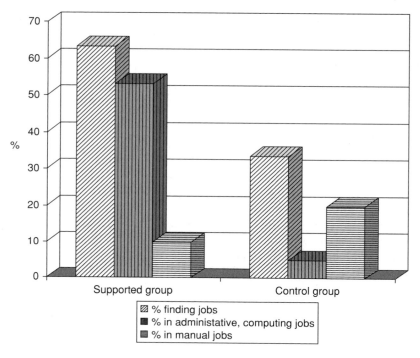

Figure 9.1 Percentage of supported and non-supported groups finding
employment during pilot project

group obtained a job at this level (see Figure 9.1). Earnings were
significantly higher in the supported group, and there was a high level
of satisfaction with the scheme both among employers and the people
with autism themselves.

In the course of the following five to six years over 200 jobs have
been found, and the scheme has expanded to cities in the north of
England and to Scotland. Sixty-three per cent of jobs are in administrative, computing or clerical positions. Other posts have included
nursery, film-processing and consultancy work; jobs in science and
government departments; and positions in housekeeping, sales, ware-
houses, and telephone and postal services (See Figures 9.2, 9.3 and
9.4). Moreover, at a time when temporary work contracts are becoming the norm, 54 per cent of these placements were permanent;
only two individuals have been dismissed from their jobs, and several
employers have offered work to more than one autistic client.

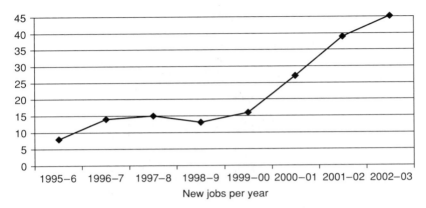

Figure 9.2 Numbers of Prospects clients finding work 1995–2003

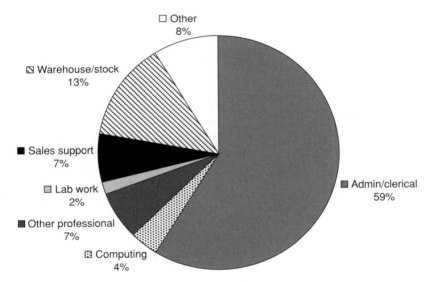

Figure 9.3 Types of jobs found for Prospects clients 1995–2003 (Total=177)

Eighty-five per cent of clients were 'very satisfied' or 'satisfied' with the jobs found, and 98 per cent considered Prospects had been 'very helpful' or 'helpful' in assisting them to find work. Managers and supervisors were also very positive about the support produced by Prospects, with almost all (99 per cent) rating the job consultant as

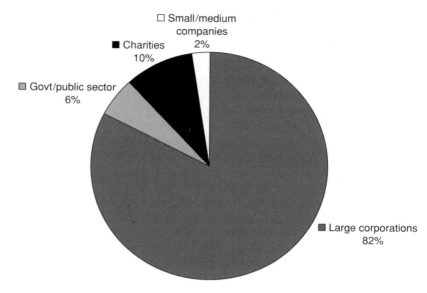

Figure 9.4 Types of companies employing Prospects clients 1995–2003

'very helpful' or 'helpful'. Over 80 per cent of line managers also felt they had gained personally from their involvement with the scheme, saying, for example: 'It has given me a greater insight into autism'; 'It has increased my ability as a manager in general'; 'I often apply many of the techniques to the rest of my team and we now use the job instruction manual (developed for the autistic employee) for all our new employees.' Although many managers had experienced some problems with the Prospects employee (mostly related to social and communication difficulties, see Figure 9.5), these improved with support from the job consultants, and almost all managers (97 per cent) stated that Prospects had supported them well in addressing these difficulties.

Based on the outcome of this scheme the National Autistic Society has recently published a number of guidelines on how to improve employment support services for people with autism, especially those who are more able or have Asperger syndrome (Powell 2002). The recommendations include:

> The development of information packs for companies on the advantages of employing people with autistic spectrum disorders, and ways of making the workplace more 'autism-friendly';

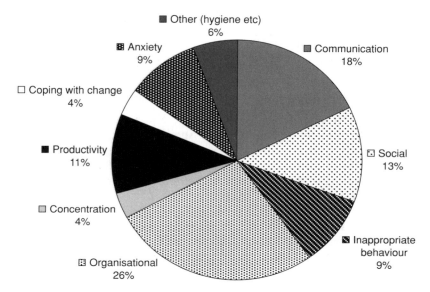

Figure 9.5 Distribution of problems reported for Prospects clients

Better information for people with Asperger syndrome themselves (how to find support; how to deal with application forms; what sorts of jobs to aim for etc);

Coordination of job support services, employers and employment agencies. The lack of a clear support pathway into work, and confusion over the role of disability employment advisors have proved to be particular drawbacks and hence much greater awareness among DEAs and the need for better training in the needs of people with autism are strongly recommended.

Specialist employment schemes should be developed on a regional basis to enable people with autistic spectrum disorders to find and keep work.

Schemes such as Prospects have demonstrated conclusively how far the employment situation for people with autism can be improved by means of specialist help. However, in the absence of such support it is all too easy for individuals to drift into a life of isolation and loneliness. Without work, opportunities to meet with peers or make friends will be severely restricted, and without money most individuals are obliged to remain living with their parents (or in some form of state-provided residential care). Leisure activities are limited, and failure to find suitable work – sometimes despite many years of trying – also results in frustration, loss of self-esteem and, for some, entry into a cycle of anxiety and depression or other psychiatric disturbance.

Other sources of support

In addition to the highly specialist service offered by Prospects there is a number of other agencies whose specific brief is to help people with disabilities find work. Whilst not having a particular focus on individuals with autism, their expertise in the field of supported employment more generally can be helpful for people with autism, although job opportunities are often restricted to less skilled work. The Employers' Forum on Disability, for example, is an organisation devoted to raising the profile of disability issues in the workplace and encouraging and assisting companies to take on clients with special needs. Some employment agencies have a particular interest in helping clients with disabilities and a web search can identify many job search and employment sites relevant for people with disabilities (e.g. www.disability.gov.uk, disability-employment.co.uk, disabilityalliance.org, support4learning.org.uk/jobsearch). Groups such as Remploy are well established in the field of sheltered employment and currently have around 11,500 employees in over eighty workshops. MENCAP's Pathway scheme, the Rathbone Organisation and the Shaw Trust also offer employment and training opportunities for people with disabilities. The Shaw Trust, for example, works in partnership with over two thousand companies, and currently supports over three hundred people in employment. The Trust offers subsidies to firms who provide employment to individuals who are unable to work at the same pace or at the same level as other employees. Sheila was a twenty-five-year-old woman with autism working as a hotel chambermaid. Because of her obsessional tendencies her work was extremely thorough and careful, but also very slow. An occupational assessment estimated that her output was approximately 60 per cent of that of other workers, and the Trust was able to provide her employers with a subsidy to cover this.

Recently, too, residential centres for people with autism have begun to offer training in job skills and support within the workplace. The Gloucestershire Group Homes Trust, for example, provides an employment training unit for adults with autism or Asperger syndrome in the Gloucestershire area, working closely with local employers and the employment service. The LEAP service (Life Education for People with Autism) in London also offers vocational training. Details of this and other support schemes can be obtained from the National Autistic Society (www.nas.org.uk).

Guidelines for successful employment

Providing information to employers

Although some individuals with autism, usually those who are most able, do manage to find employment without help, and indeed may prefer to keep silent about the nature of their disability, in the majority of cases employers will quickly become aware that the individual has 'difficulties' although they may not fully understand what these are. In view of this it is often wiser to try to explain the nature of the condition and to provide employers with information relevant to this prior to starting work. After all, if they are not sympathetic at this stage, they are hardly likely to be very tolerant if problems arise subsequently. The NAS Prospects scheme now provides detailed information packs for employers, explaining about autism, the impact this may have in the work place, and the benefits that employees with autism can bring (www.nas.org.uk). Nevertheless, as Roger Meyer (2000) notes in his employment guidebook (see below for further details), the situation concerning disclosure is different for everyone and there is no single solution to this dilemma. Disclosure, he notes, is a 'one-chance affair', and unless correctly handled it is all too easy to 'blow it' with a prospective employer. He strongly recommends professional help to guide individuals through this difficult process.

Highlighting the advantages of employing someone with autism

If placement is to be successful, the employer may well need to expend more time and effort, particularly in the early stages of the job, than might be the case with other employees. However, there are also distinct advantages in employing someone with autism. As many employers will testify, once the requirements of the job are well established people with autism often prove to be extremely efficient, competent and reliable workers. Many are happier doing routine, predictable jobs which other workers may dislike, and they are frequently able to maintain a high level of consistency in such work. Because they do not tend to seek out social interactions with others they are more likely to work steadily and consistently throughout the day without taking time off to chat or gossip. Ronnie found a job packing clothing in a small manufacturing company. When consignments arrive he is unable to relax until these are all packed and labelled, and he will readily work for up to twelve hours at a time (he boasts that his record is eighteen hours). His efforts are enhanced by the fact that he does not want the company to take on other employees as he much prefers to work alone. His work is also very accurate. After packing one assignment of eight thousand shirts, he complained to the delivery company that one was missing!

The tendency towards routine can also prove an advantage. Thus once a work pattern is established most people with autism will keep firmly to this; they will not take unnecessary breaks; they are rarely absent, and are usually very punctual. Honesty is another positive feature. Deceit, or the intent to deceive, requires considerable social sophistication, which is usually beyond the competence of someone with autism. There is little danger of dishonesty over expenses, or other infringements of office rules, because of a strict adherence to regulations, and employers often come to place a great deal of trust in employees with autism, whatever their level of functioning. The TEACCH organisation in North Carolina, which has a very successful job programme, reports that large companies turn to them time after time for autistic workers because of their low absenteeism, trustworthiness and reliability. The NAS employment service, Prospects, has also found that once companies have had a positive experience with one client with autism they are often willing to take on others. As one manager said 'I feel it is quite an accomplishment and I'd love to do it again.'

Making the job requirements explicit

It is essential to recognise that, almost inevitably, people with autism will tend to have problems understanding job requirements unless these are made very explicit; they are also likely to be poor at monitoring their own progress or behaviour. If goals are clearly set out many difficulties can be overcome; however, because autism is essentially a disorder of communication it is also important to be aware that reliance on *verbal* methods of instruction may be inadequate.

Information about the various stages of the job that must be completed, the time scale for these, or the checks that must be instituted, is often best presented in a visual form, either in writing or perhaps in pictures. The sequence in which stages are to be carried out can also be conveyed by these means. Clare's supervisor taught her to prepare a very acceptable cup of tea for other supermarket staff in the following way. First she prepared a display board on which a set of cartoon pictures illustrated the various stages involved in preparation; the board also contained photos of the other staff, indicating how many spoons of sugar each of them took. By taking Clare through these stages on a few occasions, and prompting her to follow the sequence on the board, it was soon possible to leave her alone, without supervision, to prepare drinks.

In the case of Lenny, a young man on work experience as a garage assistant, difficulties arose because of his untidiness with tools. Verbal reminders had little effect, but the problem was solved by having a large panel containing hooks and holders fixed to the wall, with the outlines of the most commonly used tools painted upon it. At the end of the day Lenny simply had to match the tools to their silhouettes. Thereafter there was no trouble with his putting them away, and the procedure also improved the tidiness of other staff members.

Leslie's idiosyncratic filing problems were solved by having him label all files according to a system first agreed between himself and his supervisor. This system was clearly displayed on the office wall as well as on the cabinets. For a short time daily checks on accuracy were made, but then random checks (at least weekly) proved sufficient to maintain standards.

Similarly, Sean's inaccuracy and slowness in entering data greatly improved when he was supplied with a simple checklist indicating the number of files he had to work through each day. He was required to tick these off as they were completed, and random checks on accuracy were also instituted. As his data entry became more accurate the daily checklists were replaced by weekly ones, though still with a clear goal for each day. However, an attempt to use monthly checklists was not successful as his speed rapidly decreased when the goals were made much longer-term.

The need for adequate supervisory and management structures

Because of the rigidity of many people with autism, once poor working practices are established these can be very difficult to shift. It is crucial to encourage good practice from the outset, and a particularly critical element in minimising problems is a clear line-management structure. This is also essential if output is to be adequately monitored. It is important, too, that the individual has a designated person in authority to turn to immediately if problems arise. Initially, supervisors may need to be prepared to monitor progress much more closely than is usual if work is to be carried out to the required standard.

They may also need to offer greater reassurance. This can obviously present difficulties at times, especially if demand is heavy or questions seem unnecessary or repetitive. However, once the basic job requirements are well established, direct supervision can be steadily reduced. Visual or written prompts or instructions may then be implemented, further reducing the need for direct contact.

The need for clear feedback

Supervisors also need to be prepared to give direct and honest feedback about an individual's performance. People with autism are not able to pick up subtle cues from others, and if not explicitly told that their work or behaviour is unsatisfactory they will tend to presume that their performance is faultless. As an example, Ben had thought that he was doing very well in his clerical job and reported that he was 'getting on fine' with the office staff. His manager had not had the heart to tell him that there were increasing complaints about his behaviour. When Ben went on holiday leave, the women in the office demanded his dismissal on the grounds of 'sexual harassment'. The offences cited included standing too close to them in the lift, spending long periods of time leaning over their desks, constantly talking of his desire for a sexual relationship, and carelessness in the way he dressed (including going around with his shirt open or his trouser zip partially undone). With Ben's permission the manager contacted his psychologist, who was asked to talk to the staff about the social problems associated with autism and ways in which they could help to deal with these. In collaboration with Ben a 'contract' was drawn up which gave clear guidelines both to him and the other employees about acceptable and non-acceptable behaviours. Ben was asked not to approach closer than within an arm's length of other staff members; if he did so, they were to tell him immediately that he was too close. The time spent talking to secretarial staff was limited to official break times only, and, to make this easier, his own desk was partially screened off from the rest of the office. Staff also let Ben know immediately if they considered the content of his conversation to be inappropriate in any way.

Making explicit the 'rules' of behaviour

As the above example illustrates, feedback alone is unlikely to be effective unless it is accompanied by clear rules regarding how behaviours should be changed. Gerald's poor hygiene problems were solved only when his manager decided to address the matter directly. For some time Gerald had been giving increasing offence to colleagues because of his failure to wash either himself or his clothes regularly. Although understandably reluctant to raise such an embarrassing issue, the manager finally decided to act. When questioned, Gerald insisted that he did *change* his clothes on a daily basis, just as his mother had instructed. However, he did not necessarily *wash* them and he regularly recycled soiled shirts and trousers. His manager explained that clothes need to be *washed* regularly as well as changed, and it was made clear that if at any time in the future his personal appearance was not satisfactory he would be sent home to change.

Like many other people with autism, Gerald was neither embarrassed nor resentful at being given personal advice of this nature. Temple Grandin (1991) recalls being given a can of deodorant by her boss and told to use it; his secretary was also instructed to take her to buy more suitable clothes. She notes 'This is part of the learning process. I was lucky enough to have people who helped me.' Because of their problems in interpreting subtle messages, or understanding the many unwritten rules by which most people function, clear and direct instructions (even if these refer to intimate topics and might seem somewhat demeaning to other people) are rarely resented. Wendy Lawson (2002) also recalls, without embarrassment, being told to buy a deodorant by a colleague. Indeed, it is *not* being able to understand what to do, *not* being informed if their actions are unacceptable, *not* being told if work is not up to standard, that give rise to problems. Often the person with autism can remain in total ignorance that they have done anything wrong until they are suddenly given a formal warning or even summarily dismissed. The resulting confusion, dismay and loss of self-esteem can be devastating.

Coping with obsessions or resistance to change

Major problems can sometimes occur if obsessional behaviours begin to intrude on normal working activities. Margaret's refusal to type more than one page at a time without being checked was dealt with by the supervisor indicating *on the work to be copied* when a check would be made. Sometimes this was after less than a page; sometimes more. By placing the emphasis on the amount of work to be copied, and by gradually extending the size of task to be completed, it was eventually possible to modify this obsession very successfully.

Dan, a trained accountant, hated change of any sort and stuck doggedly to his daily routines. This could sometimes be an advantage, but it proved a problem when a new computer system had to be installed. With the help of a social worker who had known him for many years a detailed programme was carefully introduced to explain to him what would be happening, exactly when the changes would take place, how retraining would be undertaken, and what advantage all this would offer. Because his social worker, in whom he had great trust, worked closely with his managers, reinforcing their decisions at every stage, Dan was able to accept what for him was a momentous change in his working practices.

Over time, and with such support, staff working with Dan have become very skilled in helping him to cope with change and gradually to accept more and more responsibility within the firm. Because of an increase in workload at certain times of the year, the company needs to employ a number of temporary workers. Initially, Dan had considerable difficulties in working with new staff, but as some 'temps' were employed on a regular basis, his managers tried to ensure that these were the individuals with whom he was asked to work. Despite his complaints he grew used to the annual changes in staffing, and is now able to supervise temporary workers very satisfactorily. Gradual changes to his physical environment have also been implemented. To begin with, he was unable to concentrate in a large, open-plan office and needed to work in a room alone. This was then replaced by a screened-off area in the corner of the main office. Gradually his desk was moved to a more central section, and he is now able to work successfully in a busy public area.

Personal support in the workplace

Because of the vulnerability of people with autism, employers may need to be prepared to offer more personal support than is normally expected. They may also need to ensure the cooperation of other employees and possibly, too, offer protection against exploitation, teasing or bullying.

In Ben's case, there is no doubt that the direct involvement of his psychologist was crucial. In particular, explanations of why Ben acted in the way he did, and advice on how staff might help him, had a dramatic effect on their attitudes. Sympathy, however, is unlikely to last in the absence of practical advice, and hence the additional 'contract', indicating what behaviours were or were not acceptable, was also needed. Ben is still at work with the same company after eight years.

Clare's position in the supermarket was greatly helped by her supervisor, whose own daughter had a hearing impairment and who was thus generally sympathetic towards the problems of people with communication difficulties. She kept a close watch on Clare's ability to cope with the demands of the job so that any problems could be detected at an early stage. She was also very vigilant against teasing or bullying by other members of staff. At one stage, when Clare became depressed, she was quick to recognise the early symptoms of this and to ensure that she received appropriate help. Although Clare was then off work for some time, her general reliability and accuracy were such an asset that the job was willingly kept open for her.

Making use of additional professional involvement

Although, as the examples above illustrate, many problems can be solved by relatively simple means, employing someone with autism does place unusual demands on employers, supervisors and often other employees. The value of supported employment schemes has already been noted, but support from other professionals, some of whom may well have known the individual with autism for many years, can also reduce the risk of job failure. Often it is not that the advice needed is particularly sophisticated or complex but that straightforward guidance from someone who understands the problems associated with autism can be surprisingly effective. Psychologists, social workers or psychiatrists who know the individual well may be able to supply quick and simple advice on overcoming or avoiding problems, or they may be able to offer additional practical help. Laurie's sleeping patterns were improved after his support worker offered to ring him at ten o'clock every evening and warn him to get ready for bed. This helped him to get to sleep earlier, to get to work on time – and to stay awake while he was there!

Professionals who are knowledgeable about autism can also give valuable advice, even before the job starts, about how best to structure the working environment; how to break down the different stages of the job; how to make instructions clear and explicit; how to deal with unacceptable social behaviours, the tendency to adhere to fixed rituals or routines, or problems in accepting change.

Professional advice may be helpful, too, when any major changes to working practice are envisaged. As noted earlier, a particular problem for some autistic people is that once they acquire job skills promotion to a higher level may be recommended. Unfortunately, promotion often results in increases in responsibility with which they are unable to cope. Julian was quite unable to deal with the administrative and social demands of becoming a senior lecturer and eventually required psychiatric help because of his anxiety. With his psychiatrist's support the university agreed to change his position to an 'honorary' one, which meant that he was able to maintain his status whilst avoiding the organisational responsibilities of the post. Professional guidance may also be needed to reassure worried employers. Graham had attacked the tea lady when she brought his milk in the wrong container and despite his previously gentle character his employers were worried that this incident might herald the onset of other aggressive outbursts. The psychologist involved in supporting him was able to point out that the most probable cause of the incident was the disruption of his normal routine and that such behaviour was most unlikely to recur as long as he was warned in advance about possible changes. This prediction proved true, and Graham is still at work. Although occasional difficulties occur from time to time, the company are able to contact the psychologist involved if ever they feel in need of advice.

Job retention

The involvement of outside support agencies can prove helpful in ensuring the *continuation* of good working practices. Otherwise, with time, or with changes in staffing, successful strategies originally used to minimise difficulties may be forgotten. When he was first employed in a computing company, Neil's difficulties in coping with change were fully recognised and every attempt was made to explain events to him well in advance. So successful was this strategy that after he had been in the firm for over two years his autism was almost forgotten. In consequence, no one thought to discuss with him the fact that his immediate manager was to be replaced. Unfortunately, when the new manager appeared Neil responded by threatening to bite him! Attempts to repair the relationship were not successful, and eventually Neil was once more made redundant.

Support schemes may also be helpful for people who have been independently employed initially but then need additional help when problems occur. Bradley, for example, had been employed in one of the major government departments since leaving university with a Ph.D. in mathematics. His employers were greatly impressed by his scientific skills but as time went on his problems in relating to colleagues became more and more pronounced, and as he became increasingly anxious his unusual behaviours (flapping, whistling and grimacing) were ever more intrusive. His consultant psychologist was contacted, who then explored factors affecting his social interactions and anxiety levels. Having to sit too close to others was one problem that was easily rectified. However, it also became clear that he was much more agitated on Mondays and Fridays, when his long bus journey to work tended to be particularly difficult. After detailed discussions with the psychologist, it was agreed that Bradley would work at home on these two days, and computing equipment and email links were set up for him. Bradley was then able to work on problems undisturbed for up to four days a week (he had no objections to working through weekends if he had an 'interesting' mathematical problem to solve), using his remaining time in the office to deal with routine issues or report back his findings to staff.

The right to personal dignity and confidentiality

Although liaison between professional counsellors and employers, or between management and other employees, may be crucial in minimising or avoiding problems, discussions must always be conducted in a way that is acceptable to the person with autism. If work charts or behaviour 'contracts' are drawn up, these should not be displayed in a way that is demeaning or derogatory. This should apply whether individuals are in open employment or in a more sheltered setting. If information about autism is made available to other employees, this must be done with respect to personal dignity and with the individual's consent. As noted earlier, people with autism often tend to react positively to advice about their actions or appearance rather than showing embarrassment or resentment, but this does not mean that such guidance should be given without careful thought and planning. It goes without saying that the individual with autism should also be consulted about how they wish to approach the issue of telling colleagues, and who should be told. Victor, who had just taken up a scientific post in a large chemical company, had no doubts as to the best way forward. He simply emailed everyone in the company informing them of his diagnosis, and providing details of his CV, his proposed role in the company, and how to contact him or his support worker if they needed more information; his personal website also provided brief details about Asperger syndrome and links to relevant NAS websites.

The provision of sensitive support in mainstream settings has rarely been questioned by employers, but occasional problems have occurred in placements for clients with learning disabilities. Jerome, a young man with autism, was offered employment in a small group home for people with cognitive impairments. His support worker explained that he functioned well as long as instructions were clearly written down, and he was supplied with 'reminder' cards to stick on his desk. The manager was horrified, and told the support worker that this was totally against the spirit of 'normalisation' that the organisation espoused. Signs were considered 'stigmatising' and were simply not allowed; not even the offices and toilets were labelled. Apart from the fact that this was certainly not 'normal' office practice, such rigidity denied Jerome the type of support that he needed to cope with the job. Although support should not necessarily be intrusive or highlight an individual's difficulties, a balance needs to be struck between offering excessive help and doing nothing. Taking the latter approach is unlikely to prevent others becoming aware of the disability; and in the absence of support, personal and work-related problems will almost inevitably result in social isolation or rejection and, all too often, loss of employment. Assistance may have to go beyond the boundaries of normal working practices if the individual is to be given the opportunity to demonstrate their true capacity.

Self-help

Despite the steady increase in supported employment schemes of various kinds, there are still far too few to meet the needs of all individuals with autism. Moreover, not everyone wishes for help of this kind. For those who prefer to 'go it alone' Roger Meyer (2000) has published an *Employment Workbook for Adults with Asperger Syndrome*. His experiences, as someone with Asperger syndrome, of the difficulties that can arise in the workplace, led to the production of these very helpful guidelines. He provides examples of practical exercises through which individuals can fully assess their own particular strengths, talents, individual learning styles and needs, and suggests how this self-evaluation can help them to identify the types of job most suitable for their personal profile. There is also more general discussion of how the characteristics associated with Asperger syndrome may assist or hinder work performance, and advice concerning successful (and unsuccessful) survival strategies. In addition, there is a sensitive discussion of whether or not it is wise to disclose one's diagnosis to current or potential employers. The author emphasises the point that there is no 'one size fits all' solution and that the work situation will be different for everyone, but his overall approach to assessing problems, and developing ways of overcoming these, should be of help to many who are struggling, unsupported, to meet the demands they face on a day-to-day basis in the workplace. Liane Holliday Willey, in her book *Pretending to be Normal* (1999), also provides practical suggestions, based on personal experience, on how to optimise the chances of finding and keeping work. Like Meyer she stresses the importance of self-awareness and self-evaluation in making appropriate correct career choices. She also offers hints for coping with interviews, from the value of role play and practice to more basic points such as remembering to brush teeth and hair. The issue of whether or not to inform employers about the diagnosis of autism is again raised. However, whether or not the decision to disclose is taken, she suggests asking employers whether there are any 'accommodations' to the work setting that might assist in ensuring optimum work levels. These include being able to use earplugs, headphones or dark glasses to eliminate distracting stimuli; the provision of quiet work spaces and flexible breaks, should the need for brief escapes arise; advance information about possible changes to the work routine, and continued job-skill training. These are, she notes, 'special concessions that will help you do your absolute best for the company' not 'special compensations that will release you from work responsibilities'. Indeed, she also makes explicit the responsibilities that employees with autistic-spectrum disorders have toward the company for which they work.

Many other individuals develop their own strategies for coping with difficulties. Brendan's tendency to 'daydream' (mostly about his extensive collection of Star Trek tapes) led to a very low work output, and considerable irritation on the part of his line manager. After a series of warnings, Brendan was encouraged to record the number of times he was 'off-task' during the day. This he did, but to little effect, and the frequency counts just lay in disorder in his drawer. However, after being threatened with disciplinary action he realised he would have to do something to improve the situation. Much of his work involved the production of graphs to illustrate company output etc., and he decided the same type of visual cue would be of assistance to him. Thus, instead of simply counting time off-task he plotted the data on his computer and pasted the resulting charts on his desk. Within a few weeks the frequency of periods when he was not working had significantly decreased, as Figure 9.6 illustrates.

Getting a job

So far, discussion has focused principally on the problems that are likely to arise once an individual is actually in work. However, for many people with autism, even for those who have succeeded at college or university, the preliminary stages of applying for work – filling in forms, making telephone enquiries, preparing for or attending an interview – may prove to be hurdles that they are unable to overcome.

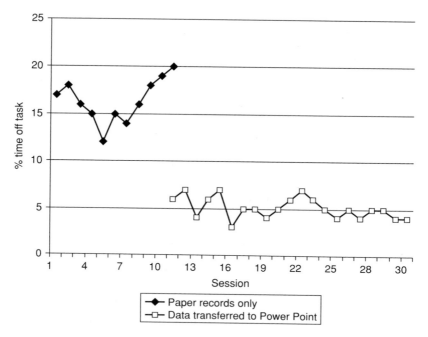

Figure 9.6 Reducing 'off-task' behaviour using computerised feedback

Justin, for example, having obtained a second-class degree in chemistry from university, sent out application forms for numerous jobs. Not one led to the offer of an interview, and finally his mother realised that in the 'health problems' section of every application form he had written lengthy descriptions of all the illnesses he had had since childhood, including every episode of flu he could remember and occasional infestations of head lice or threadworms. When she suggested that this information was not needed, he became very upset, pointing out that it could be an offence to withhold relevant information. The problem was that he had no way of discerning what was or was not relevant.

Clive, who had a higher degree in electronics, was helped to prepare an impressive CV which attracted the attention of a number of prestigious companies. None of his interviews, however, led to the offer of a job. Although he insisted that he had got on well in the interviews, his parents suspected that he had probably 'got hooked' on irrelevant topics or details of his family life. These traits, together with his poor eyecontact and poorly modulated tone of voice were, they felt, unlikely to create the right impression. However, other than trying to give him some advice on how to act they were unable to do anything to improve the situation.

Developing links between employers and schools or colleges

Just as schools may play a vital role in fostering the successful transition to college, training for pupils with autistic-spectrum disorders in job-related tasks and the social skills required to accompany these should be a central part of the curriculum. Links with employers, via job experience schemes, are also important, enabling students to familiarise themselves with different types of work environment. Indeed, much of the success of the TEACCH supported employment schemes is attributed to the emphasis on vocational training that is at the core of their educational curriculum.

Practice sessions within the school, structured by teachers who are familiar with the tasks involved, can be of great benefit, whilst the skills needed for interviews can be developed through roleplay and practice. Video recordings are valuable for giving direct feedback and allowing individuals to correct mistakes or develop more appropriate skills, and people with autism often show very little, if any, reticence or embarrassment at being recorded in this way.

College staff will also play an important role in ensuring that, once students have acquired adequate work-related skills, they are offered the opportunity to implement these in practice in the work place. However, whilst some colleges are extremely supportive of students with autism, others show far less understanding of their complex social, behavioural and educational needs. The organisation INTERACT (Graham 1999), described in the previous chapter, provides training in vocational skills such as accuracy, timekeeping and meeting deadlines, and can offer sheltered work opportunities to help students develop appropriate work skills. A similar scheme is coordinated by the employment training unit run by Gloucestershire Group Homes (Matthews 1996). Other, more general, college courses for people with special needs may also help those with autism to develop the skills needed for entering the workplace. Information about special job preparation courses can be obtained from MENCAP (mencap.org.uk); additional information can be obtained from the Family Fund's booklet *'After Age 16 – What Next?'* or the *'Directory of Opportunities for School Leavers with Disabilities*, published by the Queen Elizabeth Foundation for Disabled People. Wehman and his colleagues (1988) have also described in detail the facilities and programmes that have been used to help individuals with severe disabilities make the transition from school to employment in the United States. They stress the importance of long-term planning, the development of employment options and potential placements, the roles that teachers and parents can play in vocational training, and local state or federal initiatives that have been crucial in improving employment prospects for individuals in North America.

Applying for work

Anyone with a disability is at a disadvantage when it comes to seeking work and, whatever their level of functioning, a well-presented CV can be crucial. Appropriate help in preparing a CV or application forms can be obtained from staff at colleges, job centres or job seekers' clubs. It also helps to find out as much about the particular job in question as possible, perhaps by speaking with someone in the company, talking to someone who has done a similar job or finding out where the company's main interests or markets lie. Internet websites can be an invaluable source of information here.

It is essential, too, to be honest in completing application forms or CVs. Whilst the issue of whether or not to disclose detailed diagnostic information is a complex one (see above), some people with autism understandably feel that they should keep secret the fact that they have attended special school, been out of work for prolonged periods, been made redundant or even dismissed from previous jobs. Yet attempts to cover up such information are rarely successful. Donald, who had experienced several extended periods of unemployment and had been dismissed from two previous jobs, tried to disguise these facts on his CV by changing the dates of his times in work. This led to obvious inconsistencies in chronology, and his ineffectual attempts to explain these simply worsened his position.

If the autistic problems are relatively mild and not easily detectable by outsiders, then of course it is up to the individual to decide how open to be about the nature of his or her difficulties. However, as it is quite likely that problems will be detected at some stage, experience suggests that it may be wiser to indicate *in advance* that some concessions may be required in the workplace in order to ensure that individuals fulfil job requirements to the best of their ability. Some adults with autism tend to explain their problems in terms of having a communication or sensory disorder which may necessitate some additional support if they are to function optimally. Many prefer *not* to use the term 'autism' since they feel – perhaps correctly – that the public stereotype of autism is likely to prove a barrier to employment. Others – particularly if there has been a recent spate of positive publicity about Asperger syndrome – feel that it is more appropriate to use this label. Whatever the choice, it is essential to be able to give a brief but clear and honest explanation of what the difficulties or differences are and, if relevant, how they might have an impact on the job in question.

Preparation for interviews

Attending job interviews is a stressful experience for anyone. Interviews demand the ability to cope with unfamiliar settings and people; they require high levels of social and communication skills, the ability to think rapidly and under pressure, and to weigh up the underlying meaning behind questions, as well as to formulate appropriate answers. For a person with autism, it would be difficult to envisage a more stressful experience! The possible advantages of admitting to an existing disability have already been discussed, and in principle (although not unfortunately always in practice) anti-discrimination legislation should ensure that if potential difficulties are noted on the application form this should not reduce the individual's chances of being called for interview. Moreover, for the sake of equal opportunities the interview procedure should also be modified if there is a possibility that it might disadvantage a potential employee. If the interview panel are aware of the fact that an applicant has a disability, this may lead to their being more sympathetic: allowing more time to answer questions, being clearer in their own questioning and avoiding asking any 'trick' questions. Applicants with disabilities should also have the right to ask to be accompanied by someone who can provide additional support during the interview or help clarify questions. However, even if the interview is conducted under special circumstances, applicants still need to invest time and effort in preparation. Studies show that with the appropriate training people with autism can be helped to improve the skills needed in applying for a job or enquiring about job vacancies. Howlin and Yates, (1999), for example, found that adults attending a social skills group were able significantly to improve their 'telephone techniques' (to enquire about job vacancies) after receiving advice and practice in the correct ways to answer questions or request relevant information. Role play within the group was also effective in enhancing 'interview-type' skills. The NAS Prospects scheme also provides clients with advice about how to cope with interviews and opportunities to practice interview techniques. They may contact employers in advance to discuss any modifications to the interview that are likely to be needed, and if necessary a member of Prospects staff will attend interviews with clients needing additional support. And, as noted above, if the traditional interview format is not considered appropriate (sitting in a room with a group of strangers firing ambiguous questions is not a situation in which most people with autistic-spectrum disorders function at their best!) modifications may be requested. For example, some prospective employees have been informed in advance of the questions they are likely to be given; others have been allowed to prepare a formal presentation describing how they envisage their role within the company. Such adaptations to regular procedures have helped to ensure that interviewees with autism are not unduly disadvantaged or discriminated against at this crucial stage, and many have been successful in obtaining jobs in this way.

Even if specialist help of this kind is not available, role play with family members or friends can help to familiarise the applicant with basic interview procedures. Video recordings can be invaluable in demonstrating how the interviewee looks and sounds, the appropriateness of eye contact or 'body language', and their responses to questions. The potential candidate also needs to pay attention to the requirements of the particular job and to the more general aims of the company involved, so that replies can be appropriately structured around this knowledge. Most firms will arrange for candidates to speak informally with staff in the company prior to the interview, and this opportunity should be made use of whenever possible.

If relevant, the candidate must also be prepared to give a concise reply to questions about the nature of the disability, why special schooling was needed, or why there is a history of previous unemployment or redundancy. It is important, too, to be able to explain how the characteristics of autism may affect work (both positively and negatively) and what is needed to minimise problems. Interviewers are likely to be much more sympathetic to a candidate who recognises his or her difficulties and has taken active steps to deal with these.

If the candidate wants to ask questions at the end of the interview, a notepad with a brief, readily visible and easy-to-read aide-memoire can be useful. Again, questions should be checked with a sympathetic listener beforehand to make sure they are appropriate and neither irrelevant nor rambling. Finally, attention should be given to general appearance and to the need to turn up on time! A dummy run, to check that the journey can be made in plenty of time, is well worth the effort. Practice sessions should also cover what to wear and general grooming. Everton had spent many hours practising question-and-answer techniques with his support worker, and seemed to be fully prepared to deal with the interview. Unfortunately, he had not been given explicit instructions on his personal appearance. On the day of the interview he arrived at the city bank where he was hoping to work in old jeans and T-shirt and without having shaved. His support worker, who had arranged to sit in on the interview, had a spare razor, but the clothes were more difficult to deal with. In the end, the support worker exchanged his own suit for Everton's casual clothes – and remained acutely embarrassed throughout the interview because of his own inappropriate dress. Fortunately, however, his efforts were worthwhile and Everton got the job.

Register with disabled employment services?

In the United Kingdom, the Department for Work and Pensions offers specialist services for individuals with disabilities, and disability employment advisers (DEAs) can provide useful advice and contacts in the search for work. DEAs may be contacted through the local job centre and have direct links with companies willing to accept workers with special needs. DEAs can advise about relevant training schemes, such as the Government's New Deal Scheme for People with Disabilities and can also arrange for detailed work-skill assessments to be carried out by the nearest PACT (placement, advisory and counselling team). Unfortunately, however, few DEAs will have had training in autism, or in how to meet the needs of people with this condition. Moreover, the range of jobs to which they have access can be quite restricted and placing individuals with higher-level qualifications in jobs of an appropriate level often raises considerable problems. In addition, seeking support from DEAs almost inevitably means that the individual will have to disclose the fact that they have a diagnosis of autism. However, there are a number of reasons why the option of registering with specialist employment services should at least be considered. First, many supported employment schemes, such as Prospects, require applicants to be registered with a DEA in order to gain access to government funding for supporting clients in work. Second, registering may make it easier to apply for benefits such as the disability living allowance, and is also more likely to help individuals 'pass' the government's 'assessment of incapacity' test. If the criteria for this assessment are not met existing benefits may be lost and there may be increased pressures on individuals actively to seek work, or to accept inappropriate employment. Entitlement to 'Access to Work' funding may also result in additional financial support to enable people with disabilities find and keep employment.

Thirdly, disability employment legislation places an obligation on firms with over twenty employees to employ at least 3 per cent of people with disabilities in their workforce. Although this is rarely complied with, if a company does wish to fulfil its quota it may be prepared to view candidates with disabilities in a more favourable light, or to employ them under different conditions. Thus, certain jobs may be 'earmarked' as particularly appropriate for people with disabilities or some form of positive discrimination may operate. George, for example, worked as a computer analyst in a large construction company. As the recession progressed, the company was forced to make more and more of its workers redundant. George had always resisted admitting to having autism, although the company was well aware of his difficulties. However, as external pressures on the firm increased, the directors decided that the only way in which they could offer him protection from redundancy was for him to be supported by the Disability Employment Service.

Like George, many able people with autism feel that to seek help from disability services can lead to unnecessary stigma and misunderstanding. They may be reluctant to 'advertise' their differences in this way and fear that this could be detrimental should they choose to seek independent work at a later stage. The choice is obviously up to the individual concerned and to the particular circumstances of the job, but as government restrictions on those claiming disability benefits are steadily tightened the disadvantages of *not* enlisting additional means of support are becoming more apparent. Moreover, it is not necessary to remain with specialist employment services permanently, and if alternative employment opportunities do arise there is no reason why someone with autism should not apply for these independently.

Voluntary work

Voluntary work is often an important first step on the employment ladder and can help overcome the 'Catch-22' problem, faced by many people with autism, of not being able to get a job without experience and not being able to get the experience without a job. A substantial number of people with autism have eventually managed to find permanent employment in this way. Large charitable organisations such as Oxfam have the advantage, by virtue of their size, of being able to offer volunteers a wide range of possible activities. However, they may prove rather daunting for many people, and, for some, smaller local charities may be more appropriate. MENCAP may be able to offer advice about possible voluntary work opportunities, and other charities in the local area can also offer opportunities of this kind. Community care schemes often need voluntary workers to help with the very frail, elderly or disabled, and some individuals with autism have proved to be very patient and devoted in work of this kind. Jonathon had maintained a number of voluntary posts since leaving college, including one that involved pushing wheelchairs for people in a hospital for the terminally ill. Because of his patience and good humour and his ability to find his way through the labyrinthine mazes of the extensive Victorian site, the hospital management eventually offered him a part-time job. Stuart, who managed to find voluntary work with a major charity, was taken on to the permanent payroll there as an accounts clerk on a full-time basis after being with them for two years.

Welfare benefits

One of the inevitable hurdles that anyone who is unemployed or low paid will have to overcome is the 'benefits maze'. This *Alice in Wonderland*-like notion has a tendency to change suddenly and dramatically – and alterations can have a major impact on those already claiming benefits as well as on potential claimants. Benefits may be available for those looking for work, those needing special provision within the workplace, people on low earnings or those still involved in training. However, who can claim, what can be claimed, and whether or not it is actually beneficial to make a claim (in either the long or the short term) are all highly complex issues. Advice on benefits can be obtained from the Disability Alliance, the Disability Benefit Enquiry Line, or Ferret Information Systems. (www.ferret.co.uk), which offers extremely wide ranging advice in the field of welfare benefits and related law. Citizens' Advice Bureaux can also provide personal individual advice. Staff will need detailed information on personal and financial backgrounds in order to help, but their guidance is usually extremely competent and valuable. Nevertheless, they will almost certainly need additional information about the needs of people with autism.

Application forms for benefits tend to focus on easily recognisable handicaps, such as physical or sensory impairments, or on psychiatric illnesses, and it may prove difficult to complete the necessary forms in a way that accurately reflects the needs of someone with autism. If forms are not filled in correctly, this can easily lead to benefits being refused or stopped; hence accurate, professional advice is *crucial* before any formal documents are completed. The National Autistic Society provides an information leaflet on welfare benefits (Claiming

Table 9.2 Summary of work-based benefits that may be available to adults with autism in the United Kingdom (Figures published by the Department of Work and pensions for people under 60/65; 2003. See also Table 13.1)

Name of benefit	Who can claim	Approximate amount
Disability living Allowance	Individuals under 65 who need help with personal care or getting around; may be in work or unemployed. *Not means tested.*	**Care component**: Higher rate £56.25; Middle rate £37.65; Lower rate £14.90
	Comprises a **care component** and a **mobility component**; either or both may be claimed. Claimants can also qualify for Income support, Housing Benefit or Council Tax Benefit	**Mobility component**: Higher rate £39.30 Lower rate £14.90
Income support	Individuals whose income falls below a certain level, even if receiving other benefits. May also entitle claimants to other benefits listed below	Variable, depends on age, dependents, earnings etc Maximum £53.90; minimum £32.50
Disability premium	If receiving certain qualifying benefits	£23.00
Severe disability premium	If receiving DLA at high or middle rate	£42.85
Carer premium	If individual or partner receives Invalid Care Allowance	£24.80

Incapacity benefit	Previously in work but now incapable due to sickness/disability	Depends on age, NI payments and time out of work. Minimum £53.50; maximum £70.95
Disabled Persons Tax Credit (was Disability Working Allowance)	Individuals in work but disadvantaged because of illness/disability. May also entitle claimant to enhanced disability credits	Depends on savings etc. Minimum-maximum (exclusive of disability credits) £11.25-£62.10. Additional disability credits £11.25-£16.25
Therapeutic Earnings	Individuals who are involved in work that relates to their disability (to improve the condition or prevent deterioration etc)	Allowed to undertake permitted part-time (<16 hours) work for 26 weeks earning up to £60 per week or earning up to £20 per week indefinitely
Jobseeker's allowance	Capable of and actively seeking work. May entitle claimant to benefits below:	Depends on age and savings etc. Minimum £32.50; maximum £53.95
Back-to-work bonus	Paid if certain benefits stop because of work	Variable; one-off payment of £5-£1000
Jobfinder's grant	One off payment for people entering low paid work	Variable
Job grant	One off payment for individuals entering full time work	£100

Note: This table gives only a very brief account of possible benefits. Individual advice should be obtained (from the NAS, Citizens' Advice Bureau etc.) *before* any claims are made.

Disability Allowance, www.nas.org) that covers the criteria required for obtaining these, current methods of assessing disability or the capacity to work, advice on completing forms, dealing with the assessment process, and how to appeal against decisions. They also recommend the keeping of a DLA diary to ensure the correct level of benefits is obtained. In addition, the NAS may be able to offer some advice on a personal basis. (See also the *Disability Rights Handbook* published annually by the Disability Alliance and the guide to disability appeal tribunals by Dixon 1994). Support from the family doctor, another medical adviser or a social worker may be needed when making claims, and it is always worth letting them know in advance if their help is likely to be needed. (For a brief summary of possible benefits, see Table 9.2). There are also a number of charitable organisations that may be able to assist with a one-off grant. They vary greatly in terms of the amount of money they have, and in their eligibility criteria, and some may only be available to people living in a particular area. A useful reference book summarising these possible sources of help is *A Guide to Grants for Individuals in Need* (Smyth and Wallace 1997).

Despite the range of potential benefits available, many individuals with autistic-spectrum disorders, especially those who are more able, face considerable problems when they attempt to claim the support to which they are entitled. Powell (2002) notes three particular areas where people with autism receive poor service. First and foremost is the lack of understanding of autism amongst staff employed in disability benefit centres. This can result in job-centre interviews being highly stressful, with clients with autism frequently being unduly pressurised to accept unsuitable work, and/or refusal of the disability living allowance. Second, the work test for incapacity benefit is often applied inappropriately, so individuals who are unable to work – for example due to social anxiety – are deemed ineligible to receive financial help. Third, the system by which a claimant loses benefit if he or she leaves a job 'voluntarily' works against those who may in effect be forced out of work because of stress, teasing or bullying.

The following solutions are recommended:

1   Training in autism-related issues for staff in the Department of Works and Pensions (DWP), so that the process of 'signing on' for benefits is made more tolerable.
2   Training is also needed to ensure that staff can properly assess the eligibility of people with autism.
3   Social and health care services should also be involved in supporting people with autistic-spectrum disorders in their dealings with

DWP staff, and in advising clients on how to claim benefits. For this, a thorough understanding of the information requirements of the DWP is essential, and forms must be filled out correctly and in a way that adequately represents the individual's needs. It is particularly important to make sure clients do not unwittingly complete forms in such a way as to jeopardise their claim.

Summary

Thirty years ago there was almost no specialist provision for young children with autism, but the combined efforts of professionals and parents have resulted in the development of widespread, varied and effective educational programmes. Today the need is for a similar expansion in vocational training and occupational provision for adults with autism, especially those for whom modifications within the normal working environment could offer far greater opportunities for social integration and personal development.

10 Psychiatric disturbances in adulthood

A personal view

Wendy Lawson, now an extremely successful writer and teacher with Asperger syndrome, was twenty when she attempted suicide. Her apparent apathy towards life and her desperate confusion (she had just lost her job as a trainee nurse) resulted in her admission to psychiatric hospital. She writes, 'A deep dark awareness of depression and nothingness over took me. . . . Completely withdrawn and feeling I had fallen into a bottomless pit, I was placed on a program of medication'. She was diagnosed as having schizophrenia, a diagnosis that took her twenty-five years to overturn. It was only after one of her own children was found to have an autistic disorder that she finally received the diagnosis of Asperger syndrome (Lawson 1998).

Therese Jolliffe, a young woman with autism, also writes about the difficulties that she and others like her may face on a daily basis:

> Most people find that they can at least share their physical suffering with others, but no-one really understands what the emotional suffering of a person with autism is like, and there is no pain killer, injection or operation that can get rid of it or even . . . relieve it a little. Autism affects everything all the time [even] your dreams . . . People with autism get very angry because the frustration of not being able to understand the world properly is so terrible. Life is such a struggle; indecision over things that other people refer to as trivial results in an awful lot of distress. . . . If someone says 'We may go shopping tomorrow' or 'We will see what happens' they do not seem to realise that the uncertainty causes a lot of inner distress. . . . I constantly labour, in a cognitive sense, over what may or may not occur . . . It is the confusion that results from not being able to understand the world around

me which I think causes all the fear. This fear then brings a need to withdraw. Anything which helps reduce the confusion has the effect of reducing the fear and ultimately reduces the isolation and despair, thus making life a bit more bearable to live in.

(Jolliffe *et al.* 1992)

Being forced constantly to confront such problems, often with little help and support, it is hardly surprising that people with autism may also suffer additional psychiatric difficulties as adults. However, for a number of reasons, the nature of the association between autism and other disorders – particularly schizophrenia – is often misunderstood.

Autism and schizophrenia

The terms 'early childhood schizophrenia' and 'infantile psychosis' were originally used as alternative labels for autism (Creak 1963, Eisenberg 1972), and for many years there was ambiguity as to whether autism was, in fact, a psychotic disorder. Kanner himself initially considered that autism would probably turn out to be an early manifestation of schizophrenia, writing in 1949: 'I do not believe that there is any likelihood that early infantile autism will at any future time have to be separated from the schizophrenias'. Somewhat later, Szurek and Berlin (1956) claimed that it was 'clinically fruitless, even unnecessary, to draw any sharp dividing lines between . . . psychosis, autism, atypical development, or schizophrenia'. This belief in the association between autism and schizophrenia was further strengthened by a number of studies between 1970 and 1980. Bender and Faetra (1972) suggested that as many as 90 per cent of a group of children diagnosed as autistic were considered to have developed schizophrenia in adulthood. Dahl, in a later study (1976), quoted figures of 50 per cent. Watkins and colleagues (1988) found that 39 per cent of children with a diagnosis of schizophrenia (assessed on a number of separate scales as well as by clinical interview) had shown 'autistic symptoms' when younger. Sula Wolff and colleagues in Edinburgh also suggested a link between Asperger syndrome and schizoid disorders, and that this group may be more at risk of developing schizophrenia in adult life (Wolff and Chick 1980, Wolff and McGuire 1995).

However, in a seminal paper published in 1972, Michael Rutter was among the first to highlight a number of crucial variables relating to onset, course, prognosis, treatment and family history that differentiated between autism and schizophrenia. Wing (1986), too, has questioned the diagnostic criteria employed in these early studies, and certainly it is far from clear that all cases fulfilled criteria for autism as children. Ghaziuddin and colleagues raised particular concerns about co-morbidity in cases diagnosed as having 'Asperger syndrome' (Ghaziuddin *et al.* 1992a), whilst Werry (1992) discusses in some detail the problems inherent in making a diagnosis of early-onset schizophrenia or of schizotypal/schizoid disorders.

Subsequent diagnostic classification systems, such as ICD-10 or DSM-IV, now make clear the distinction between the two conditions but that is not to say, of course, that autism and schizophrenia never coexist. Wolff and McGuire (1995), found that two out of seventeen females and two out of thirty-two males with a possible diagnosis of Asperger syndrome (they were initially diagnosed as 'schizoid') later developed schizophrenia. Clarke and colleagues (1989) report on one case of schizophrenia in a group of five young men with autism who also developed psychiatric symptoms. Petty *et al.* (1984) describe three cases in whom early-onset schizophrenia seems to have been preceded by autism. In addition, there have been occasional single-case reports of the association between autism and later schizophrenia (Szatmari *et al.* 1986, Sverd *et al.* 1993).

However, larger-scale studies of individuals with autism have failed to find any evidence of increased rates of schizophrenia. (Chung *et al.* 1990, Ghaziuddin *et al.* 1998). None of the cases followed up by Kanner, over a period of forty years, was reported as showing positive psychiatric symptoms (delusions or hallucinations), and Volkmar and Cohen (1991) found only one individual with an unequivocal diagnosis of schizophrenia in a sample of 163 cases. Similarly, Gillberg and colleagues (Billstedt *et al.* 2003) report on one case with a diagnosis of schizophrenia in their follow-up of eighty-three people diagnosed with autistic disorder.

Schizophrenia also appears to be relatively uncommon amongst more able individuals or those with Asperger syndrome. Asperger (1944) noted that only one out of his 200 cases developed schizophrenia, and Wing (1981), in a study of eighteen individuals with Asperger syndrome, describes one with an unconfirmed diagnosis of schizophrenia. Rumsey *et al.* (1985), in their detailed psychiatric study, found no evidence of schizophrenia. None of the relatively able subjects in the studies of Mawhood and colleagues (2000) or Howlin *et al.* (2004) had developed a schizophrenic illness, and only one individual in a similar group studied by Szatmari *et al.* (1989b) had been treated for chronic schizophrenia. Tantam (1991) diagnosed three cases of schizophrenia amongst eighty-three individuals with Asperger syndrome, but these were all initially referred for psychiatric reasons.

Volkmar and Cohen (1991) have concluded that the frequency of schizophrenia in individuals with autism is around 0.6 per cent (roughly comparable to that in the general population) and that 'it does not appear that the two conditions are more commonly observed together than would be expected on a chance basis'. Similar findings were reached in the more recent overview by Lainhart (1999). Thus, although some studies have suggested that there may be 'an excess of schizophrenia in later life', at least among individuals with Asperger syndrome (Wolff and McGuire 1995). Wing (1986) criticises such extrapolations as being 'distressing without being constructive'.

Affective disorders

In contrast to the relatively small number of cases with a formal diagnosis of schizophrenia, there are very many more case reports of individuals with affective disorders. As early as 1970 Rutter noted the risk of depressive episodes occurring in adolescents or older individuals with autism, and subsequent reviews have reported a high frequency of affective disorders both amongst individuals with autism (Lainhart and Folstein 1994) and within their families (Bolton *et al.* 1998, Piven and Palmer 1999, Smalley *et al.* 1995). Abramson and colleagues (1992) suggest that around one-third of people with autism suffer from affective disorders and high rates of depression are found amongst high-functioning individuals, as well as those of lower ability. Thus, Tantam (1991), in his study of eighty-five adults with Asperger syndrome, noted that 2 per cent had a depressive psychosis and 5 per cent had a bipolar disorder. A further 13 per cent suffered from non-psychotic depression and/or anxiety. In the study by Rumsey *et al.* (1985) of fourteen relatively high-functioning individuals, generalised anxiety problems were found in half the sample. Similar figures were reported by Wing (1981), who found that around a quarter of her group of eighteen individuals with Asperger syndrome showed signs of an affective disorder. Bipolar affective disorders or mania without depression tend to be reported less frequently than depression alone, although Wozniak *et al.* (1997) found that up to 21 per cent of their autism/PDD sample had been diagnosed as having mania.

Because none of these studies is based on representative samples of people with autism, the resulting estimates of the prevalence of psychiatric disturbance must be treated with caution. A preliminary study by Abramson and colleagues (1992) suggests that the rates of affective disorder may be as high as 33 per cent, i.e. around twice the lifetime prevalence in the general population. Tantam's findings indicate overall rates for mania of 9 per cent, 15 per cent for depression and 7 per cent for clinically significant anxiety disorders, whilst the rates for schizophrenia are much less, at around 3.5 per cent. In the absence of larger-scale studies, such statistics must remain tentative, but it has become increasingly clear that problems related to depression and anxiety are a significant risk for people with autism as they grow older.

Other psychotic conditions

Although the occurrence of first rank schizophrenic symptoms is relatively infrequent, there are reports of individuals who show isolated psychotic symptoms, including delusional thoughts. Tantam (1991) suggests that the delusional content is often linked with autistic-type preoccupations. For example, one young man described by Lorna Wing (1981) could not be deterred from his conviction that some day Batman was going to come and take him away as his assistant. Ghaziuddin and his colleagues (1992b) describe another who was unduly concerned about the ozone layer and believed the air in Michigan was not pure enough to breathe. Bruno, a patient of the author's, was threatening to take revenge on the United States president and the United Kingdom prime minister because he believed the American and British air control authorities had conspired to prevent him from qualifying as an airline pilot. Another young man had, since childhood, had 'voices' to whom he could talk when he was particularly angry or upset. He believed firmly that the voices were real, but they did not provoke any distress or make him do things that he did not wish to do. Instead they appeared to offer him a means of working through difficult situations, and if he became particularly agitated his parents would send him off to 'talk to his voices'.

A number of other authors have described cases of delusional disorder, various unspecified psychoses (occasionally associated with epilepsy), paranoid ideation, catatonia and hallucinations (Clarke *et al.* 1989, Ghaziuddin *et al.* 1992b, Rumsey *et al.* 1985, Tantam 1991, Szatmari *et al.* 1989b, Wing and Shah 2000). Obsessional compulsive disorders have also been reported (cf. McDougle *et al.* 2002), although it can often prove very difficult to distinguish between these and the ritualistic and stereotyped behaviours that are characteristic of autism. Thus, in their study of more able individuals Szatmari *et al.* (1989b) caution: 'We found it very difficult . . . to distinguish between obsessive ideation and the bizarre preoccupations so commonly seen in autistic individuals'.

Tourette syndrome is another disorder that has been linked with autism (Baron-Cohen *et al.* 1999 a and b, Ringman and Jankovic 2000). However, again there can be difficulties in reliably distinguishing the involuntary movements associated with tic disorders with the stereotyped motor movements that characterise autism, and co-morbidity findings vary markedly. In the follow-up study of Howlin *et al.* (2004) for example, no one was diagnosed as having a tic disorder, whereas 23 per cent of the individuals followed up by Billstedt *et al.* (2003) were reported to suffer from motor tics, and one woman had a severe case of Tourette syndrome.

Epilepsy

As noted in the earliest descriptions of autism (Lotter 1966, Rutter 1970, Kanner 1971) epilepsy is another complicating psychiatric factor, occurring around 25 per cent to 30 per cent of cases (Lord and Bailey 2002). Onset is frequently in adolescence or early adulthood. The risk of developing fits appears to be higher amongst those who are profoundly retarded, but there does not seem to be a marked difference between groups of normal IQ and those with mild to moderate retardation. Eleven of the adults with an IQ of 50 or above assessed by Howlin *et al.* (2004) had had at least one fit. In four of these cases IQ was between 50 and 69; in seven IQ was within the normal range. Occasionally the onset of epilepsy is associated with marked behavioural changes and regression in adolescence (see below) although this is by no means always the case. The pattern of seizures in autism can take many different forms including infantile spasms, atonic seizures, myoclonic seizures, absences (petit mal), complex partial seizures (psychomotor epilepsy) and generalized tonic clonic seizures (grand mal) (Gillberg and Coleman 2000).

Suicide and other causes of death

Long-term follow-up studies of children and adolescents with psychiatric disorders have demonstrated above-average mortality rates compared to age- and sex-matched controls, especially with regard to death from 'unnatural causes' (suicide, accidents etc., Kuperman *et al.* 1988, Larsen *et al.* 1990; Östman, 1991). Research also suggests that death rates are higher in individuals with autistic spectrum disorders (Gillberg and Coleman 2000, Shavelle *et al.* 2001). Isager and colleagues (1999) followed up 207 cases with autism or autism like conditions over a twenty-four year period and found that seven individuals had died, giving a crude mortality rate of 3.4 per cent – approximately double the expected rate. Mortality was highest in those with severe to profound learning disabilities, or those of higher intelligence. In the former group (n=4), all of whom were in residential institutions, two deaths were attributed to choking while unsupervised, one to pneumonia and one to meningitis. In the more able group (n=3), who lived either independently or with parents, one death followed an epileptic attack and two were due to drug overdoses (one deliberate, the other *probably* accidental). Occasional deaths, due to a range of different causes, have been reported, too, in long-term follow-up studies (Lotter 1978). Causes of death include car accidents (Kanner 1973, Larsen and Mouridsen 1997), encephalopathy, self-injury, nephritic syndrome and asthma (Kobayashi *et al.* 1992); unrecognised volvulus (in a woman in a long-term psychiatric institution, Larsen and Mouridsen 1997), status epilepticus (Howlin *et al.* 2004), and cases of drowning, pneumonia and complications arising from long-term psychotropic medication (Ballaban-Gil *et al.* 1996).

The largest single study of mortality rates (Shavelle *et al.* 2001), based on over 13,000 individuals with autism registered on the California Department of Developmental Services' database, concluded that 'on average . . . mortality was more than double that of the general population'. In individuals with mild mental retardation or those of normal IQ, deaths from seizures, nervous system dysfunction, drowning and suffocation were three times more common than in non-disabled controls. Amongst individuals with more severe mental retardation there was a threefold increase in deaths from all causes (other than cancer).

Suicide as a cause of death has been noted in a number of studies. Amongst the 'schizoid' individuals (several of whom appeared to meet criteria for Asperger syndrome) studied by Wolff and McGuire (1995), ten out of seventeen women and seventeen out of thirty-two men had attempted suicide. Tantam (1991) described the case of one man who threw himself into the river Thames because the government refused to abolish British Summer Time and he believed that watches were damaged by the necessity of being altered twice a year. In Wing's group of eighteen individuals with Asperger syndrome three had attempted suicide although, fortunately, their attempts had not been successful. One young man, who had become very distressed by minor changes in his work routine, tried to drown himself but failed because he was a good swimmer. When he tried to strangle himself the attempt also failed because, as he said, 'I am not a very practical person.'

Nordin and Gillberg (1998) have suggested that higher death rates of individuals with autistic-spectrum disorders may be due to the association of autism with severe mental retardation and epilepsy. However, the examples cited above indicate that many other causes are also operating. Although the number of deaths related to the inadequate medical and physical care of individuals living in institutions is a particular cause for concern, it is evident that better understanding of the difficulties that lead some young people to attempt suicide could also avoid unnecessary loss of life.

Case studies of psychiatric disorder amongst individuals with autistic-spectrum disorders

Because data on mental health problems in autism are based on clinical case reports or small group studies there are no systematic studies of prevalence and estimates of the frequency of co-morbid psychiatric disorders vary from 4 per cent to 58 per cent, (Lainhart 1999). A systematic search for case reports of psychiatric disorder in individuals with autism (see Table 10.1) resulted in the identification of thirty-five different studies involving 200 patients aged fourteen years and older. Eighty-six cases were diagnosed with autism or PDD; 114 were described as having Asperger syndrome or were within the high-functioning range of the autistic spectrum. As is apparent from Figure 10.1 by far the most frequent psychiatric diagnoses given (in 56 per cent of cases) related to depression or anxiety disorders (including major and minor

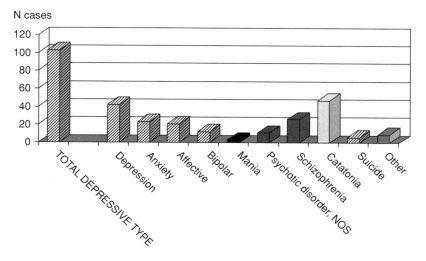

Figure 10.1 Psychiatric diagnoses in case studies of individuals with autism (N=200)

Table 10.1 Case studies of psychiatric disorders in individuals with autistic-spectrum disorders (includes only reports involving patients in mid-teens or older)

Study	Date	Age	Sex	PDD diagnosis	Psychiatric diagnosis
Asperger	1944	Adult	m	1 Asp/HFA	Schizophrenia
Darr and Warden	1951	33	f	1 Autistic	Low mood/delusions
Mittler et al.	1966	?	m	2 Autistic	2 × Schizophrenia
Reid	1976	32	f	1 Autistic	Depression
Wolff and colleagues	1980/1995	17+	m+f	13 Asp/schizoid	6 × Suicide;
					3 × Depressive disorders
					4 × Schizophrenia
Wing	1981	16+	m	10 Asp/HFA	4 × Affective
					1 × Psychosis
					1 × (?)Schizophrenia
					4 × Severe withdrawal
Petty et al.	1984	17	m	1 Autistic	Schizophrenia
Komoto et al.	1984	13+	f+m	2 Autistic	Depression
Gillberg	1985	14+	m	Asp/HFA	Bipolar
Sovner	1986	24	f	1 Autistic	Bipolar
Akuffo et al.	1986	40	f	1 Autistic	Bipolar
Rumsey et al.	1985	18+	m	7 Asp/HFA	7 × Anxiety disorder
Linter	1987	16	m	1 Autistic	Bipolar
Steingard and Biederman	1987	24	m	1 Autistic	Bipolar
Sovner	1988	26	f	1 Autistic	Depression
	1989	31		1 Autistic	Bipolar
				1 Autistic	Depression

Table 10.1 (cont'd)

Study	Date	Age	Sex	PDD diagnosis	Psychiatric diagnosis
Clarke et al.	1989	18–44	m	2 Asp/HFA	Delusional disorder
					Schizophrenia
					Depression
				1 Autistic	Psychosis nos
Szatmari et al.	1989b	17+	m+f	1 PDD	4 × Anxiety disorder; OCD
				6 Asp/HFA	Schizophrenia
Kerbeshian et al.	1990	33	f	1 Aut+SLD	Bipolar
Ghaziuddin et al.	1991/2b	16+	m+f	1 Aut + Down's	Depression
				3 Autistic	Depression
					OCD*
					Mood disorder
Realmuto and August	1991	16–21	m	2 Autistic	2 × Catatonia
				1 HFA	
Tantam	1991	18+	m	30 Asp/HFA	4 × Mania
					4 × Bipolar
					1 × OCD*
					2 × Depression
					3 × Schizophrenia
					1 × Psychosis (epileptic)
					4 × Hallucinations
					4 × Anxiety disorder
					7 × Depressive symptoms
Volkmar and Cohen	1991	15	m	1 Autistic	Schizophrenia
Sverd	1993		m	1 Autistic	? Schizophrenia
von Knorring and Hägglöf	1993	Adult	m	1 Autistic	Schizophrenia
Ghaziuddin et al.	1994			1 Autism/MR	Mood disorder
Kurita et al.	1997	?	m	1 Autism/MR	SADS
Kerbeshian and Burd	1996	15–38	m&f	4 Autistic	4 × Tourette* and bipolar

Table 10.1 (cont'd)

Study	Date	Age	Sex	PDD diagnosis	Psychiatric diagnosis
Larsen and Mouridsen	1997	16	m	1 Autistic	Schizophrenia
Ghaziuddin et al.	1998	13-adult	m+f	12 Asp/HFA	8 × Depression
					OCD*
					2 × Tourette*
					2 × psychiatric nos
Howlin et al.	2000	21+	m	2 HFA	Catatonia
					Depression?
Wing and Shah	2000	15–50	m+f	14 Asp/HFA	14 × Catatonia
				11 Autistic	11 × Catatonia
				5 PDD	5 × Catatonia
Konstantareas and Hewitt	2001		m	7 Autistic	7 × Schizophrenic symptoms
Perry et al.	2001	16–29	m	3 Atypical aut	3 × Depression
				4 Autistic	4 × Depression
Billstedt et al.	2003		m	19 Autistic	Schizophrenia
					Bipolar
					Depression
					4 × Affective
					12 × Catatonia
Howlin et al.	2004	21+	m	5 Autistic	2 × Anxiety disorder
					2 × Depression
					Catatonia
				5 HFA	Anxiety + depression
					2 × Anxiety disorder
					2 × Anxiety + depression

* Studies reporting only cases of Tourette syndrome or OCD and no other psychiatric disorder are not included here because of problems of diagnosis/definition in autistic populations.

depression, mood disorders or bipolar affective disorder; depression and anxiety; severe social withdrawal and attempted suicide). Mania alone occurred much less frequently, in under 2 per cent of the total. The relatively high number of cases of catatonia reported largely reflects the special interest in this disorder of Lorna Wing and her colleagues. Billstedt *et al.* (2003) also specifically probed for this disorder in their follow-up. This illustrates how case reports cannot be used to determine the prevalence of psychiatric illness since the researchers' particular area of expertise or interest will lead to systematic bias in the types of cases seen. However, these figures do provide a *rough* guide to the relative frequency of different disorders, and data from this and other reviews consistently suggest that whilst depressive types of disorder are relatively common, schizophrenic illness is much less prevalent.

Are higher-functioning individuals at greater risk of psychiatric disturbance?

It is often suggested that the risk of psychiatric disturbance, especially related to depression and anxiety, is particularly high amongst more able individuals with autism, or those with Asperger syndrome. There are several reasons for this view. First, because of these individuals' relatively good cognitive ability and *apparently* competent use of language, they frequently fail to receive the level of support they need. Second, despite their superficially good expressive skills, many have extensive linguistic and comprehension difficulties (especially involving abstract or complex concepts) and their understanding of the more subtle aspects of social interaction is often profoundly limited. Such deficits frequently prove an almost insurmountable barrier to social integration. Third, others' expectations of their social and academic potential are often unrealistically high and there may be constant pressure for them to 'fit in' to society's 'norms'. Finally, their own awareness of their difficulties and of the extent to which they are isolated from others can result in great sadness and low self-esteem. All these factors can place enormous pressures on the individuals concerned, and sometimes result in intolerable levels of anxiety and stress. Nevertheless, there is little evidence of differential rates of mental health problems amongst subgroups within the autistic spectrum. On the whole, the findings from the case studies summarised in Table 10.1 did not indicate a higher prevalence of such problems in higher-functioning as compared to less able individuals. And, although the former group were somewhat more likely to be diagnosed as having

% cases

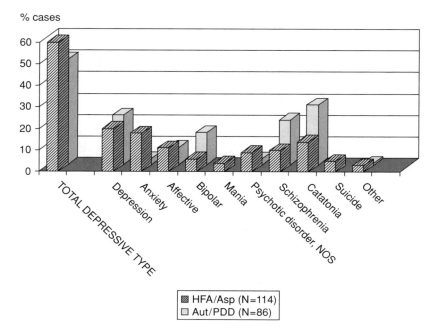

Figure 10.2 Psychiatric diagnoses reported in individuals with autism/PDD and those with Asperger syndrome or high-functioning autism

mania or anxiety disorders, this may be because it is much more difficult to diagnose these conditions in individuals who have little ability to describe their moods and feelings effectively (Sturmey 1998). In their case the problems may simply be labelled as unspecified 'mood disorders' (see Figure 10.2).

However, many of the clinical case studies reviewed did not distinguish clearly between high-functioning and low-functioning individuals, or between those with autism or Asperger syndrome. Indeed, diagnostic criteria were often not specified, and very few reports provided information on the IQ levels of the individuals concerned. Szatmari *et al.* (1989b), in one of the few well-controlled studies in this area, failed to find any marked differences in rates of psychiatric disturbance between adults with a diagnosis of Asperger syndrome and those with high-functioning autism, although the autism group tended to show more bizarre preoccupations.

In summary, crucial data on the prevalence and nature of mental health problems across the autistic spectrum are still lacking and there is a particular need for epidemiological studies in this area. Better research is needed, too, into ways of improving the identification and treatment of psychiatric disorders, for many clinicians working in adult psychiatric services often know relatively little about people with autism. Thus, the obsessionality, flattened affect, poor eye-contact, unusual body movements and echoed speech that are typical of autism may be misinterpreted as symptoms of psychosis (Volkmar and Cohen 1991). Impoverished language (Howlin 1996b), literal interpretation of questions (Wing 1986) and concrete thinking (Dykens *et al.* 1991) are all additional sources of confusion. It is also important that isolated 'symptoms', such as the unusual ideas or fixations noted above, are kept in perspective. For example, when a psychiatric nurse heard of the voices experienced by the young man described earlier, his parents were told that he was seriously mentally ill. Their attempts to persuade medical staff that this was not a crisis but typical behaviour were dismissed as collusion and denial, and it was with great difficulty that they prevented his being compulsorily detained in a psychiatric hospital.

Failure to understand the characteristic communication and social difficulties associated with autism can give rise to potentially serious misunderstandings and misdiagnosis, even in the case of relatively able individuals. For those with little or no speech the risks of an incorrect diagnosis (or failure to diagnose when problems do exist) are even higher.

Finding the appropriate treatment for people with autism who develop additional psychiatric disorders can also prove difficult. Clinical experience suggests that delays in diagnosis and treatment are particularly undesirable within this group as behaviour patterns that are established during the course of the illness (e.g. disturbed waking and sleeping patterns) can then be very difficult to alter, even when the patient's condition generally has improved (Howlin 1997b). Medication can be helpful (McDougle 1997) but rarely works in isolation. There is no evidence for the effectiveness of psychoanalytically based interventions (Campbell *et al.* 1996). Individual psychotherapy or counselling may be beneficial for some higher-functioning people but clinical experience suggests that these approaches *must* be combined with direct practical advice on how to deal with problems. If appropriately adapted, cognitive behavioural strategies seem to be of potential benefit (Hare *et al.* 1999, Reaven and Hepburn (2003), Stoddart 1999) although there is very little systematic research in this area, and even single case studies are rare.

Problems of diagnosis

Diagnosing schizophrenia in people with autism

One of the difficulties in reaching consensus about the prevalence of psychotic illness lies in the unusual patterns of communication and social behaviour found in autism. Because of this the application of conventional diagnostic systems can lead to considerable problems. Dykens and colleagues (1991), in a study of thought disorder in intellectually able people with autism, found that many gave abnormal responses on the Thought, Language and Communication Disorder scale (Andreasen 1979). 'Poverty of speech' was particularly marked, and Rorschach responses were also odd, with many idiosyncratic and unusual expressions occurring. For example, when describing what the ink blot looked like, one subject reported: 'just the human heart in black and white'. Dykens and colleagues note that thought disorder is generally considered to be a first-rank symptom of schizophrenia and diagnosis is often made on the basis of this. If the unusual language of individuals with autism makes them *appear as if they have thought disorder* then there is a serious risk of misdiagnosis.

Misinterpretation of this kind might well explain the higher rates of schizophrenia reported in some studies. Lorna Wing (1986) suggests that individuals with autism or Asperger syndrome may be incorrectly diagnosed as having a psychotic illness because of the way in which they respond to questions about their mental state. Thus, responses may be very slow and often tangential to the question asked. However, although unusual, concrete and pedantic, they do not show the characteristic vagueness of schizophrenic thought. Wing quotes the answer of one young man to a general-knowledge question about charities: 'They provide wheelchairs, stilts and round shoes for people with no feet.' She also notes that people may well answer 'Yes' to any question asked, simply to cut short the conversation, or they may pick up and repeat phrases used by other patients on the ward (particularly unusual ones) which can further complicate diagnosis.

The literal interpretation of questions may also lead to problems. If someone with autism is asked a standard diagnostic question, such as 'Do you ever hear voices when no one is in the room?', most will answer 'Yes' – for of course we *all* hear voices when people are not actually in the same room. If asked 'Do you ever think people are talking about you?' the majority of people with autism are likely to answer in the affirmative, since people have probably been talking about them for as long as they can remember! This failure to interpret the underlying meaning of the question is likely to lead to a positive response by someone with autism, even though there is no real evidence of delusions or hallucinations.

Other problems can arise from individuals' concrete use of language or their inability to describe abstract or emotional concepts. Danny, a nineteen-year-old who had just started college, developed symptoms of severe anxiety, including headaches, stomach aches, and a variety of other signs. When referred to a psychiatrist he insisted that his stomach pains were caused by a 'shark in his insides'. This explanation was interpreted as a delusional symptom; he was admitted to hospital and placed on long-term medication for schizophrenia. However, his mother explained that as a young boy he had had a favourite book where illnesses were described in this way: such as a crocodile in the head giving people headaches, a mouse chewing at the root of a tooth causing toothaches, or a monkey with a hammer producing pains in the ear. In his attempts to explain his physical symptoms he had reverted to these childish symbols, with little understanding of the impact that this might have on clinicians.

Diagnosing affective disorders

The inability of people with autism to communicate feelings of disturbance, anxiety or distress can also mean that it is often very difficult to diagnose depressive or anxiety states, particularly for clinicians who have little knowledge or understanding of developmental disorders. Even parents may explain changes in behaviour as being 'just a phase' that their son or daughter is going through, especially if they have experienced previous periods of withdrawal, slowness or 'odd' behaviours in childhood. In many cases it is only when the illness becomes very marked that the severity of the disorder is recognised. By this time the individual may have become very withdrawn, often refusing to leave the house, giving up work or other activities and failing to take care of themself adequately. Martin, a twenty-one-year-old living alone, was not recognised as being ill until a visit from his brother revealed that he had no food in the house, had not eaten for days, had not paid his rent for weeks and had been failing to collect his welfare benefits.

Jonah's mother knew that he had been having difficulties at work, but she was not aware of any major problems. He continued to visit on a regular basis and kept to all his other set routines. She was distraught to receive a rather formal note informing her that he intended to commit suicide the following week. He added: 'I am sending you this note because I did not want you to go around to the flat and be upset if I had left it in a mess' (there was no recognition that she would be devastated by finding him dead). Diana's mother had assumed that her growing reluctance to leave the house was just another of her obsessional phases, and it was only when she became increasingly distressed and withdrawn that psychiatric help was sought. Steven, a young man in his early twenties, was referred for behavioural treatment because of his increasing 'rigidity'; he could not bear to be touched, refused to let anyone close to him and became virtually mute. Although a behavioural programme was attempted, this had little effect and it was only when his symptoms were recognised as depressive and antidepressant medication was introduced that his behaviours slowly began to improve.

The diagnostic process may also be complicated by the fact that stress and depression can sometimes manifest themselves as aggressive or even paranoid behaviours. Douglas (who is also described in the next chapter) had become increasingly upset by the pressures of work. He had no one to talk to except his elderly mother and finally, when she failed to respond to his pleas for help, he attacked and injured her. It was only then that the need for psychiatric help became apparent, although he himself continued to deny any need for this. Martine was arrested by the Metropolitan Police for loitering in the early hours of the morning in an area where there had previously been terrorist attacks. She lashed out at anyone who approached her and steadfastly refused to tell the police where she lived or even to give her name. At the same time, she muttered constantly to herself about 'the other forces' that had carried her off before. She was rapidly admitted to the nearest hospital on a section, and only later was it realised that the forces referred to were other *police* forces, who had acted in similar ways towards her in the past. The fact that she had not given her name and address, she subsequently explained, was because her mother had always instilled in her the importance of never telling strangers where she lived!

The inability of many individuals to talk about feelings or emotions is also a major problem for clinicians. Diagnosis and treatment for mental disorders rely heavily on the ability to describe feelings, and if this is lacking it can be very difficult to offer appropriate help. Stuart's parents were convinced that he was becoming very withdrawn and depressed, but when they eventually managed to obtain a referral to a psychiatrist Stuart sat with a fixed grin on his face, repeating 'Everything is fine.' His parents were dismissed as over-anxious and intrusive, and it was only when he became overtly psychotic that their concerns were finally taken seriously.

Moreover, as noted above, even if a diagnostic assessment is attempted, the very concrete and unusual way in which people with autism talk about their feelings can easily lead to errors and misunderstandings. Elaine was a thirty-year-old woman whose daily life had been severely disrupted by the death of a favourite care worker. Initially she showed little response to this, but progressively became more and more distressed. When asked what the matter was, she could only repeat: 'The cabbage was burnt on Tuesday.' Cabbage, particularly if burnt, was a particular hate of hers, but as this was her only way of expressing her emotional distress it very much hindered attempts to assess her mental state.

Understandably, many psychiatrists working in the field of adult mental health know relatively little of the problems of people with autism. It is therefore crucial that when carrying out a diagnostic assessment the physician involved is fully informed about the individual's usual style of communication, both verbal and non-verbal, so that symptoms are neither overlooked nor misinterpreted. Many parents, especially of more able individuals, report that they are often discouraged or prevented from speaking to the professionals concerned in the treatment of their son or daughter. Whilst respecting the right of the person with autism to be treated like an adult, it is also vital that the information received is reliable. Szatmari and colleagues (1989b), for example, in their study of high-functioning adults with autism, found that the history given by parents indicated the presence of psychiatric disturbance much more frequently than information based on the individuals' own reports. Communication deficits are so central to autism that it will almost always be necessary to seek help in 'interpreting' what is said from someone who knows the individual well. The need for an 'interpreter' may be just as great as for someone who is deaf, yet access to such assistance is often denied to people with autism.

Diagnosing psychiatric disturbance in less able individuals

There have been relatively few studies of mental health problems in individuals with severe to profound intellectual impairments. Although some case studies of co-morbidity have involved individuals of very low ability (e.g. Kerbeshian and colleagues 1987, 1990, Perry *et al.* 2001), many have focused on those who are higher-functioning. Around 57 per cent of the cases included in the review cited above, for example were described as having Asperger syndrome; many other reports gave no details of IQ, and only a few involved people with a measured IQ of 30 or below. Volkmar and Dykens (2002) suggest that standard psychiatric diagnostic procedures work reasonably well for individuals whose cognitive abilities lie within the mild to moderate range but there is little systematic research in this area and certainly for those with limited verbal ability other strategies are required. The short version of the Psychiatric Assessment Schedule for Adults with Developmental Disability (the Mini PAS-ADD; Prosser *et al.* 1998) is a useful screening tool when psychiatric disorder is suspected. Information from this may also be backed up by use of a rating scale, such as the Developmental Behaviour Checklist (Einfeld and Tonge 1995), which provides a measure of behavioural disturbance. The full version of the PAS-ADD (Moss *et al.* 1998), which uses information from both respondents and informants, can then be used to gather more detailed information about psychiatric problems.

Lainhart (1999) also provides a number of useful guidelines that may be of value in assessing psychiatric difficulties in people with autism. First, she suggests that the starting point for making a diagnosis is the assumption that psychiatric disorders in developmentally disabled individuals are conceptually the same as in any other groups. Thus, signs of the full clinical syndrome should be present during at least one episode. For example, for a diagnosis of depression there should be evidence of a sustained *change* in mood, attitudes towards self and/or others, mental and bodily energy, and psychological and general functioning. Second, it is essential to be informed about the patient's mood, thinking and behaviour when they are functioning at their best, and to assess how these have changed. For example, for a diagnosis of affective disorder it would be critical to compare *current* mood, sleep patterns, communication, thought processes, mood, distractibility, and enjoyment of activities etc. with 'best baseline' in order to understand if and how the features have changed over time. Third, diagnosis, especially in people with autism of cognitive low ability, will be based more on observed changes in thinking, behaviour and mood rather than on patients' own descriptions of their difficulties. As noted above, even very able individuals with autism are likely to have problems describing emotions and internal feelings. Thus, a parent, other family member, or someone who has known the person well for a long time should always be involved in the diagnostic process, both in order to provide information on past functioning but also to act as an 'interpreter'. Finally, when the diagnosis of an additional psychiatric condition is made, this should be carefully monitored over time. Possible medical and neurological causes should be investigated, and Lainhart also suggests that the diagnosis of schizophrenia should never be made until other alternative conditions such as delirium, dementia, seizure disorders, sensory impairment, mood disorders and stress-related disorders have been excluded.

A detailed developmental history is also a crucial part of the diagnostic process. The Autism Diagnostic Interview (ADI-R, Lord *et al.* 1994), for example, can be used to provide information about past functioning, which can then be compared with the current state. Nevertheless, it has to be recognised that the diagnosis of psychiatric disturbance in individuals with severe to profound learning disabilities can pose a major problem for clinicians and although attempts have been made to adapt current diagnostic systems to meet the needs of this group the situation remains far from satisfactory (See Bregman 1991 and Bernal 1994 for helpful discussions of these issues). One problem arises from the fact that, because individuals with autism are often so immersed in their routines, certain aspects of their daily functioning may remain apparently intact even when they are severely disturbed or depressed. Parents often report a determined insistence on carrying out daily rituals or routines, and the characteristic symptoms of depression – such as changes in eating or sleeping – may be slow to emerge because of this. Instead, important indicators are increases in aggression to self or others, unprovoked attacks on people or property, agitation, withdrawal, or a marked increase in obsessional and ritualistic behaviours. Behaviours of this kind may be the individual's only means of communicating disturbance or distress, and it is therefore essential to try to establish the reasons underlying them. Particular heed should be taken if the emergence of such behaviours is associated with significant life events or changes. However, depressive and other illness may not necessarily be related solely to external factors, and failure to identify possible environmental causes obviously does not rule out the possibility of a psychotic illness. Detailed assessment and observation of the individual and his or her environment will be required if the correct diagnosis, and consequently appropriate treatment procedures, are to be formulated.

Treatment

Just as the recognition of mental illness in people with autism can present many problems, so, too, can the provision of appropriate help and intervention.

Medication

Although there are some useful reviews of the drugs that can be used in the treatment of behaviour problems in autism (Campbell and Cueva 1995, McDougle 1997) there has been relatively little systematic study of the effectiveness of pharmacological treatments for psychiatric disturbances in this group. In United States surveys of drug treatments, parents report a bewildering variety of interventions and an equally wide range of drug effects (Rimland 1994b), and medication is used routinely with both high- and low-functioning individuals (Martin *et al.* 1999). Clarke (1996) presents a balanced and informative account of pharmacological interventions for psychiatric disturbances in people with autism, and it is clear from this that, despite claims for the effectiveness of certain drugs, the data in support of such claims are often limited. McDougle (1997), for example, suggests that drugs that increase 5-HT uptake neuro-transmission, such as 5-HT (5-hydroxytryptamine) inhibitors, (clomipramine, fuvoxamine, fluoxatine, sertraline), and 5-HT agonists, such as buspirone, may help to reduce symptoms such as aggressive or repetitive behaviours, or to improve social functioning. However, the author also notes that only two controlled studies of this class of drugs have been published. The situation is much the same with other drugs, such as DA (dopamine) receptor agonists (e.g. haloperidol); drugs that modulate DA, such as risperidone, and drugs that affect NE (norepinephrine) function. There are also concerns about the safety of some of these agents. Until, recently, for example, fenfluramine, an indirect 5-HT agonist, was widely recommended as a treatment for many different problems associated with autism, but anxiety about long-term adverse effects is now such that its use, especially with young children, is strongly discouraged. There is little information on the types of drugs that are most effective in treating psychiatric disorders in people with autism; medication may have very different effects on different individuals, and needs to be carefully monitored. For example, amongst twelve patients with autism and affective disorders, who were prescribed either antidepressants or mood stabilisers or both, Perry *et al.* (2001) found that two improved almost immediately (i.e. within two weeks), seven responded within two to seven weeks and three showed no improvement.

The wide spread of ability in people with autism, and the presence of associated problems such as epilepsy, can mean that their response to medication may be even more variable than in the general population. Paradoxical responses to medication (becoming very overactive and agitated when prescribed a tranquilliser, for example) are an additional risk. Certain drugs, such as neuroleptics, which may be helpful in the treatment of schizophrenic disorders, may also have untoward effects. Some, for instance, may reduce facial expressiveness and therefore contribute to the social difficulties of someone who already has impairments in this area (Tantam 1991).

In the case of marked psychiatric disturbance, however, delays in prescribing appropriate medication can have serious effects. If it is decided that pharmacological treatments are to be employed, carers should be fully informed about possible side effects so that signs of any negative reactions can be dealt with quickly and effectively. Clear guidelines should be agreed *in advance* as to how progress will be monitored, how long the drug will be given before its efficacy is assessed, and how long medication should continue before the drug is discontinued, recommended for longer use, or gradually withdrawn.

All too frequently one comes across cases of individuals with autism who have been on the same drug, or cocktail of drugs, for many years, with little obvious benefit. Often medication continues because carers are frightened about what will happen if it is withdrawn, whether or not there is any evidence that it is – or ever has been – effective. Other individuals, particularly those in long-stay hospitals or institutions, are simply prescribed one drug after another in the apparent hope that eventually 'something' might work. The result is often to make their lives even more impoverished than they were initially, without providing any obvious benefits.

Some individuals with autism may refuse to take medication at all because they are convinced this will be damaging to their health, and a great deal of persuasion may be required to overcome this resistance. Others who suffer unwanted or expected side effects may discontinue treatment, no matter how essential this is. Sarah, a young woman in her mid-twenties, had been prescribed medication for severe depression for several years. This had little apparent effect other than an increase in weight. Her mother requested a review of the medication in order to explore possible alternatives but was told this was unnecessary. However, Sarah had always had an obsession with her appearance, and when strict dieting had no impact on her weight she abruptly stopped taking the medication, without her doctor's knowledge. After a short time she had to be admitted as an emergency to her local psychiatric hospital.

It is essential to predict possible side effects, as far as possible, for if the individual is prepared for these in advance they may be able to tolerate them more willingly. If such effects are not tolerable, for whatever reason, then unnecessary delay in seeking an alternative may result in total refusal to accept further treatment.

Avoiding the development of further behavioural disturbance

A particular problem that arises in treating people with autism stems from their adherence to routine. Once they become set in a particular pattern of behaviour it can be very difficult to shift this. Hence, if unwanted behaviours become established during the course of a psychiatric illness it can prove almost impossible to change these later, even when mental health has significantly improved.

Steven, whose withdrawal and muteness are described earlier, was not recognised as having a depressive illness for many months. A behavioural programme was implemented to reduce his 'obsessional' behaviours, but this proved both ineffective and inappropriate. Finally, he was placed on antidepressant medication and showed slow but steady improvement. However, even when he seemed much recovered he still refused to let anyone approach him and remained virtually mute. A subsequent behavioural programme, carried out at home and at his day centre, very slowly helped to increase his tolerance of being touched, but he continued to avoid speaking. His mother, knowing that his reading and writing skills were good, suggested that he should be encouraged to reply to questions in writing. This he seemed to enjoy, and he also began, occasionally, to use writing to communicate spontaneously. Over the next few years his written communication became more extensive and his self-confidence in social situations seemed to increase until, eventually, he began speaking freely once more.

James, now in his thirties, became very housebound during his late teens, when he was depressed. By the time his parents sought help his reclusiveness was well entrenched, and although his mood state is now much improved he is still resistant to leaving the house. If he does go out this is only for a short walk with his mother, and he is far more dependent on his parents than he was when younger. Moreover, because of his dependence on them the quality of life for the entire family has greatly deteriorated.

Psychological approaches to intervention

This tendency for 'ill' behaviours to persist, even when the disorder is in remission, makes early diagnosis and treatment particularly crucial. It also means that psychological treatments, to re-establish appropriate behaviour patterns, should be employed as an adjunct to pharmacological interventions as early in the recovery stage as possible.

Prior to a brief period of inpatient treatment for depression, Sally had developed many obsessional behaviours, refusing to leave the house or to talk to anyone outside. On her return home a careful programme was planned in order gradually to encourage a wider range of activities. Initially the demands were very limited: one walk with the dog in a week and one visit to the hospital hydrotherapy pool (she enjoyed swimming but could not cope with the crowds at the local leisure centre). Her mother took time off work to be with her at such times and, by degrees, with help from social services, the frequency of outings was increased. She is still unable to go out unaccompanied, but at least no longer spends all her time in bed as she had done before her admission.

Psychological therapies, particularly those using a cognitive-behavioural approach (Sheldon 1995, Haddock and Slade 1995, Greenberg and Beck 1990), may be used to repair the loss of confidence and self-esteem that often follows illnesses of this kind. However, because such strategies traditionally focus on internal cognitions or emotional states and feelings, they will need some modification. Encouraging someone with autism to *write down* positive things that have happened is obviously more helpful than simply instructing them to restructure negative thoughts. Following a short depressive illness Damien remained convinced that his life was one of great deprivation and misery. In fact, because he had a small legacy from his parents he had far more opportunities than many other young men of his age. In counselling sessions he would always concentrate on his inability to find a job (which he did not really need) or a girlfriend (with whom he could never have coped). Although allowing some time for his complaints the therapist began to insist that he kept lists of 'good things' that had happened between sessions. Initially he had difficulty finding even one positive event to report, but as time went on he was encouraged to produce increasingly longer lists, which then became the focus of therapeutic work. Reaven and Hepburn (2004) also illustrate how visual representations (of degree of anxiety/improvement etc.) can help even children with autism monitor their own progress and steadily gain control over their lives.

When working with less severe problems, or with individuals of lower ability, more direct behavioural strategies can be very effective. Relaxation and distraction techniques, such as thought-stopping, have been described in some detail in the chapter on obsessional behaviours and are often particularly successful in dealing with anxiety-related problems. (See also Clements and Zarkowska 2000 for strategies for working with more severely cognitively impaired adults.) But it may be necessary to address environmental factors too. George, for example, had a marked fear of dogs, which at one stage almost prevented his leaving the house. A desensitisation programme which aimed gradually to reduce his fear of dogs was implemented, and his anxieties were slowly reduced. He also learned to avoid certain places, such as the local park, where dogs were likely to appear without warning.

However, problems arose once again when he started work and had to pass a factory where guard dogs roamed the grounds. His anxiety increased rapidly until it reached a stage where he was unable to go to work unless accompanied by his mother. She learned that the dogs' barking was also upsetting other residents, and in the end they campaigned to have the dogs better restrained and kept well away from the road. Once this was accomplished she began systematically to reduce the distance she accompanied him, until eventually he was able to walk to work alone as long as she stood and watched until he passed the factory gates.

Sometimes behavioural approaches alone cannot be implemented, particularly if the anxiety or agitation is very severe. In such cases anxiety-reducing medication may improve the response to psychological intervention, or encourage the individual concerned to attempt alternative strategies for dealing with difficulties (Ghaziuddin *et al.* 2002).

Responses to loss

Grief reactions following the loss of a relative, a favourite staff member or another resident often prove particularly difficult to recognise or to treat. The person with autism may seem apparently unconcerned, even by the death of someone very close, and if they do mention it are likely to concentrate on tangential, even seemingly callous, issues such as how much they have been left in the will. Even if asked directly they will often deny any upset. Other individuals may show no reaction initially but then, sometimes after several weeks or months have elapsed, become tearful or show other signs of distress. Maria, a woman of forty with superficially good communication skills, when asked if she was sad about the death of her father insisted she was 'glad he's gone to heaven and is out of pain'. However, a few weeks later she began to embark on bizarre monologues about punishment and pain, murder and the police, and was clearly extremely disturbed. It proved very difficult to help her cope with her grief (and probably anger) because of her lack of ability to express her feelings. Although reflective methods were tried, suggesting how other people would feel in these circumstances, it was doubtful that these sessions meant very much to her, and usually they ended with long discussions about her obsession with the weather. Eventually she did emerge from this period of disturbance, but this seemed to be in the absence of any real support. In contrast, Colin, in many ways less able, was helped to talk more constructively about the death of his father. His mother was anxious that explanations should be kept as concrete as possible since once, when he was a child, she had made the mistake of pointing upwards and telling him that his grandad had 'gone to heaven'. For many months afterwards he would persistently try to get into the attics of houses, apparently under the impression that that was where heaven was. On this occasion she used booklets specially designed for people with learning disabilities, which illustrate clearly the events surrounding a parent's death and how people react and feel (Hollins and Sireling 1994). How much he really understood was never clear, but he seemed to enjoy 'reading' these books (they have no words) and discussing how and why those left behind reacted as they did. Although such materials are not specifically written for people with autism, because of their directness and clarity they can be a useful aid to carers in their attempts to offer comfort and support. Other books in this series can also be used to help people deal with traumatic events such as leaving home (Hollins and Roth 1994, Hollins and Hutchinson 1993), coping with severe illness (Donaghy *et al.* 2002), or the experience of sexual abuse (Hollins *et al.* 1992, 1994).

Another potentially valuable approach involves the use of 'social stories' (Gray and White 2002). By means of cartoon-type drawings and simple scripts the relevant events can be illustrated, feelings and emotions explored, and possible solutions presented. Because the materials are constructed individually to suit the person and situations involved they can be adapted for use by those who are non-verbal as well as by those who are of higher ability and have relatively good language skills.

Psychotherapy and counselling

Counselling to deal with the impact of trauma or bereavement may be an important adjunct to therapy, particularly for older or more able individuals. Although there is little experimental validation of these techniques, experience suggests that in order to succeed such intervention needs to incorporate direct, practical advice about strategies for change. Introspection alone, even for very able clients, is rarely effective, and may well prove counterproductive. Douglas was an eighteen-year-old who had received analytically based psychotherapy for some years. Early sessions had focused on his relationship with his mother and the role this may have played in his subsequent problems. Douglas became obsessed with this 'explanation' and was convinced that his mother was entirely responsible for all his difficulties, including his late development of language and occasional seizures. Because of this he made no attempts to modify his own behaviour, and even when he got into trouble with the police for following young women he insisted that this was all his mother's fault.

Group therapy also seems to have little positive value. Groups for individuals with psychiatric disorders are generally based on the premise that therapy can help to *repair* damaged social functioning and that interaction with others sharing the same problems may help to speed recovery. However, this process will not help people with autism to gain skills that they never had; communication is rarely adequate for expressing complex emotions, and their ability to share ideas and experiences is likely to be extremely limited even when they are functioning at their best. Exposure to groups of this kind can in fact exacerbate anxiety and distress. Moreover, the inability of people with autism to 'cooperate' in group therapy sessions can lead to their further rejection by both staff and other patients.

Inpatient hospital treatment

Many families, and individuals themselves, may be resistant to inpatient hospital treatment. There are understandable fears that the person with autism may be misunderstood or become even more distressed by this major upheaval; there may be concerns, too, about the use of prolonged or inappropriate medication. Thus, it is essential that those dealing with patients with autism are aware of the implications of this condition for diagnosis, assessment and treatment. If mental health professionals themselves are inexperienced, it is vital that they consult with and take advice from others who do have expertise in this area. The problems that arise in hospital tend to occur because neither staff nor other patients are able to understand the behaviours of someone with autism. Even on wards for people with acute psychotic conditions, there will generally be some relationships formed between staff and patients, some displays of humour and some sharing of experiences. However, a patient with autism is unlikely to be able to take part in any such interactions, and their lack of response is often a source of considerable irritation both to staff and fellow-patients. Even their failure to respond to therapy may somehow be viewed as deliberate and because of their fundamental lack of interpersonal skills the quality of their treatment is often far from optimal.

Martine, for example, after another confrontation with local police because of her night-time wanderings, was placed on twenty-four-hour supervision in an isolation ward and, because of her failure to 'cooperate' with staff, was deprived of any privileges. The nurses had complained because she did not have any nightwear or toothpaste/ brush etc., and demanded that she tell them where she lived and who cared for her. They refused to believe her when she said she lived alone and that there was no one whom she could contact to obtain these items. Having searched her belongings (thereby adding further to her distress) they found her address and phone number and left endless messages on her answerphone informing the owner (i.e. Martine) that she was in hospital and needed someone to take responsibility for her.

Parents whose sons or daughters require admission to a psychiatric hospital frequently complain that the information they could give is ignored, even though only they are able to give a clear account of which behaviours relate specifically to the autism and which are likely to be features of a psychotic disorder. They are also likely to be far more knowledgeable about situations or strategies that increase or decrease stress and anxiety, or exacerbate behavioural disturbance. However, because their son or daughter is an adult (and particularly if they have superficially good language) parents' attempts to be involved tend to be viewed as inappropriately intrusive or as breaching patient-doctor confidentiality.

It is crucial that if admission to hospital is required, therapy is not undermined because of a lack of knowledge or understanding amongst staff. Harry, for example, was admitted on a section, having been found wandering half naked in the streets at night, muttering to himself about aliens and apparently talking to disembodied voices. When his parents finally found out where he was (which was only when they contacted the police), he had been heavily sedated with medication to which they knew he was allergic. Moreover, although they were aware he was very depressed, his preoccupation with aliens had existed since childhood and was not an indication of psychotic thought processes; and because his speech tended to be very echolalic when he was anxious, he would often repeat past conversations. The doctor in charge refused to take their concerns or explanations seriously, and Harry's condition, both physical and mental, rapidly deteriorated. He required intensive medical care because of his abreaction to the medication, and when he was finally released from hospital the first thing his parents did was initiate legal action against the staff there.

Such stories, or previous personal experience, may result in some parents doing their utmost to avoid hospital admission. Janie was a young woman whose autism had not been diagnosed until her twenties. She then suffered a period of severe depression, constantly talking about her wish to die and making several unsuccessful suicide attempts. However, because she was unable to express her feelings adequately, and because she always had a determined smile on her face, local psychiatric services dismissed her problems as 'hysterical and attention-seeking'. Her mother recognised the severity of her depression, but at the same time was convinced that if Janie went into hospital 'she might never come out again'. Over several months Janie became progressively more withdrawn, reclusive and paranoid. Finally, she stopped eating and sleeping and became so disturbed that she was admitted to hospital. By this time the severity of her problems was such that it required many months of treatment and medication before any improvement occurred. Delays in receiving hospital treatment, should this become necessary, also increase the risk of developing maladaptive behaviour patterns (such as never leaving the house or sleeping only during the day and playing records all night long) that will later prove very difficult to modify.

The treatment of epilepsy

Epilepsy, of course, is not a psychiatric disorder as such (although occasional cases of epileptic psychosis have been reported, Tantam 1991), but it may require treatment by psychiatrists or neurologists in adulthood, and hence is included here. Treatment will clearly be determined by the nature and frequency of the seizures, and there is no evidence to suggest that successful control is particularly difficult to achieve for people with autism (see Gillberg and Coleman 2000). However, because individuals are unlikely to report unwanted side effects themselves, careful monitoring of their response to treatment, and readiness to change medication if necessary, is particularly important. Otherwise, physical or behavioural difficulties may escalate. Alternatively, in the case of more able individuals, they may refuse to continue with medication.

Some adolescents or young adults have one or two isolated fits but no more, and because of the side effects of much anti-epileptic medication it is now generally agreed that drugs should not automatically be prescribed in these cases. Instead, the decision to treat with antiepileptics should be made on a case-by-case basis (Hirtz *et al.* 2003).

The need to be aware of behavioural change

Although much remains to be understood about the nature and treatment of psychiatric illness in people with autism, it is apparent that the risks of disturbance, particularly related to anxiety and depression, are substantial. For those who are more able, and hence more aware of their difficulties, such responses are hardly surprising. They may fully recognise their limitations, and acknowledge the many differences between themselves and their peers, yet have virtually no means of altering this situation.

Even these individuals are unlikely to communicate their distress, or express their need for help in an effective way, and for the less able this may be almost impossible. Thus, the early detection of mood disorders, and the provision of appropriate treatment may depend heavily on the vigilance of carers. Sudden changes in behaviour, a loss of interest in previously enjoyed activities, swings of mood, unexplained outbursts of rage or anger, aggressive or self-injurious attacks, increasing withdrawal, can all be indicators of emotional stress. Undiagnosed physical or medical problems, such as infections, or inappropriate medication, may also be a cause of behavioural disturbance. It is crucial always to take these signs seriously, to explore why such changes have occurred, and to examine possible physical, emotional and environmental factors (especially those related to loss or change) as thoroughly as possible. In this way it may be possible at least to minimise the impact of psychiatric disturbance on individuals who already have to contend with the burden of their autism.

11 Legal issues

Is there a link between autism and criminality?

Although there is little evidence of any significant association between autism and criminal offending, occasional and sometimes lurid publicity has led to suggestions that there may be an excess of violent crimes amongst more able people with autism or those diagnosed as having Asperger syndrome. Certainly, tragic events do sometimes occur. In the United Kingdom in 1994, for example, a thirteen-year-old boy diagnosed as having Asperger syndrome murdered an eighty-five-year-old woman on her way to church, apparently without any motivation. In 2001, a London newspaper reported the case of a seven-year-old boy with Asperger syndrome who had killed his six-month-old brother, stabbing him seventeen times and cutting off his left hand. He had then gone to the police to tell them what he had done. The first his mother (who had been at home all the while) knew was when the police arrived at the house.

A number of reports has also appeared in the academic literature from time to time. In her original account of thirty-four individuals with Asperger syndrome Lorna Wing describes the case of one man who had injured another boy whilst at school, apparently because of his obsession with chemical experiments (Wing 1981). Mawson and colleagues (1985) report on a forty-four-year-old man with Asperger syndrome who was committed to Broadmoor Special Hospital after attacking a baby. This followed a series of other attacks, including stabbing, on young women or children, which had begun in his teens. The attacks seemed to be related to his obsession with getting a girlfriend, his dislike of certain styles of dress and his dislike of the sound of crying. He also had a fascination with poisons. Simon Baron-Cohen (1988) describes the unusual case of a twenty-one-year-old man who had, over a period of several years, violently assaulted his seventy-one-year-old 'girlfriend'. Offences of a sexual nature have also been reported. Chesterman and Rutter (1994) describe a young man with Asperger syndrome who had been charged with a number of sexual offences. These seemed to relate mainly to his obsession with washing machines and women's nightdresses. The case was complicated by the fact that he struck the interviewing police officer when it was suggested that he might also have been contemplating burglary; as far as he was concerned 'he was merely intending to make use of the occupant's washing machine'. A history of sexual offending and unusual sexual interests is described by Milton *et al.* (2002) in their case report of a man with Asperger syndrome detained within a secure mental health unit. Kohn *et al.* (1998) also describe an adolescent with Asperger syndrome with convictions for sexual violence.

A number of cases involving arson is also recorded. Everall and Le Couteur (1990) describe a case of fire-setting in an adolescent boy with Asperger syndrome, and Digby Tantam (1991) mentions five cases of fire-setting, four of which occurred when other people were in the building. Tantam also cites another case in which someone had killed his schoolmate: 'probably as an experiment'. Nevertheless, he also adds that violence, in a fight, in an explosion of rage or in sexual excitement, is rare. Amongst the men with Asperger syndrome whom he studied sexual offending was relatively infrequent, although some got into trouble for indecent exposure. Property offences were also rare except as the 'side-effects of the pursuit of a special interest'.

Other, mainly anecdotal, reports of offending by people with autism or Asperger syndrome suggest that inappropriate social responses, especially to strangers, may result in police involvement, and crimes may also be linked to obsessional interests. Because of this, offending may well be of an unusual or even bizarre nature, such as attempting to drive away an unattended railway engine because of an obsession with trains, or causing explosions and fires because of an obsessional interest in chemical reactions (Wing 1986).

Estimates of offending by people with autism or Asperger syndrome

On the basis of their single-case report, Mawson and colleagues suggest that many people placed in secure units because of violent offences may have Asperger syndrome. In fact, evidence in support of such a statement is extremely limited. Scragg and Shah (1994) assessed the entire male population of Broadmoor Special Hospital, using case notes to identify possible autistic cases. Then, by means of the Handicap, Behaviour and Skills schedule (Wing and Gould 1978) and personal interviews, they identified three cases with autism and six with Asperger syndrome. Out of a total of 392 patients this represented a prevalence rate of just over 2 per cent. Although the numbers are small, this is clearly a much higher figure than the rates for autism or Asperger syndrome in the general population. The offences committed included violence or threats of violence (five cases), unlawful killing (three cases, including one of matricide) and fire-setting (one case). Solitariness or lack of empathy was noted in each case. Six of the cases had a fascination with topics such as poisons, weapons, murder books or combat. Because the prevalence of Asperger syndrome in this special hospital setting was higher than predicted Scragg and Shah concluded that there is a significant association between Asperger syndrome and violence. Nevertheless, as Ghaziuddin and his colleagues point out, the number of reports of violence or offences by people with autism or Asperger syndrome is actually very small. In 1991 they reviewed accounts of offending by people with Asperger syndrome. Out of a total of 132 cases, only three had a clear history of violent behaviour (these are the cases described by Wing 1981, Baron-Cohen 1988 and Mawson *et al.* 1985, noted above). The low incidence of violence found by Ghaziuddin is compared with a rate of 7 per cent for violent crimes (rape, robbery and assault) in the 20–24-year age group in the United States (United States Bureau of Justice Statistics 1987).

As Scragg and Shah (1994) suggest, there may well be more people with autism in prisons or secure accommodation than is realised, and it is clearly important that such individuals are correctly identified and treated. However, estimates of the prevalence of violence in this group can only be made on the basis of community studies. Until then speculation on the alleged links between violence and autism or Asperger syndrome is only likely to increase the stigma and distress of individuals and their families. Currently there is no reason to suppose that people with autism are more prone to committing offences than anyone else. Indeed, because of the very rigid way in which many tend to keep to rules and regulations they may well be more law-abiding than the general population.

Causes of offending

Although it has been suggested that a lack of empathy may be a significant factor in violent attacks by people with autism or Asperger syndrome, other significant variables include their lack of social understanding, the pursuit of obsessional interests and a failure to recognise the implications of their behaviour either for themselves or others. Rigid adherence to rules may also give rise to problems. Occasionally, too, crimes may be unwittingly, or unwillingly, committed at the instigation of others. Very often, of course, a combination of these factors is involved, but rarely does there appear to be deliberate intention to hurt or harm others.

Failure to recognise the impact of behaviours on others

Douglas was a man in his forties who, despite numerous problems since childhood, had not previously been diagnosed as autistic. He was arrested after attacking his eighty-year-old mother. Apparently he had been under considerable stress at work, and had tried, he said, to make his mother understand his problems. Finally, in desperation he had hit out at her. He insisted that 'she was not badly hurt . . . nothing broken . . . just a bit bruised', and that he had 'only shaken her about a bit'. He expected their lives to return to normal after her return from hospital and could not understand why it was necessary for the police to be involved. His apparent lack of remorse led to criminal proceedings, his placement in a bail hostel, where he was very badly treated, and subsequently probation, which he greatly resented. He continues to believe that his mother will return to live with him, despite her removal into social services care many miles away, and remains bitter that so much should have been made of 'such a trivial incident'.

Obsessional pursuits

Sandy, a young woman who since childhood had had an obsession with matches, had spent many years in a residential school. Staff there were well aware of the potential dangers of her obsession and ensured that matches were never available. Throughout her school years no problems occurred and eventually, in her late teens, she left to live with a foster family who cared for a number of other disabled people. After only a few days she found a box of matches and set fire to the bed of another foster child while he slept. Serious damage was caused, and it was only with luck that no lives were lost. Sandy showed no remorse for her actions, and it was felt by all concerned that if she had access to matches on other occasions the same behaviour would occur. The only alternative was to remove her from the foster home to a unit where much greater supervision could be guaranteed but where access to 'normal living' was far more restricted.

Max, a boy in his mid-teens, became fascinated with reading accounts of death and destruction, and the Bible and stories of the Holocaust in Nazi Germany occupied almost all his time. One night his parents awoke to the smell of gas and found the oven full on. He admitted he had done it 'to see what happened to people if they were gassed', but showed no intent to harm or any realisation that what he had done could cause death.

Clive, aged thirty-five, had been placed in a high security hospital after police, investigating complaints by neighbours about his verbally threatening behaviour, found a large number of guns in the house. On interviewing his mother it emerged that his father had also collected guns since his time as an army officer. Ever since he was a small child, Clive had been encouraged to spend his pocket money on toy guns, and as soon as he was old enough he began to collect shotguns, replica weapons and eventually pistols. Although initially he had obtained licences for these, many of his later acquisitions were not licensed, hence his arrest and subsequent committal to special hospital. Despite his frequent verbal outbursts, Clive had never been physically violent (except to his elderly mother) and had never threatened anyone with a gun. Nevertheless, his psychiatrist was seriously concerned that were he to become particularly agitated he might well use a gun. Clive's later appeal against being held in hospital failed because, despite the seriousness of his situation, he was unable to disguise his love of guns, and talked about them almost constantly to members of the panel reviewing his case.

Chapter 6 describes the case of Joey, whose long-time obsession with washing machines, and his tendency to find his way into houses where they were being used, led to the police being called. The situation became much worse after an incident when he punched the arresting officer. The policeman had accused him of 'breaking and entering', and Joey was outraged! Whilst he might *enter* properties without permission the last thing he would ever do was break anything and his only way of dealing with such a 'false accusation' was to hit the officer concerned.

Sarah (also described in Chapter 6) had always had a fascination with babies since she was a toddler herself, and as she grew older would try to cuddle them whenever she could. As a young adult, however, her tendency to lift them from their prams and carry them around began to lead to serious problems, especially as she was unable to understand why a behaviour that had been allowed in childhood now resulted in such attention.

Obsessional pursuits also seem to have been involved in the case described by Mawson and colleagues. As a teenager he was described as becoming 'girl-mad' and would carry around pictures of naked females, openly and without embarrassment. He once tried to strangle a girl 'because he had lost control of himself' and he developed 'a frank sexual interest in a female teacher', following her about and getting close to her at every possible opportunity. He was eventually admitted to Broadmoor.

Lack of social understanding

Louis, a young teenager, had great difficulties understanding facial expressions, particularly those of children. He would try to touch the faces of young children, and if he felt a facial expression was not friendly he was likely to become quite aggressive. Attempts to help him appreciate the danger of this behaviour, both for himself and others, failed, and after an attack on a young girl he was eventually placed in secure hospital care.

Eric, a youth of eighteen, tended to be badly teased by youngsters in his nearby town, and would get very upset by this. His parents had grown used to him coming home and kicking doors and furniture when this happened. However, one night when they were not in he decided to kick the neighbour's car instead. This he did in full view of the owner, a policeman, who immediately arrested him.

Ivan, a twenty-year-old living a life of almost total isolation with his elderly parents, was desperate for friends, and having been badly bullied in the past by his peers began to seek out the company of much younger children. He particularly liked young girls, because they tended to be quieter and gentler, and he would frequently approach them in parks or shopping malls. Local mothers became increasingly concerned, and the situation came to a head when a small group of older girls deliberately followed him home and then complained that he had enticed them in. Although the police decided not to pursue the case, the family became the focus of hate mail, threats and abuse, and eventually had to leave the area altogether.

Gerry was another young man whose lack of social awareness had serious repercussions. Although very high-functioning, he would become very agitated if his plans were disrupted in any way and particularly distressed if trains or buses were late. On one occasion when the last bus home was delayed he began shouting, pushing aside the other person at the bus stop, a young woman, in order to check the timetable. She had believed he was about to attack her, physically and/or sexually and, terrified, had sought safety in a nearby shop. The police later picked up Gerry on the bus, but he, having no idea that he had upset anyone, denied the whole incident. This denial was viewed as evidence of his guilt, and when the case came to court the magistrate was far from sympathetic, especially as Gerry showed no empathy for the woman's evident distress. Only the intervention of his lawyer, who had considerable experience of helping clients with learning difficulties, helped him to avoid a custodial sentence. Unfortunately, around two years later, a very similar incident occurred, but with a much younger girl, and he was placed on the sex offenders register.

Misuse by others

A particularly sad case was that of Darren, who had been thrown out of his home by his father at the age of sixteen after being used by a local gang of youths as an unwitting agent in various petty thefts. He was placed in a social services hostel, where he seems to have suffered prolonged sexual abuse from other residents. On one occasion he ended up in hospital having been forcibly injected with drugs. Eventually he was arrested by the police following a robbery in which he had been made to drive the stolen goods away in a 'getaway' vehicle whilst the others disappeared. He was initially picked up because the car he was driving had no tax disc, no lights and no bonnet, but he was quite unaware that these deficits were bound to bring him to the attention of the police. Fortunately, one of the arresting officers, who had a relative with autism, suggested that he might be autistic, and psychiatric services were called. After the diagnosis of autism was made the case was dropped and Darren was finally returned home to his family.

Young people with autism living in areas with high rates of street crime may be at particular risk. Berty, for instance was frequently used by a local gang to deliver drugs, or to keep stolen goods in his house. He was picked up after the police saw a collection of recently stolen items neatly lined up in the front window of his house. However, victimisation can occur in many other settings, including the workplace. Chapter 9, for example, cites the example of Jo, a man who had worked in a jeweller's shop for some time and was often trusted to lock up the safe at night. A new nightwatchman, recognising Jo's innocence, simply asked him to hand over the keys one night. The resulting robbery led to his arrest as an 'accomplice', and although this charge was dropped he inevitably lost his job.

Victimisation may also lead to other problems. Thus, Raymond, having been constantly teased, harried and bullied by groups of local children, became increasingly reluctant to leave the house. One day, when his parents were out, stones were thrown through his bedroom window. At his wits' end, he marched into the street and grabbed the first (and smallest) child he saw. Although this boy had nothing to do with the incident, Raymond attacked him and was charged by the police for causing grievous bodily harm. He was sent to a psychiatric hospital because of the apparently motiveless attack, although, of course, to his parents the motives were only too clear. They had been seeking help for their son ever since he had left school but their fears that something like this could easily occur had never been taken seriously.

In a very different case, Mark, a middle-aged man with autism, who had fallen out on numerous occasions with his siblings, was offered several thousand pounds by his brother if he would 'just sign a bit of paper'. Being very poorly paid (he worked for the family firm), he willingly signed. Only later did he learn that he had signed away his share of the property that was to be left to them after their father died. In that his IQ on formal tests was over 140 and he was fluent in several languages, attempts by his lawyer to persuade the court that he had acted without understanding of what he was doing met with little sympathy.

Misinterpretation of 'rules'

Trouble may also ensue if 'rules' are misunderstood, or interpreted too rigidly. Martine, described in Chapter 10, got into serious trouble, when stopped by the police for loitering in an area that was on terrorist alert. She refused to give them any information, on the grounds that her mother had told her never to talk to strangers. Jonathan, who had been working in a central London office for several years, lost his job after attacking a cloakroom attendant with his umbrella. She had given him the wrong ticket and he believed himself to be perfectly justified in acting in this manner, as 'she was not doing her job properly'. Had he shown any remorse it is possible that he would have been given a formal warning but allowed to stay on. However, he was adamant that it was she who had 'broken the rules' and like many autistic people he was not able to recognise that even if he felt no remorse it might be useful at least to pretend.

There are also likely to be problems when social 'rules' change, as, for example, because of heightened public anxiety over certain issues. Thus Martine's tendency to wander round buildings in the centre of the city, closely examining the brickwork, had initially been dismissed as rather eccentric. When the area became the focus of possible terrorist activity, the same behaviour was viewed very differently. Bruno's declaration that he was going to 'deal with' the president of the United States and the British prime minister because he had been refused a commercial pilot's licence was treated with some amusement by most of his neighbours. After the 2001 attacks in New York such threats became unacceptable, but Bruno had no idea why he could have got into trouble for talking in this way. Similarly, Jim's collection of replica weapons had been the one topic that he was able to discuss even with strangers. Again, after fears of terrorism increased, talk of this kind became far less socially appropriate. Such cases illustrate only too well that it is not necessarily the behaviour of the person with autism per se that gives rise to problems but changing societal attitudes, in the wake of external events.

Approaches to intervention

The way in which dangerous or potentially criminal behaviours are dealt with will depend on individual circumstances and the underlying causes of the behaviour. If obsessional, social or communication deficits are at the root of the problems, then these will need to be addressed in the manner suggested in earlier chapters. However, again, a few basic guidelines should be remembered.

Begin early

In the discussion of obsessional and social problems in earlier chapters, emphasis was placed on the need to be aware that behaviours that seem innocuous, innocent or even charming in young children may take on a very different perspective when adulthood is reached. Although figures are not available, clinical and anecdotal evidence suggests that many of the actions that lead people with autism into trouble as they grow older are not new but simply developments of behaviours established in childhood.

As a child, Christopher was fascinated by the activity of copying words and pictures. He became accomplished at copying other people's handwriting, and his parents were quite proud of the way in which he was able to copy their signatures. By the age of fourteen he had managed to open several bank and building society accounts in the local town and would cash money by forging his parents' signatures on cheques. He obtained several hundred pounds in this way, which in turn he used to feed his other obsession with railways and travelling. By the age of fifteen he was totally beyond the control of his gentle but ineffectual parents, and by seventeen had been arrested on forgery charges.

Joey, mentioned earlier, had had a fixation with washing machines since a very young age. Having become used to wandering in and out of neighbours' houses he later widened his horizons and would enter any house where he heard a washing machine in action. The sight, on returning home, of a well-built, silent young stranger sitting on the kitchen floor on is not one that most people expect, and after the police became involved his family had to try to put a stop to this behaviour. This proved an almost impossible task for them, and greatly frustrating for him. Input from a clinical psychologist was successful in diverting his obsession (mostly to websites of washing-machine manufacturers), but it was still many months before the problem could be brought under control.

Inappropriate sexualised behaviours, resulting from obsessional interests, can also give rise to problems. Although many of these, such as touching women's tights or breasts, may be perceived as innocent enough in a three-year-old, they may well be viewed very differently in a thirteen-year-old and could result in placement either in prison or a special hospital by the age of thirty.

Establish consistent rules

Awareness among carers of the potential dangers of such behaviours, and the imposition of appropriate limitations from an early age, could often prevent serious difficulties later. Without help a person with autism is unlikely to be aware of the possible implications of his or her actions or of their impact on other people and – even with help – understanding may remain very limited. Prevention is by far the most effective strategy and instilling the basic rules of social behaviour from an early age is crucial. Teaching children to say 'No' if they are asked to do anything that they know is wrong is also important.

Although, as pointed out in previous chapters, rules can be problematic, it is generally better to establish firm ones in early childhood which can then be relaxed, if appropriate, later. The imposition of new or stricter guidelines on adults is likely to prove very difficult and will almost certainly be much resented.

Social skills training

In some instances, additional training in social awareness may offer help. In the case of the young man with an obsession with faces, described earlier, attempts were made to improve his ability to interpret facial expressions more accurately and thereby to reduce his aggressive outbursts. The interactive DVD programme devised by Baron-Cohen and his colleagues (2002) is potentially of considerable value in enhancing the ability to 'read' faces and emotions, and is currently being evaluated. The scenarios used in various social skills packages for children with autism (e.g. Howlin *et al.* 1998) can also be adapted for use with older or more able individuals. Research materials developed for high-functioning individuals are also valuable, both for assessing and for modifying difficulties in social understanding that can lead to more serious problems. These include the 'Reading the Mind in the Eyes' Test (Baron-Cohen *et al.* 1997), the 'Strange Stories' Test (Happé 1994), and the 'Awkward Moments' test (Heavey *et al.* 2000). Baron-Cohen (1988), in his account of the young man who regularly beat up his seventy-one-year-old partner, also suggests that a social-cognitive approach to intervention may be of value.

While these approaches seem promising, there are no long-term evaluations of the effectiveness of such methods, and in some cases the profundity of the social impairment is such that attempts to improve social understanding are almost certain to be of limited effectiveness. Indeed, in a few cases – such as that of Sandy's fascination with firesetting or Clive's obsession with guns – it may be necessary to ensure that the individual is no longer exposed to the situation in which the problems occur or that others are protected from the risk of danger: decisions that may have profound effects on personal liberty.

Pharmacological treatments

Although Posey and McDougle (2000) report some favourable effects of medication for people with Asperger Syndrome, Milton *et al.* (2002) found little evidence for the effectiveness of drug treatments for offences of a sexual nature. Their patient, a thirty-year old man with a history of attacks against women and thefts with a sexual motive from the age of thirteen, had previously been unsuccessfully treated with anti-libidinal medication. However, a subsequent management programme combining environmental and cognitive-behavioural approaches with fluoxetine treatment (to reduce the obsessional nature of the problem) also failed. Exposure to a more structured environment seemed to have little effect; aspects of the cognitive behavioural programme used with other men on the ward were clearly not appropriate for him, and the fluoxetine resulted in the development of facial tics but no reduction in his sexual activities. The authors discuss the problems inherent in dealing with problems such as this and note that lack of effective treatments may result in people with Asperger syndrome being unnecessarily 'trapped' in high- or medium-secure facilities. They conclude that specialist provision, which is probably only feasible at a national level, may be the only real option.

The response from the criminal justice system

A further important issue is the way in which serious or dangerous behaviours are handled by the police and the courts. Although individuals with mild learning difficulties are known to be a particularly vulnerable group (Clare and Gudjonsson 1993), personal experience suggests that the judicial system can sometimes be very lenient towards those with obvious disabilities. At times, police responses to dangerous or illegal behaviours have been rather too gentle and kindly, thereby inadvertently giving the message that the behaviour is not particularly serious. Indeed, a lift home in a police car following a misdemeanour may well prove a considerable incentive to repeat the action. If it is necessary for the police to be involved – perhaps following an aggressive attack on staff or peers – it is essential that the matter is dealt with formally and seriously so that the individual concerned fully recognises the implications of his or her actions and is discouraged, as far as possible, from repeating these.

If court action is required, it is important that all involved are fully aware of the social and communication deficits of the individual with autism, and that an expert assessment is sought in order to determine the extent of his or her problems, and the type of intervention that will be required. Accused individuals must also be given every help to understand what is happening as well as to appreciate the seriousness of their actions. The series of books written by Sheila Hollins can help prepare everyone involved for what will happen (Hollins *et al.* 1994). Very often an expert assessment will prevent the case from coming to court or help to remove the need for punitive action. However, in certain circumstances such assessments may conclude that, because of the lack of social awareness or the severity of obsessional behaviours (or a combination of the two), individuals are of such risk to themselves or others that a custodial sentence is deemed necessary.

Custodial treatment

There are no data on the numbers of people with autism or Asperger syndrome who are given custodial sentences. However, if this option is considered necessary then it is crucial that all those involved in management are made fully aware of the needs of someone with autism. Lack of social understanding, isolation, vulnerability to abuse, inappropriate behaviour, due either to failures of comprehension or obsessional tendencies, are all likely to single out the person with autism. For some, the set daily routine of secure establishments may well have benefits, but if treatment or therapy is offered they may be unable to make use of this. When Andrew was placed in a secure unit for 'sexual offending' (continually exposing himself in public despite warnings), staff learned that he had been previously abused as a child. Group therapy, with similar victims, was arranged, but Andrew was unable to contribute to the group and was frequently disruptive. Another therapist realised that he was most willing to talk about his problems when alone in woodwork sessions, and she had begun to make some progress with him. However, woodwork was considered a privilege, privileges were withdrawn because of his disruptiveness in the group, and hence his one opportunity to take advantage of therapy was effectively denied.

Unless an informed and flexible approach to management can be developed, what is meant to be, at least partly, a therapeutic regime can be highly punitive and completely counterproductive for someone with autism.

12 Sexual relationships and marriage

Marriage and parenthood

Until relatively recently, the issues of marriage or other close sexual relationships among adults with autism had received little attention. It was generally assumed, either implicitly or explicitly, that intimate relationships simply did not occur or if they did were so rare as to be of little general interest. Among the sixteen follow-up studies reviewed in Chapter 2, for example, only 6 per cent of the individuals involved were reported to be married and only in two studies were there accounts of individuals with children of their own. Generally, if sexuality were written about at all, the accounts mostly concerned inappropriate or unacceptable sexual behaviours and how to deal with these. However, given that autism is, in the majority of cases, a genetic disorder, it is clear that within the families of many (possibly most) children with autism there will be mothers and/or fathers who share the same condition. Genetic family studies have confirmed that close relatives are very likely to manifest some components of autism, including problems related to language (from articulation disorders through reading and spelling difficulties), social relationships, and/or rather rigid patterns of behaviour, interests or beliefs (see Lord and Bailey 2002). Clinically, many professionals working in this area have become aware that one or other (and sometimes both) of the referred child's parents share characteristics in common with their offspring. More recently, too, there have been published accounts by individuals (mostly women) whose partner has autism or Asperger syndrome. Many of these accounts have focused on the difficulties of being married to someone with autism, and a number of self-help or professional support groups have been set up in order to help women in this situation. Websites for partners of people with autism are also on the increase (see www.nas.org.uk for further information).

The problems generally experienced by partners are typically those described in Chapters 4 to 6: namely problems in communication, in sharing, in understanding, expressing or responding to feelings and emotions, and difficulties relating to inflexible, stereotyped and repetitive patterns of behaviour. In her recent book on this topic Ashley Stanford (2003) writes specifically about how the core diagnostic symptoms of Asperger syndrome impinge on relationships. As Stanford's book also illustrates, however, in many cases marital discord can be significantly reduced once the diagnosis is recognised, and the 'unfeeling' or 'eccentric' behaviours of the spouse are accepted as part of the condition, not as deliberate attempts to hurt or wound. The types of strategy that are generally effective for people with autism – consistency, clarity, predictability, direct guidelines, minimisation of stress, and a gradual (and mutually agreed) approach to behavioural change – if adapted to the family setting can also have a significant and positive impact.

For partners of someone with autism, the discovery that they are not alone in their situation and that there are numerous others who have to deal with the same puzzling dilemmas can come as an enormous relief. Support and self-help groups for partners can also be invaluable. However, one question that is rarely addressed is: if life with someone with autism is so intolerable, how is it that so many do get married? Gisela Slater-Walker, co-author with her husband of '*An Asperger Marriage*' (2002), notes that when he was first diagnosed she 'found little solace in the literature that I read from other women in a similar situation. . . . I sensed a great deal of bitterness'. However, both she and others have pointed out why, at least initially, certain characteristics that are typical of autism can be so appealing. Gisela Slater-Walker recalls her husband's gentleness, lack of prejudice and calmness in dealing with very difficult situations (such as when she had an epileptic attack). His lack of conformity to the 'macho' norms of many male students was also an attraction to her when they were at college together. His outstanding skills in certain areas tended to disguise his problems in others, and his immense knowledge of particular topics was particularly impressive. Other behaviours, such as never walking alongside her when they were out, were viewed, then, as amusing eccentricities. In writing about her initial meetings with her ex-husband, Wendy Lawson (1998) remembers:

> He was a man of few words but his commitment to keeping the church clean and getting the fire going to warm the building impressed me. He seldom complained, gossiped or criticised other people. . . . We could not communicate in any depth but it seemed

enough to be in each other's company, and so the relationship continued.

In my own clinical experience, I have had several women tell me that they chose their husband because he was so different from what they had experienced in the past. Some, for example, reported having fathers who were very emotional, unpredictable and sometimes violent. For them, meeting a man who was calm, predictable and rarely expressed irritation or anger was a major attraction. 'He was the archetypal strong, silent stranger,' said one. Others, whose previous partners had proved unfaithful, devious or violent, were delighted to find at last someone who seemed so loyal, devoted, honest and gentle. Still others who were single mothers at the time were relieved to find a man who got on so well with their young child. In a few cases, too, the financial security offered by a man who has an apparently stable career (typically in computing or engineering) is a considerable draw. Only later in the marriage do cracks appear, for example: when the lack of emotionality seems more like insensitivity or harshness; when the absence of any social interests or activities becomes oppressive; when the tendency always to be honest and direct has alienated a whole network of old friends; when the initially comfortable silences become unbearable; when the predictability of behaviour becomes terminally boring, or when the lack of 'macho' competitiveness leads to failures at work.

However, as Chris Slater-Walker's account of his marriage illustrates, for a person with autism being married to someone who is 'neurotypical' also has its difficulties. Untidiness, unpredictability, unnecessary socialising, indulgence in small talk, illogical arguments and, at times, what seems to be unremitting criticism are but some of the problems he describes.

One of my own patients, a very intelligent and in many ways successful man, could not understand why his wife wanted him to say, at least occasionally, that he loved her. 'I said it when we married,' he insists, 'and I've never changed my mind, so why should she need me to say it again? Of course, I would tell her if I stopped loving her!'

Nevertheless, as the recent books by Stanford and the Slater-Walkers illustrate, few problems are insoluble if the problems associated with autism/Asperger syndrome are acknowledged and if the mutual will to deal with these exists. Compromise is clearly needed on both sides, and solutions to difficulties may need to be somewhat unusual. For example, Gisela Slater-Walker describes how Chris's lack of communication and his monosyllabic replies to questions became increasingly difficult for her to tolerate and were one of the main factors almost leading to the breakdown of their relationship. They discovered the solution in email. This they use to communicate on a daily basis – even at home – as it allows Chris the time to 'collect his thoughts and express them without any external pressure'. The fact that his wife tends to be more precise in what she writes than in what she says has also helped, and their exchanges are more fruitful – 'even witty'. Nevertheless, she notes, 'I have still found it of limited use in sorting out areas of disagreement: Chris has the ability to push away unpleasant issues, and it is very easy to ignore emails that you do not want to answer!' The value of emails and text messages in improving joint communication is also noted by Stanford (2003), who provides many other practical suggestions for understanding and dealing with the complexities of autism within a relationship. Further advice as how to make relationships work is provided by Aston (2003) in her book *Aspergers in Love* and by Patrick, Estelle and Jareb McCabe's *Living and Loving with Asperger Syndrome* (2003).

There is now a growing number of other accounts by or about married people with autism or Asperger syndrome, some involving several individuals within one family. Liane Holliday, for example, is the mother of three daughters, one of whom – like her – has Asperger syndrome. She has written extensively about family life, marriage and parenthood, and the adaptations that have been required in order for them all to coexist happily and, on the whole, peacefully (Holliday Willey 1999, 2001). Needless to say, not all marriages are so successful, Wendy Lawson (1998) writes of how her problems with emotional and social understanding led to her sliding almost unawares into an unsatisfactory relationship that later terminated in acrimony and divorce. In contrast, some parents' personal experience of having autism can be very valuable in terms of understanding their children who are similarly affected, Both Wendy Lawson and Liane Holliday Willey provide many examples of how they were particularly sensitive to the difficulties of their children with autism and hence better able to offer the support and structure they so needed. Similarly Marion, one of my own patients and the mother of five children, at least three of whom are on the autistic spectrum, said that she found it much easier to cope than she would have done had they all been 'normal':

> I understand them and they understand me, and the sorts of explanations other people need just aren't necessary. . . . I couldn't cope if I thought they needed me to be talking to them all the time. . . . And anyway, having the same interests saves us a lot of time and money.

The family are all intensely interested in church bells and are the mainstay of the local bell-ringing group!

Other authors in writing about their child with autism note how they, too, began to recognise similar features in themselves or in other family members. Valerie Paradiž (2002), for example, when coming to terms with her son Elijah's autism, realised for the first time that the behaviours she had found so difficult to understand in her father when she was younger (obsessionality, self-focused monologues, narrow interests) were almost certainly related to autism. Her grandmother also seems to have shared several of these traits, and certain characteristics of the author's own – such as her preference for solitary activities as a child, her need for sameness and the intense preoccupations that lasted into adulthood – were, she realised, all part of the autistic spectrum. Thus, the jigsaw pieces of her life – the bits that had never quite seemed to join up – gradually began to fit together as she traced her son's development.

Clearly, although in its more extreme form autism can be very difficult to live with and relate to, many characteristics that are part of the 'broader phenotype' can, in the right circumstances, actually help family life to proceed more smoothly. Shared interests can obviously strengthen the bond between partners or between children and parents as, for example, in the case described above of Marion and her children, whose lives all revolved around bell-ringing. In her book *Hitchhiking Through Asperger Syndrome* Lisa Pyles (2002) notes tendencies in both herself and her husband that, being similar to those of her son, make it easier for them to 'connect' with him. Checking, counting, list-making, problems in dealing with anything new, difficulties in recognising faces, logical 'black and white' thinking and a great need for order are all family characteristics, as is a relative indifference to social company: 'Our idea of a nice Friday night is . . . sharing a thermos of coffee between our two side-by-side computers'. Similarly, Liane Holliday Willey's need for routine was evidently reciprocated by her husband:

> When any one of my children begins a new routine, my husband and I encourage it. We believe the adherence to a routine encourages an adherence to a schedule. . . . We know that a house filled with chaos is difficult on all of us. . . . My husband only feels safe and confident when he has woken up to his morning routine which begins with a cup of coffee and ends after two hours on his computer. Anything from that norm makes him squirm all day.
>
> (Holliday Willey 2001)

The same author also notes that for thirty-five years her father ate the same meal at the same time (four-thirty p.m.) in the same restaurant. 'The waiters . . . respect his routine and even they have come to depend on it. In fact, they call should he miss a few days to be certain he is not at home ill'.

It is clear from these and many other accounts, together with the extensive research on the genetics of autism that – contrary to popular belief – people with autism are capable of forming romantic attachments, marrying and raising families of their own, often very successfully. As in any relationship, problems can occur, but in many cases, if the diagnosis is recognised and the implications of this better understood, major difficulties can be resolved. However, often the onus is on the non-autistic partner to adapt to the person with autism rather than the other way round, as is apparent from the many personal examples sited by Stanford (2003). Attempts radically to change the personality and habits of the autistic partner are unlikely to be particularly successful. As Wendy Lawson (2002) warns,

> I would suggest that any individual contemplating a long-term relationship should take the time to get to know their prospective partner. Ask yourself the question 'Am I happy to be waking up next to this person in fifty years' time?' With so many of us, as individuals with ASD, what you see is what you get!

But, then, perhaps such advice would not go amiss in any relationship.

Stanford (2003) describes many of the ways in which non-autistic individuals can help to make life easier for their partners with autism.

> If you start bemoaning the numerous allowance that you're making for your AS partner it may help to think of the number of allowances that the typical Aspie has to make every day just to survive in a non-Aspie world. Try this exercise: ask your partner, 'What specific things do you have to force yourself to do?' It will probably give you valuable insight into the massive amount of effort your partner is already making just to survive day-to-day. Your efforts to work around a few nonfunctional routines won't seem quite so daunting.

> I tried the above exercise with my typically quiet husband. He launched into a long list of tasks that he had to do to get by in the world, listing probably 30 details such as 'touch dirty things', 'look at people,' and 'move my body'. Over the next few days he thought

of other tasks he had to do just to survive. As he shared these with me, I was stunned. I realized that if I were him, I probably wouldn't want to get out of bed in the morning. It helped me see the depth of his tenacity and willpower.

Difficulties in making close relationships

The earlier chapter on social functioning explores the general difficulties that people with autism face in relating to others. Failure to understand the nature of relationships, the skills required for developing these or the rules governing social interactions can all cause difficulties, even in the most superficial of contacts. When more intimate relationships are involved, the problems may be even more profound.

Wanting to be like everyone else

In many cases, children with autism who are aloof and socially isolated when very young begin gradually to take more interest in the world and the people around them as they grow older. More able children, in particular, may become very aware of what others of their own age are doing, and as teenagers they too feel it is time to accompany their peers to clubs and discos. The wish for a sexual partner may also be overwhelming. However, the situation may be compounded by rigid attitudes or beliefs about what is 'normal'. When Joel, for example, reached the age of twenty-one he announced that he would have to find a girlfriend because 'everybody of twenty-one or over has a partner'. He was convinced that not to have one would lead to his being ridiculed by his fellow students. He also developed an obsession with getting married at the age of twenty-eight, as his brother had done, and insisted that 'time was running out' for him. The topic of his forthcoming marriage dominated every conversation, and he was only persuaded not to book a wedding venue when his father told him that that was the job of the bride's family.

The firm belief that everyone else has successful relationships, finds girlfriends and gets married can lead to considerable dissatisfaction and frustration. It can be extremely difficult to convince young adults with autism that other people manage to attain fulfilment without intimate relationships; their view of everyone else living 'happily ever after' may also prove remarkably resilient to factual information.

Even for those individuals who have a more realistic view of intimate relationships the need to be loved and accepted is a very powerful force, and there may well be a conflict between the desire for the comforts of intimacy and recognition of the problems that a close relationship are likely to entail. Gabriella, a young woman in her twenties, had been very close to her mother, and was devastated when her parents decided to move abroad for health reasons. She greatly misses the comfort her mother had always provided, but at the same time admits she would be unable to cope with an intimate relationship with anyone else. She says, very seriously: 'I'd really like to find a gay man to be my friend, someone who I could talk to and cuddle sometimes, but without any risk of demands for a sexual relationship'.

Other individuals, such as Temple Grandin, have deliberately avoided intimate or sexual relationships because they find them far too confusing.

> She was celibate. Nor had she ever dated. She found such interactions completely baffling, and too complex to deal with. 'Have you cared for somebody else?' I asked her. She hesitated for a moment before answering, 'I think lots of times there are things that are missing from my life'.
>
> (Sacks 1993)

For some individuals with autism, same-gender sexual experiences have proved more rewarding. Toby, for example, noted: 'It's hard enough for me to understand people generally – but even my dad says he can't understand women – I think I'll stick with men for the time being.' Jerome found himself particularly isolated at school, not solely because of his general social difficulties but also because his interests and behaviour were so different to those of other boys. Feeling that he was a 'misfit' at college he became involved in a 'gay rights' group where he made a number of good friends of both sexes. Finally he settled into a mutually supportive relationship with another young man which has now lasted over a decade. Gerry-Lyn, after the breakdown of her miserable and violent marriage, joined a women's self-support group, where she met another woman with very similar interests and background and they, too, have now been together for many years.

However, in certain areas, gay meeting places can place young men, in particular, at risk of sexual exploitation or violence. Thus, before venturing into clubs or other centres it is essential to find out as much as possible about the types of clients or activities they attract, and – as with any new situation – it is always wisest to go accompanied. Basic safety rules such as not giving one's address to strangers, not going to an unknown house with someone after a single brief encounter, and above all being able to say 'No' when necessary, should always be borne in mind.

Impairments in social understanding

In autism, the complex skills required for developing and maintaining social, emotional or sexual relationships are almost always affected, and thus attempts to acquire a partner are often inappropriate and may sometimes lead to serious problems. For example, it is not uncommon for young men with autism to get into trouble because of inappropriate approaches to women. Clifford was a very tall and attractive twenty-year-old whose somewhat eccentric style of dress caused rather a stir at college. However, whenever he saw a female student looking at him he would rush up and ask her to be his girlfriend, demanding to know the reason if (as invariably happened) his offer were refused. In other cases approaches may be even less subtle. David, who had been attending a special college course, was sent home by the principal after a few weeks because he had been seen exposing himself to female students. He had done this even when a member of staff was close by, apparently having no realisation that his behaviour was totally unacceptable. When asked why he said he had been studying a magazine article on the size of penises. Having measured his own, he was happy to learn it was of above-average size and he thought the female students would be pleased to see it. Julian, who had recently left boarding school to attend college, was also suspended after he and a female student had been found having intercourse during the lunch break. Neither he nor the young woman concerned (who had quite severe learning disabilities) had made any attempt to stay hidden, much to the amusement of the other students. Knowing of his social difficulties, the principal warned him that such activities could not be tolerated and that he would have to leave if he were found in similar circumstances again. That very same afternoon he was observed in similar circumstances with another female student, having apparently little understanding that the embargo applied to all females, not just the one he had met that morning.

Difficulties understanding and coping with emotions

For other individuals it is not so much their lack of social understanding that is the primary problem but their inability to cope with the emotional demands of a close relationship. In his interview with Temple Grandin, Oliver Sacks questioned her about love and sex:

'What do you imagine falling in love is like?' I asked.

'Maybe it's like swooning – if not I don't know. . . . I've never fallen in love . . . I don't know what it's like to rapturously fall in love. . . . When I started holding the cattle I thought "What's happening to me?" Wondered if that was what love is . . . it wasn't intellectual any more.'

She is wistful about love, in a sense, but cannot imagine how it might be to feel passion for another person.

(Sacks 1993)

Genevieve, an intelligent woman with autism in her early thirties, was happy to find a man who shared interests very similar to hers, and for some months the relationship blossomed. However, she then began to find his need to see her every evening almost 'suffocating' and was unable to understand his distress when she said that once a week was quite enough. Henry, a man who had married in his late thirties, seemed very happy in the relationship, but when his wife went to work abroad for some weeks shortly after their marriage, he immediately asked an ex-girlfriend to move in with him, as 'he didn't like cooking and cleaning very much'. When his wife returned, he seemed to have no idea why this situation so outraged her. Gerard, whose marriage was going through a very bad stage, had agreed to a year's separation from his wife in an attempt to repair their crumbling relationship. He managed to father a child by another woman during this time, and could not understand why this resulted in the end of the marriage as he thought he and his wife had started to get along much better together.

A rather different problem stems from the inability to understand that the non-autistic partner may need the company of other people from time to time. Greg, who disliked change of any kind, became very distressed if his wife's friends 'popped in' unexpectedly, and insisted that all such visits should be by appointment only. He even tried to prevent the midwife from visiting when his wife had a baby. Barty hated visitors under any circumstances but became very angry when his wife began going out alone because of this, insisting that she could not love him any more.

Obsessions and infatuations

The obsessional tendencies associated with autism can also sometimes lead to major difficulties when these extend to social interactions. Oliver, aged twenty, whilst on a work experience placement in his father's office, became besotted with the daughter of the company director. He began to follow her everywhere, telephoned her constantly and lay in wait for her outside her home whenever he had any free time. The police were called on several occasions, and eventually a legal injunction was sought against him. Oliver refused to accept this, believing that since the young woman always spoke to him kindly she wanted a more intimate relationship with him. Because he refused to comply with the injunction and showed absolutely no understanding of the serious nature of this offence he was eventually admitted, on a compulsory section, to a psychiatric hospital. Clara, a young woman in her early twenties who also had visual problems, became infatuated with a fellow student at her college for the visually impaired. In vacations she would travel miles across the country, turning up at his parents' home at all hours of the day or night and demanding to be allowed to stay. His parents were eventually obliged to take out an injunction in an attempt to prevent these visits, but Clara then resorted to constant phone calls and emails instead, and at home talks about him incessantly.

Social naivety

Problems can also arise if the person with autism misinterprets others' expressions of affection or kindness. Roland, who was visiting relatives in America, was delighted to find a young female cousin in California who was very demonstrative towards him. Feeling rather sorry for him, she would cuddle him and tell him how sweet he was. The situation changed suddenly when her fiancé came home and her attentions were directed elsewhere. Roland continued to seek kisses and cuddles and, in the end, because of the fiancé's displeasure, it was 'suggested' that he move on to visit another branch of the family. This he did, somewhat puzzled, but on his return to England was still convinced of her affection towards him. He wrote endless letters, most of which went unanswered. He was certain that she would soon ask him to return and became increasingly despondent when she did not.

Because Anthony, a first-year university student, was recognised as having special problems, a female student was asked to 'befriend' him and offer help or support as necessary. Totally misinterpreting the motives behind her kindness, Anthony became convinced that she was in love with him and pursued her relentlessly until staff were forced to intervene, much to his resentment and incomprehension. Such naivety can at times be exploited by other people. Daniel, working in a computer office, was told by other staff that the boss's daughter 'really fancied him'. They persuaded him that if he telephoned her several times a day she would eventually admit to her feelings. After a few phone calls of this kind Daniel found himself in serious trouble, and it was only through his manager's intervention that he kept his job.

The Internet is a further possible source of problems for the unwary seeking companionship. Theo became involved with a young woman in America, with whom he chatted on a daily basis. She had suggested that he might come over to visit 'some time', and his parents were horrified when they learned that he had cashed in his various bank accounts in order to buy a plane ticket. Fortunately they were able to contact the young woman, who said the invitation was just a polite gesture, not an offer of accommodation or anything more. They explained the situation and she wrote back to him saying that, unexpectedly, she would be away when he visited. In recompense his parents managed to organise a package tour for him to Disneyland instead. Gerard, however, was less fortunate. He had been chatting with a 'nice man' on the Internet, and again had decided to go to the United States to visit him. However, when he arrived the address given was found to be false, and he became so agitated that the police were called. After a night in gaol he was put on the next plane back home, at considerable expense.

Women with autism can also find themselves in unexpected difficulties because of their failure 'to read' the necessary social cues. Judy, in her thirties, has a tendency to pour her heart out to anyone who will listen, giving intimate details of her past emotional, social and sexual life. On several occasions she had been happy to have men accompany her home in order that she could continue with her tales – but was then horrified if they made any sexual approaches. They, in turn, could become very unpleasant if they believed she had simply been 'leading them on'. No matter how she tried, she said, she could not work out whether people were trying to be sympathetic or wanting to exploit her, and she had reached the conclusion that it would be best for her never to talk to strangers again – a decision that would severely limit her social activities.

Another young woman Janice, was an expert swimmer and had absolutely no embarrassment about stripping off in public. In her rush to get into the swimming pool she was quite likely to change into her costume with little attempt at modesty. Moreover, even if she were fully dressed she had no hesitation in showing people her appendix scar or demonstrating bruises or marks anywhere on her body. Because she was physically attractive such behaviours often gave very misleading signals to her instructors or other people using the pool.

Donna Williams (1992) also recounts the time when she met a young man at the skating rink. After he had walked her home a few times he had kissed her and told her 'he wanted me to come and live with him one day'. Being rather tired of living at home, she piled her belongings into a taxi and arrived at his house.

'What!' he exclaimed in disbelief.
'You said you wanted me to live with you,' I explained.
'One day, I said,' he stressed.
Nevertheless I was there and that was that.

Social naivety, of course, is not confined to women. Marcus, a man in his thirties, horrified his parents when he told them that he always went to a certain city pub after he left work as the people there were so friendly. The pub was a well-known meeting place for gay men, but, although there was no indication that he had been taken advantage of in any way, his parents insisted that he stopped going.

Sandy, also in his thirties, was given a great deal of support from his cousin, who was an active campaigner for gay rights. On one occasion a friend of the cousin's made sexual advances towards Sandy, who complied with these. Later Sandy admitted that he had not wanted to do what was asked nor had he found it a pleasant experience; but he had not liked to say 'No' for fear of upsetting his cousin.

Other sexually unacceptable behaviours

In the case of less able people with autism, sexual problems tend to be associated with socially unacceptable behaviours. Ruble and Dalrymple (1993), found that that among a group of individuals, aged between nine and thirty-nine years, over half exhibited behaviours such as masturbation in public, taking off clothes, touching others in an unacceptable way, developing fierce attachments to particular members of staff, discussing inappropriate topics or looking up shorts or down shirts. If not dealt with appropriately, behaviours of this kind can lead to exclusion from a wide range of activities; there may also be repercussions for others. Josh, for example, would go through phases when he seemed to masturbate almost constantly. After an incident at the local swimming pool when he removed his bathers in full view of a mothers' and toddlers' club, all the clients at his day unit were banned from using the pool. Paul had had a fascination with female breasts since he was tiny, and as a grown man he still continued to try to stroke any 'well-endowed' women. On a day trip to the beach he had wandered up to a couple of elderly women in swimming costumes and caused such a furore that the whole group had to leave rapidly.

Infatuations with particular individuals can also give rise to problems. Jenny, a young woman in her late teens, developed a marked attachment for one of the male care workers at her day centre. If he were not there for any reason she would become extremely distressed, and whenever she saw him would rush up and embrace him, attacking anyone who tried to remove her. The care worker was moved to another centre in order to try to defuse the situation, but, enraged by this, Jenny then began accusing him of sexual abuse. It took many months before these accusations were completely disproved, but by then the man's career as a care worker was over.

Of particular concern is when the focus of attraction is young children. Realmuto and Ruble (1999), for example, describe a young man who was sexually aroused by young children, leading to his gradual exclusion from community activities and, ultimately, arrest by the police.

Dealing with problems of relationships

Choosing to be alone

Despite the frequent difficulties encountered in making and maintaining relationships, many people with autism – particularly those who are more able – do manage to develop effective coping strategies over time. Sometimes these simply involve *avoidance* of potential problems. Kanner, in his follow-up study, describes the types of rationalisations made by individuals to explain their lack of close relations. Activities such as dating were said to 'cost too much' or be 'a waste of money'. One man said he felt that perhaps he 'ought to get married but can't waste money on a girl who is not serious'. Kanner notes, too, that many seemed to feel frightened by any intimacy and that there was a 'sense of relief' in being able to excuse themselves in this way. Oliver Sacks also describes Temple Grandin as choosing to avoid close relationships rather than dealing with the confusion they would inevitably bring (Sacks 1993).

Donna Williams's precipitate move into her boyfriend's house led to both physical and sexual abuse, and for many years afterwards she avoided sexual relationships. She was also horrified if close friendships – which to her had no sexual component – became more serious. Describing the point at which her friendship with a boy called Tim suddenly became much more intense on his part she writes: 'It was like a slap in the face . . . he had killed off the sense of security I had found in him in one fell swoop' (Williams 1992).

Extending social contacts

One important way of reducing feelings of isolation and rejection is to try to improve general social contacts as far as possible. For many individuals the opportunity to mix more with people in their own age group, particularly if they include the opposite sex, can defuse the urgency for a close relationship. A focus on increasing the opportunities to make *contacts* with other people rather than directly on *relationships* offers a much greater chance of enriching the quality of people's lives. Often the apparently overwhelming desire for 'a girlfriend' can be substantially diminished as long as the individual concerned has more contact with people generally and is encouraged to fill their time as usefully as possible. Social-skills groups specifically for people with autism may also help those with shared interests to get together. Julian and Serena, for example, were both members of a social group for adults with Asperger syndrome. They discovered a mutual interest in landscape gardening, and now spend much of their free time visiting National Trust gardens together, an activity they had previously avoided because of the anxiety they had felt when visiting alone. Self-help groups such as Asperger's United or Internet sites specifically for people with autism and Asperger syndrome can also play an important role. Even if the individuals involved have few other social contacts, in this way they are at least enabled to relate to a small number of other people with similar problems and interests.

Avoiding potential problems from childhood

Many difficulties in adulthood could in fact be avoided if potential difficulties were recognised earlier in childhood. All too often it is behaviours that have been condoned or even actively encouraged in a young child with autism that give rise to major challenges in later life. Childish habits, such as taking off one's clothes in public or a fascination with others' feet or women's breasts, may be regarded with some indulgence in a three-year-old. In a 23-year-old they are likely to be viewed as sexually inappropriate or threatening. Such behaviours may continue either because the child or adolescent has no perception of their social unacceptability or, conversely, because they become aware of the attention that inevitably ensues. It can be difficult to find a more effective way of getting attention, for example, than marching up to an elderly woman on the bus and fondling her breasts!

Firm and consistent limitations on behaviours of this kind in childhood are the most effective way of avoiding problems in future. Clear and unambiguous policies on dressing or undressing in public, topics that should not be discussed with strangers, rules on when and where to masturbate, should all be introduced as early as is appropriate for the individual concerned. For example, Marcus's parents recognised that his fondness for touching women's earrings (whether he knew the individuals in question or not) could give rise to problems as he grew older. They did not wish to eliminate the behaviour completely as he seemed to gain so much pleasure from it. Instead, strict rules were laid down about *whose* earrings he could touch (mother's, aunt's grandmother's etc.) and *when* and *where* he could do so. Knowing that the behaviour was allowed under certain circumstances, he complied with these guidelines, and subsequently the behaviour has never given rise to particular problems. However, the first thing he did after getting a job as a paper boy was to pay for his own ears to be pierced!

Simple rules of this kind might also have avoided problems in the case of Adrien, a young man with no sense of personal space. Leaning up against people or pushing into them on his way to do something else caused only minor problems when he was small. However, when he became a well-built young adult, the same behaviours were viewed very differently. He has been arrested by the police on several occasions for alleged 'sexual assault', which have actually been incidents when he has pushed up against young women waiting at bus stops (either to get to see the timetable or 'Because I was cold').

Understanding sexual needs and sex education for people with autism

Surprisingly little research has been conducted into the sexual needs – or indeed the sexual understanding – of people with autism, but the studies that have been done suggest that sexuality is a far more important issue than is often recognised. Ousley and Mesibov (1991) found that among a group of high-functioning individuals with autism, males expressed more interest in dating and sexuality than females, although in fact 70 per cent of women had engaged in some degree of sexual activity with a partner compared to only 9 per cent of the men. Amongst groups of intellectually impaired adults with autism, masturbation tends to be the most common sexual activity, but sexually oriented behaviours involving other people have been reported in around 30–40 per cent (Haracopos and Pedersen 1992, Van Bourgondien *et al.* 1997, Realmuto and Ruble 1999). Nevertheless, Van Bourgondien *et al.* (1997) noted that many group homes forbade behaviours such as hugging and kissing among their residents. Konstantareas and Lunsky (1997) found that it was possible to obtain information regarding the sexual knowledge, understanding and experiences of individuals with autism and intellectual disabilities using appropriate questionnaires, and clearly this is an area that needs to be researched in much greater detail if the sexual needs of young people and adults with autism are to be better understood.

Although individuals' understanding of sexual issues is correlated with their intellectual ability (Konstantareas and Lunsky, 1997) even amongst more able adults there may be confusion about what is or is not sexually acceptable behaviour. This is hardly surprising, since as children and adolescents they are likely to learn little from their peer group (the source of most children's sexual knowledge) and parents tend to be occupied with too many other problems to devote time to their sexual education. However, because of their fundamental problems in *social* understanding, sex education may be even more important for them than for other children. The problem is that the instructional methods or materials that are appropriate for normal youngsters may be worse than useless for children with autism. Many mothers, for example, can recount tales of their autistic child divulging the contents of a 'sex lesson' loudly and publicly in the middle of a crowded store or bus.

Some of the sex education programmes that have been developed for use with people with more general learning disabilities may be adapted to meet the needs of children and adolescents with autism, and a variety of books and resource packs is available. Most attempt to teach students to recognise when behaviours are acceptable or not and when they might be in a vulnerable situation and need to say 'No', as well as providing basic information about preventing disease or unwanted pregnancy. *Sexuality and Mental Handicap* (1990) by Hilary Dixon is a useful source of teaching ideas and strategies, as is the picture guide by Hingsburger and Ludwig (1992) and the illustrated course by Atkinson *et al.* (1997) *I Have the Right to Know*. The themes covered in these manuals include recognition and awareness of body parts, menstruation and the menopause, masturbation, sexual relationships (including how to say 'No'), and sexual health, using contraceptives and avoiding the risk of AIDs and other infections. A particular advantage of many of the materials designed for people with intellectual impairments is that they are set firmly within the context of developing other social skills such as improving self-esteem, making decisions, understanding social roles, making friends and dealing with emotional feelings generally. Many make use of video instruction and include exercises involving role play, group discussions, practical advice and problem-solving, which can be helpful for people with autism.

When working with people with autism it will also be necessary to help them develop awareness of areas that present few difficulties for non-autistic students of similar intellectual levels. Why certain behaviours, such as following people or removing clothes in public may offend or frighten others; *what* other people will think of them if they do; *what* unwanted consequences may follow; all these will need to be made clear and explicit. Although written over twenty years ago, Melone and Lettick's (1983) very practical sex education programme for moderate to more severely impaired adults with autism can be very helpful. This focuses on basic topics such as the identification of body parts, aspects of personal hygiene, and appropriate social behaviours, ranging from how to relate to strangers and familiar adults to dressing appropriately or using public lavatories. The programme also covers issues such as physical examinations, so that if routine health checks are required the student knows what is expected and how to cope.

Teaching of this kind should, ideally, be offered on an individual basis, but it is also crucial that the fundamental rules about what is or is not acceptable be endorsed by everyone involved. If parents, staff and other carers keep consistently to the same guidelines, then it will be much easier for the person with autism to learn what is required. Structured teaching, clear guidelines and direct feedback combined with behavioural approaches when necessary, are the best means of avoiding major difficulties and establishing appropriate behaviours. It is important, however, to recognise that mistakes will occur from time to time. Instead of despairing when this happens, such occasions can be used as practical teaching sessions. Indeed, these may prove much more effective than abstract instructions. For example, after Josh was barred from the swimming pool for masturbating he became much more aware of the likely consequences of this in the future and the problem showed some reduction. Geraldine, a young teenager with a tendency to strip off all her clothes, also showed a reduction in the frequency of this behaviour when it resulted in her being temporarily banned from her favourite activity, horse riding.

Other more recent books about puberty, sex and sexuality that may be valuable for carers of children and young adults with autism include those by Scott and Kerr-Edwards (1999, *Talking Together about Growing up*, published by the Family Planning Association), and *Holding on, Letting Go* (Drury 2000).

Jerry and Max Newport's book *Autism/Asperger's and Sexuality: Puberty and Beyond* (2002) also helps to explode the myth that somehow people with autism are not sexual beings. Written by authors who themselves have Asperger syndrome it describes the problems that may be faced in this area – and more importantly – ways of overcoming them.

Improving the general quality of life

As is the case when dealing with many other social difficulties, a crucial aspect of any intervention programme for sexual problems is to improve the quality of life generally. Explaining to an adolescent youth that sexual relationships are not necessary for happiness and that many people live fulfilled and happy celibate lives is not likely to have a great impact, unless satisfaction can be gained in other ways. As well as making rules and regulations it is important to increase the number of alternative leisure activities as far as possible, especially those that offer the opportunity for meeting others. Clubs for people with disabilities, as well as mainstream activities suited to the individual's own special skills or interests, can prove remarkably helpful. Rupert a man in his early forties, eventfully joined a silverwork class and found he had a real gift in this area. He says he finds the activity 'far more therapeutic than going to see a psychiatrist', and because of the attention he gets from the rest of the class his oft-stated wish 'to find a good woman who will look after me' now seems to have subsided. John, a teenager whose pursuit of female companions led to his exclusion from a number of local clubs, eventually enrolled in karate classes in which he did extremely well. Again, the admiration he obtained from other members of the group seemed to diffuse his previously overriding goal of 'getting a girlfriend'.

For less able individuals, too, attention to the daily programme may have far greater impact on the frequency of unacceptable behaviours than any attempts at direct intervention. Observational studies, even of highly specialist and well-staffed units, often reveal that life for those attending or living in them is remarkably bleak (Murphy and Clare 1991). Under these conditions of deprivation it is not surprising that behaviours such as masturbation, tearing or stripping off clothing, or even sexual harassment of others, occur. An individually designed timetable, with attention to the structure of each part of every day, can be a crucial factor in reducing difficulties. Focus needs to be placed on the whole life of the individual, not on specific 'undesirable' or 'challenging' behaviours, which in many cases are indicators of deprivation and understimulation rather than pathology.

Dealing with sexual abuse

It is generally acknowledged that there is an increased risk of sexual abuse towards individuals with intellectual disabilities (Turk and Brown 1993, Baladerian 1991). Although there are no studies specifically assessing the frequency of abuse among those with autism such people may in fact, be particularly vulnerable because of their difficulties in fully understanding even the simplest of social interactions whilst at the same time appearing entirely normal. The ease with which such abuse can occur and the vulnerability of the victims is aptly illustrated in this quote by Wendy Lawson (1998).

> One day, in the autumn of my 9th year, I was on my way home from school. . . . The man came towards me and began to talk to me. . . . but I did not understand what he was saying. He mentioned a boy named Ben . . . and said that Ben was his son. Ben was one of the boys who bothered to talk to me at school. The man, probably around 30 years of age, asked me to do things that seemed strange to me. I wanted to go home.
>
> For several days after this the man met me on my walk. About a week later he took me to his house . . . (it) was dark and smelt musty. 'Why are the curtains closed?' I asked, 'Everyone knows that you don't close the curtains in the day time.'
>
> The man signalled me to come closer to him. While standing still he took my clothes off. 'It's too early for bed and my programs are on,' I said.
>
> 'This is a special time, just for us' the man said. 'When we have finished you can have a ride on my motor scooter.'
>
> This man took me to his home on several occasions. I don't know why I didn't say no, or why I didn't tell my parents. I think it had something to do with him being a grown up and me being a child. It felt good to have someone's attention, even though the things he did with me were strange. Somehow, I knew my behaviour was inappropriate but I did not know why. I did know that children did what grown ups told them to do.

The strategies described in this chapter and elsewhere, of developing appropriate 'rules' of social behaviour from an early age, and teaching individuals to 'say no' to suggestions they know to be wrong, can help to reduce these risks a little. Nevertheless, if abuse does occur it may be very difficult for someone with autism to explain what has happened or to prevent its reoccurrence, and even more difficult for them to talk about their feelings of distress. Often the only indication that abuse has occurred may be a sudden or marked deterioration in the individual's behaviour or mood. Howlin and Clements (1995) identified ways in which the trauma resulting from physical abuse might be better recognised in people with autism, and they describe a number of characteristics that were compatible with a diagnosis of post-traumatic stress syndrome. More recently, Sequeira *et al.* (2003) found that individuals with intellectual impairments and autism who were known to have experienced sexual abuse also exhibited symptoms associated with post-traumatic stress. Their symptoms were very similar to those shown by non-disabled victims of abuse and included social withdrawal, aggression, temper tantrums, agitation, a lack of interest in the environment, restlessness and overactivity, mood swings and self-injury. There was also a rise in stereotypes, including rocking and repetitive behaviours. It is clear that the sudden emergence of behaviours of this kind should be treated very seriously. Unfortunately, establishing exactly what has happened or who the perpetrator might be can pose enormous problems, especially if the victim is non-verbal. And, as is often the case with children, even if abuse is suspected it may be very difficult to prove. The picture books designed by Sheila Hollins for people with learning disabilities can be helpful in exploring some of the practical and emotional issues surrounding abuse, but professional help should always be sought in such circumstances. If abuse has occurred, counselling techniques developed for people with learning disabilities may help to minimise the resulting confusion and distress. If, as often happens, firm evidence is lacking, efforts may have to concentrate instead on ensuring that the environment is made as safe and secure as possible. Because the person with autism may be unable to explain what has happened, or to prevent it happening again, the onus of protection lies entirely on the carers, and this responsibility should never be treated lightly.

13 Enhancing independence

Variability of outcome

As is evident from previous chapters, the outcome for people with autism or Asperger syndrome is extremely variable. Some may spend all their lives in educational and residential accommodation with other autistic individuals; others continue to live a life of isolation and exclusion; still others go through university, find jobs, marry and raise families of their own. Innate linguistic and cognitive skills are major factors in influencing outcome, with good intellectual and language abilities being crucial predictors of outcome. However, these alone are not enough. In order to maximise opportunities for people with autism appropriate support structures are required to circumvent problems related to social and communication difficulties, to reduce the negative impact of ritualistic behaviours, and to enhance the potential value of special skills or interests. Recent research has identified strategies that can be used to improve functioning in these areas, and also provides evidence on how occupational and educational facilities can be improved in order to optimise assets and modify deficits.

There are a number of other aspects, not previously addressed, that are also important for outcome.

Raising expectations and changing attitudes

An article in the London *Times* some time ago (December 4 2001) discussed various case studies of individuals with autism or Asperger syndrome. However, these were not reports of disturbed children or adults with severely challenging behaviours but descriptions of world-famous individuals such as Albert Einstein, Andy Warhol, Ludwig Wittgenstein and Glenn Gould, all of whom appear to have shared the characteristics associated with autism. This article – and indeed a growing number of other accounts (cf. Paradiž 2002) – focuses on the *gifts* rather than the disadvantages associated with autism and Asperger syndrome and how, given the right circumstances, such gifts can be nurtured and encouraged. Articles such as this and the personal autobiographies of autistic people are, very gradually, beginning to change society's view of autism and how much can be achieved by individuals with this condition. Nevertheless, there is still a long way to go. Many of the contributors to Clare Sainsbury's recent book *Martian in the Playground* recall how at school they were assumed to be 'dumb', emotionally disturbed or just plain lazy by teachers and classmates alike. A large number of them were removed to classes for slow-learning children even though, in fact, their abilities frequently outstripped those of their mainstream peers. Wendy Lawson, Donna Williams and Temple Grandin all recall that as children they were considered 'weird', 'crazy' or 'stupid' by their peers and teachers, although eventually all went on to achieve highly successful careers. Even those who should know better are not immune to underestimating the skills of people with autism. Thus, Jim Sinclair, a man with autism who is now a powerful advocate for others with this condition, notes in his chapter for the book *High Functioning Individuals with Autism* (Schopler and Mesibov 1992): 'In May of 1989, I drove 1200 miles to the 10th annual TEACCH conference, where I learned that autistic people can't drive'!

Sinclair warns how the progress of people with autism may be severely restricted by the mistaken expectations, assumptions and prejudices of others – assumptions that often prove extremely difficult to shift. Thus, whilst it is important to avoid excessive demands or to have unrealistic expectations of what individuals are able to achieve, undervaluing their potential ability may do even more damage. The balance between under- and over-pressurising can be a difficult one to attain, but can be helped by thorough assessments of the individual's skills and deficits. Language and IQ tests alone are not sufficient (although they may be crucial in changing attitudes to individuals who have been mistakenly regarded as 'backward' or 'retarded'), and it is important to be aware that different tests may produce very different estimates of ability. Temple Grandin (1991), for instance, describes how although she scored at the ceiling of certain tasks, she performed at only average levels or below on those requiring speed of processing or symbolic functioning. Similar problems related to their very uneven profiles of skills and difficulties are also highlighted by many of the contributors to Clare Sainsbury's book. Assessments of social functioning and of the environmental factors that appear to enhance or limit learning are also required before any conclusions about potential abilities or appropriate placements can be made.

Lack of self-drive and initiative

At a recent meeting in London for people with Asperger syndrome organised by the National Autistic Society it was suggested that some of the individuals there might make their own arrangements to meet on a regular basis without the facilitation of Society staff. The suggestion was greeted with much incredulity, and as one young man, an undergraduate student, commented, 'You should know that you might as well ask us to go to the moon.' Even Temple Grandin describes how dependent she was on her mother and governess for developing her early abilities and on gifted, experienced teachers for teaching her to make the best use of her skills at school and college. 'Passive approaches', she asserts, 'don't work'.

Again, whilst it is important to avoid over-dependence on parents or teachers, unless the push for action – for achievement, for success – comes from other people it is unlikely to emerge spontaneously. Just as those who are least able will, if left to themselves, spend their time in stereotyped and ritualistic activities, so those who are more gifted may do little to utilise their gifts profitably unless directed how to do so.

It is important to recognise that this somewhat didactic approach sits rather uneasily within the current philosophy of care for people with disabilities. Normalisation principles of 'choice' and 'self-direction' may help typically developing individuals or those with learning difficulties to mature and flourish. For someone with autism, they may prove a major disadvantage. Clara Park (1992) describes how her daughter made no use of her exceptional drawing skills for many years. Only when she was given small amounts of money for each picture did her interest revive. It was not even that the money meant much to her, 'but numbers did, and she liked to see them rise in her checkbook'.

In order to be able to exercise choice individuals must understand what options are available, and in the case of people with autism it may well be necessary for families, teachers or carers to help them experience, first, what these options are.

Flexibility of provision

The importance of flexible and individualised educational and employment programmes has been discussed in earlier chapters, but a far

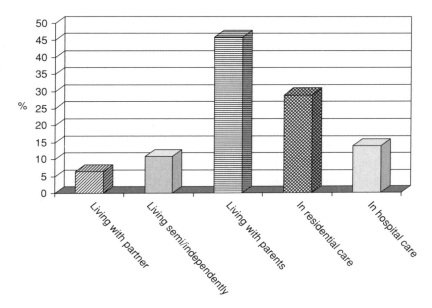

Figure 13.1 Residential outcomes in studies of adult outcome

wider range of supported and semi-independent living accommodation is also badly needed. The follow-up studies described in Chapter 2 indicate how few young adults are ready to leave home and live independently once they reach the age of eighteen, and even the most able tend to require some continuing support before they are able to cope alone. Among the sixteen follow-up studies included in that review the proportion of individuals living either alone or in semi-supported accommodation was only around 11 per cent, with 6 per cent being married or living with a partner; in contrast, the proportion still living with their families was 46 per cent, just under a third were in some form of residential facility and 14 per cent in long-term hospital care (see Figure 13.1).

There has undoubtedly been a steady growth in specialist provision for adults with autism over recent years. Recent information from the National Autistic Society in the United Kingdom, for example, lists over 130 different establishments that are either run by or affiliated to the NAS or which offer specialist provision for people with autism. Many more facilities for people with disabilities including those with autism can be traced via disability websites. Provision includes rural- and urban-based centres, offering day, weekly, respite or fully residential care. Some are designed specifically for individuals who are more able; others offer care to a wide range of clients within the autistic spectrum. Some are exclusively for people with autistic-spectrum disorders; others cater for a range of other conditions too. The following scenarios give examples of different types of provision and the success or failure of these, depending on the ability of the individuals concerned and the amount of support offered.

Autistic communities

In the 1960s and 1970s autistic communities offered the chance of a new life for many young adults who otherwise would have had little option but to go into hospital care. Such provision proved invaluable for many individuals and their families, offering for the first time environments that were uniquely able to cater for the needs of people with autism. The focus was on structured environments that could enable the young adult to continue to grow socially and emotionally whilst at the same time minimising behavioural disturbance. Generally there would be a few houses on one site, with up to thirty or forty autistic residents in total. Many were sited in extensive grounds in the countryside, offering opportunities for working in quiet horticultural settings. Examples are Somerset Court in southern England, some of the TEACCH centres in North Carolina, Benhaven in Massachusetts, and Bittersweet Farms in Ohio.

In recent years, however, there has been a swing away from facilities of this kind – partly because of their size, but mostly because of their isolation from ordinary community life. The possible disruption of family ties is also an issue. Gregory was a young man who had spent all his life in a small inner-city apartment with his family. On leaving his local 'autistic' school he moved to a community for adults with autism almost two hundred miles away, in the middle of the countryside. His parents had no car and could barely afford the cost of the trains and taxis required to visit him. The situation became particularly difficult after the sudden death of his father; and although his now elderly mother remains devoted to him, visits to her son have become progressively more difficult and are now only possible once or twice a year.

Small group homes for people with autism

Because of such problems large communities have tended to be replaced by specialist but smaller-scale housing for people with autism in communities offering better opportunities to develop links with local work and leisure facilities, and to maintain family ties. Again, the TEACCH organisation in North Carolina was at the forefront of such developments, which have now spread widely, both across the United States and many other countries.

For people with autism such units can offer many advantages and a great sense of security, as well as enabling them to develop new contacts outside. Even so, they are not without their difficulties. Because of their small size staffing can be a problem; the organisational structure may be too loose to allow the development of consistent management strategies; and staff may lack the skills to deal with more complex problems. For example, Anthony, a young man with a degree in mathematics, was admitted to a new group home for people with Asperger syndrome. The staff there had all previously worked with autistic clients but were not particularly familiar with the needs of individuals who were more able. Anthony, who had previously lived with his father, resented any attempts by staff to direct his activities, and there were also tensions between him and another resident. She would deliberately provoke him when no one was around, and he would respond by smashing crockery. Although no one was ever hurt, and despite the fact that his outbursts only occurred when he was distressed, he was warned that no further incidents would be tolerated. Some months later, goaded beyond endurance, he smashed another set of crockery and was immediately told to leave.

With adequate training and support for staff, and access to a wide range of educational, occupational and leisure facilities within the community, problems of this kind need not arise, and for many people with autism such provision offers the best opportunities for continuing development. However, because facilities of this kind are relatively expensive places remain limited and are currently available to only a minority of people with autism.

'Mixed' communities or group homes

One criticism frequently levied against autism-specific provision is that individuals with autism are unlikely to provide one another with much social stimulation, and therefore placement within a mixed client group is likely to be of greater benefit. In fact, there is little evidence to support the view that simply mixing with non-autistic, learning-disabled residents will enhance social functioning. Nevertheless, there is often considerable pressure from social services to 'integrate' people with autism into small, mixed group homes. This is obviously a much cheaper option than providing specialist autistic provision, but the lack of structure, poor understanding on the part of staff, emphasis on group activities, inadequate or inappropriate daily programmes and, often, lack of space can result in major problems.

Jane, for example, was moved by social services – and much against her parents' wishes – from a large but well-known residential establishment for people with autism on the grounds that it was too far from her local community. In her new placement, in a small group home in a run-down area of South-East London, she hated the lack of space, the noise and most of the other residents, and because of the proximity to her parents' house was constantly absconding back to them. In the end her behaviour became so disruptive she had to be excluded, and after lengthy and drawn-out battles with the local authority her parents eventually managed to have her transferred back to her initial placement, where she rapidly settled down once more.

Sometimes, however, mixed provision may be entirely suitable for someone with autism. Brendan was a young man who had became very disturbed in a large but rather noisy unit for people with autism. He had been transferred to a small group home where the staff, despite knowing little about autism, recognised his need for isolation and routine. His day, although not particularly stimulating, was very predictable, and he was befriended in the house by two middle-aged women with Down syndrome who took it upon themselves to look after him, checked that he did some routine chores and were not in the least disturbed by his obsessional behaviours. The lack of pressure resulted in a marked reduction in stress and anxiety, and after a while Brendan was able to regain some of the skills he had formerly lost.

Larger communities such as those run by the Home Farm Trust, Camp Hill, or other Steiner organisations may also be able to offer a supportive environment for people with autism. The calm atmosphere, variety of activities and sense of space can be very beneficial and, because residents have a mixture of different disabilities, there may be more opportunity for social interaction. Darren had been in one such establishment for several years, and over time had developed a very close relationship with a female resident of his own age. The staff, recognising the strength of their mutual attachment, provided them with plenty of opportunities to be together, and when the couple decided to get married they were given all the help they needed to move into a small apartment of their own on site. They now live happily together but with continuing support from the main centre whenever this is required. Unfortunately, the fact that people with autism can develop close relationships is not always recognised, or particularly welcomed.

Dave and Andrea, who lived in another group home, also announced their wish to become engaged. Andrea was rapidly moved to another residence in a different county, and the only time they were able to meet was when Dave went back to his parents' house at weekends. His father would drive many miles each weekend to pick up Dave and then Andrea, and then take them back to their respective establishments. Both became increasingly distressed by their enforced separation, but it was several years before their families were able to organise the practical and financial help needed for them to live together in a supported flat of their own.

On the whole, residential placements will only succeed if staff take seriously the necessity of understanding the special problems of people with autism as well as respecting an individual's specific needs; there must be recognition, too, of the importance of adapting the environment to meet these needs, and of the necessity for an appropriate degree of support and structure.

Living at home

Because of a lack of – or a dissatisfaction with – available provision, many adults with autism continue to be dependent on their parents long after most young people are likely to have left home. Although such arrangements may have short-term advantages, in the long term they can prove destructive for all concerned. Over-dependency can foster resentment and numerous relationship problems. It may restrict family life to an unacceptable degree. And, even if the arrangement is successful in most cases, it will not be possible for this to continue for ever. George was a man in his forties whose attempts to move into sheltered accommodation had always terminated after a few weeks. At the slightest problem his parents would suggest he move back home again, and once there the habitual patterns of arguments, nagging and occasional violence would resume.

In contrast, Jenny lived happily with her seventy-five-year-old mother, and they were a mutual source of companionship to each other. Although Jenny had a part-time job, her mother did all the cooking and housework, and at the age of thirty-five Jenny was unable to either make a cup of tea or use a washing machine. Tragically her mother died suddenly of a heart attack leaving her daughter entirely alone and unable to cope. Social services, who had had no previous contact with the family, were obliged to try to find her somewhere to live, but without any knowledge of her special needs organising a suitable placement proved extremely difficult.

Susie's parents had refused to let her go away from home after a brief and disastrous stay in a residential unit at the age of twenty. As the years went by she became more and more obsessional; self-stimulatory and self-injurious behaviours increased, and it was impossible to leave her alone at any time. Although social services offered some financial support, her parents have only a few hours of help a week at home and, as time passes, despite being virtually housebound and becoming increasingly anxious about what will happen to her when they die, they still cannot bear to let her go.

Brien also lived with his elderly mother after his father died. His father had always insisted that Brien 'would never go into a home' and that his brothers or sisters would ultimately take care of him – a wish none of them dared to contradict. However, his mother was much more realistic and began to arrange for brief periods of respite care in a nearby group home. Brien began to enjoy his weekends away, and gradually spent longer periods there each week. As his mother became more infirm he was able to move into the new home without distress, developing a close relationship with several members of staff. When his mother eventually died, not only was Brien well settled but he was surrounded by people whom he knew and trusted and who could offer him the consolation and support he needed.

Independent living

It is important to recognise that living independently is not synonymous with living without support. Most adults without a disability live independent lives, but they will nevertheless generally rely on a complex network of peers, family, work colleagues and neighbours in order to survive. However, unless a similar support network can be built up for people with autism living in the community, independence can in fact mean isolation, loneliness and rejection. Jenny was left financially secure by her parents when they died, and they had been promised by her social worker that she would continue to be offered support in her own flat. Nevertheless her social worker then left, financial cutbacks resulted in almost all non-emergency services being withdrawn, and it was only when an aunt visited and found Jenny to be living in filthy conditions, with hardly any food, that some minimal support was reinstated. However, because she is able to support herself financially, is of normal IQ and has a permanent job her need for ongoing help has never been acknowledged and major crises continue to occur at regular intervals.

Prior planning may help to overcome some difficulties of this kind. Matthew lived with his widowed mother until his thirties, but she then decided he had to become more independent. She bought him a small flat a few streets away where initially he just spent his weekends. As time went on he began to sleep there during the week, and gradually started to eat a few meals alone. His mother has built up a network of 'friends' and supporters for him locally, and although she continues to be very involved, she now feels that if she were to die he would be able to cope with this additional support. Gerald's parents knew that they would have to leave London because of health problems, but before they left they worked together with their son and local services to find him somewhere to live. Accommodation was provided by an organisation that supports people needing rehabilitation (for example, after a psychiatric illness). Although he has an independent apartment, a warden is available to check that all is well, and if problems arise these can be quickly dealt with. Gerald's parents remained living close by for a year or two after he moved, but were then able to move to the country without further difficulty.

Daniel, a thirty-year-old clerk, was not considered capable of living in a flat of his own, but a charitable organisation run by the church provided a bedsitter in a house for residents with other disabilities. Residents are taught to cook and care for themselves, as well as to cooperate in necessary group activities such as cleaning and shopping. A 'support tenant' lives on-site to provide help if necessary. After ten years there Daniel was able to move a flat of his own.

Although *gradually* increasing independence by such means is desirable, this may not always be possible. Although she was highly intelligent, Anna had always lived at home with her mother and was very dependent on her for all her needs. When her mother died suddenly social services became involved, although they had never previously been aware of her needs. They found her a tiny flat, helped her to furnish this and taught her basic cooking, shopping and cleaning. Surprisingly she coped very well, but as they became aware of her social isolation and vulnerability a key worker was allotted to 'call in' every few days and keep a check on possible problems. This degree of supervision was neither expensive nor time-consuming but, because it was offered *before* problems arose, has undoubtedly helped to prevent major difficulties.

The road to independence can also be helped by recently developed 'supported living' schemes. Although financial restraints on social services mean that such schemes are far less widely available and more limited than they should be, in principle they are designed to allow people with disabilities to choose where and with whom they will live, and, with help, to negotiate the package of support they will need in order to achieve independence. This may involve help with finances, shopping, domestic arrangements or travel; access to work, training or leisure opportunities; counselling or emotional support. Financial support is provided through statutory benefits, and a number of agencies can now offer assistance with supported living schemes of this kind. Further details should be obtainable from local social services, and Lowndes (1994) and Morgan (1996) describe how some such schemes have worked in practice.

Letting go

As the above examples indicate, there is no one ideal form of provision for people with autism. Different environments will be needed to suit different needs. Moreover not only is there a need for a wide range of provision but, it should also be possible for individuals to change their living environments as their needs or skills change.

A few basic guidelines can help to ensure that the transition from home to other accommodation is accomplished as smoothly and with as little disturbance as possible:

- Plans for adult life should be made as early as possible, preferably by the mid-teens. It is also important to ensure that planning meetings actually result in appropriate action. Anita's parents had been involved in formal planning meetings with local education and social services from the age of fourteen. In view of her very special needs (she also had physical and sensory problems) her key worker had guaranteed that suitable residential accommodation would be provided when she reached school-leaving age. Her parents spent a considerable amount of time exploring possible provision, and having found a unit that seemed fully to meet her needs had understood that a place would be available. A month before she was due to leave school at eighteen they were informed that the placement was too expensive and, anyway, being too far from home it no longer met social services' requirements. Her parents were told that as there was no local unit that could offer her an appropriate standard of care Anita would have to remain at home, with only part-time attendance at a day centre. It was almost two years later when Anita finally moved into residential care.
- In order to aid the transition from home, respite provision should be accessible, if needed, from an early age. This will enable the individual and his or her family to get used to separations, as well as providing a welcome break.

- There should be *no* expectations that other family members will take on the role of caring for the person with autism when parents die. No matter how willing they may be when younger, changing circumstances can make this impossible as they grow older, and expectations of this kind will only generate unnecessary guilt and possibly resentment.
- Social services *must* be made aware of the individual's potential need for care from an early stage. Usually this is not a problem in the case of those who are more handicapped and have always needed special provision. In the United Kingdom, for example educational and social services are obliged, officially at least, to begin joint planning for transition from the age of fourteen years. However, if someone has been through mainstream education, perhaps gone to university and had a job, it can be very difficult to persuade hard-pressed social services that, in their mid-twenties, they suddenly need special support or accommodation. Thus, even if there seems to be little reason to request help in the foreseeable future, it is important that the *potential need* is formally recognised.
- Seek out additional support networks. Somewhat paradoxically it is often most difficult to provide very able people with the help they need. Specialist provision is rarely appropriate, but living alone such people are at risk of being very isolated and may be vulnerable to abuse and prone to depression. If their parents are alive and well, they will generally be able to help out if problems occur. If they are not available, this role will need to be taken on by others. Again, social services support should be enlisted well before problems emerge. Charitable or religious groups, other family members, or a 'circle of friends' may also be able to offer ongoing help, as long as the basic support systems are already well established. Encouraging activities and interests outside the home can also help to ensure against loneliness and isolation.

Marriage and family relationships

It is clear that, although many people with autistic-spectrum disorders do marry and have children of their own, life as part of a couple can be difficult for them, their partners, their children and other family members. Reciprocity in relationships is particularly difficult to achieve when one of the partners is autistic, or both of them. However, better understanding of the nature of the problems and the genetic background to autism, and information about ways of minimising difficulties on both sides, can help to repair damaged relationships and to minimise – if not completely avoid – future problems. The books cited in Chapter 12 provide much practical advice and explanation, and have certainly been found helpful by couples seeking to understand and improve their relationships. Support groups for non-autistic partners (usually women) have also proved useful for some. In families where children *and* parents are within the autistic spectrum their shared experiences can mean that problems are better understood and tolerated, and mutual understanding may help to develop more effective – if sometimes rather unusual – management strategies.

In the case of someone with autism who is considering having children, it is important that they are advised about the genetic risks since there is evidence that a parent with this condition may well have an affected child. What the exact risks are is unclear, as is the likely severity of the disorder in offspring. Sometimes children may be more severely affected than parents, sometimes less so, but currently there is no way of predicting this. Some married individuals with autism (or their partners) make a deliberate decision not to have children because of the practical problems involved; child-rearing is difficult at the best of times, but for someone with social and communication problems, who is likely to be greatly disturbed by disruption to routine, the difficulties may be just too much. There are clearly no right or wrong answers here, but counselling may be useful in evaluating the practical and genetic implications of such a decision.

Developing other social networks

Many individuals with autism will not marry, but nevertheless this does not mean that life should be lonely and without interests. Sport and other leisure activities can be an important source of interpersonal contacts, and social interactions often develop more easily if built around specific activities that require cooperation and sharing. More able people with autism often find the activities provided by the local gym or sports clubs a helpful source of relaxation as well as offering the opportunity to meet other people with similar interests. Special-interest groups (which can involve anything from TV test cards to woodlice) also enable people to share their particular interests/skills with like-minded individuals. For those who are less able, sporting activities may need to be carefully modified but can lead to impressive gains in independence and social interactions. (See Evans 1995 for programmes especially adapted to meet the needs of people with autism.)

For many, church or religious groups can also provide much-needed support and social contacts. They offer the opportunity to be with other people but in a relatively structured, protective and predictable environment, with a common source of interest. High-functioning adults often express their relief at feeling they can trust people within the church group in a way they are unable to do outside and clearly feel much more at ease in these surroundings. For those who are less able, church groups may also prove more tolerant than society as a whole. Diana's constant chanting was quite accepted by the Jehovah's Witness congregation which she attended each week, and in her calmer moments they would also invite her to play the piano, much to her own and her parents' delight. Shared beliefs can also be a basis for long-term relationships or marriage, and a number of my own patients have met their partners through church organisations.

However, it is also important to be aware of the potential vulnerability of someone with autism to unscrupulous manipulation. Jonas, for example, collected information about religions of all kinds. When he wrote off to a new sect that had recently settled in his area, he was quickly encouraged to leave his parents and move in with them, handing over all his financial affairs to the control of the group. Despite his unhappiness he was unable to resist the psychological pressures they placed upon him to stay, and it was only with great difficulty that his parents were eventually able to get him away. Abuse by other extreme pressure groups can also be a risk. Janice, who loved animals, became involved in a local anti-vivisection organisation and was so distressed by their propaganda that she began to give them all her money. Despite the fact that she rapidly got into serious debt, it proved very difficult for her family to persuade her to discontinue her membership. The family were also very concerned that she might become involved in the violent protests that were the hallmark of this particular group.

Financial support

Finally, whatever plans for living, daily occupation or leisure are formulated, the one sure thing is that these will require financial support. For anyone with a disability resources are likely to be very limited, and this may well restrict their opportunities to make use of the facilities that are available. It is therefore essential that individuals, and their families or carers, are fully aware of the range of benefits to which they are entitled, and are given appropriate assistance to claim these. The Department for Work and Pensions now provides a very helpful website (and links to other relevant sites) explaining what benefits are

Table 13.1 Summary of other benefits that may be available to adults with autism in the United Kingdom (Figures published by the Department of Work and Pensions for people under 65, 2003. See also Table 9.2)

Name of benefit	Who can claim	Approximate amount
Invalid care allowance	Individuals spending at least 35 hours per week caring for someone receiving DLA at higher or middle rate	Depends on income, can affect amount of other benefits received. Currently £42.25 per week
Housing benefit	Paid by local councils to individuals who have problems paying rent	Variable, depends on earnings/savings etc. Maximum level is equivalent to 'eligible' rent
Blue badge scheme	Entitles owner to free parking in metered areas/yellow lines; and designated parking place outside own home	
Vehicle excise duty	Exemption for individuals receiving higher rate of DLA mobility component, or for vehicles used solely by that individual	
Council tax benefit	Rebates (or help with payment) for individuals with a disability and/or their carers	Variable, depends on earnings/savings etc. Maximum is full cost of tax
Social fund	DSS grants or loans to help with purchase of items that cannot be paid for out of regular earnings (bedding, laundry, cooking equipment etc)	Variable
Budgeting loans	DSS loans that help individuals to spread the cost of more expensive items (cookers/removal expenses)	Variable
Crisis loans	DSS loans for emergency payments when there is serious risk to family health and safety	Variable

Note: this table gives only a very brief account of possible benefits. Individual advice should be obtained (from the National Autistic Society, Citizens' Advice Bureau etc.) before any claims are made.

available, who is eligible to claim them, how much can be claimed and what restrictions etc. exist (www.dwp.gov.uk). Citizens' Advice Bureaux are also invaluable sources of advice on how and what to claim. Social security offices, too, should also be able to advise on entitlements (but see Toynbee 2003). Benefits that may be particularly relevant to people with autism are listed in Table 13.1 and work-related benefits in Table 9.2. Further details can be obtained from the National Autistic Society, who can also advise those wishing to draw up wills or trust documents in order to protect the financial interests of someone with autism.

Conclusions

Although in the course of this book a great deal has been written about the problems faced by individuals with autism, hopefully it is also clear that much can be done to overcome or minimise these difficulties. Despite sometimes overwhelming odds, many such individuals manage to achieve a great deal in their lives. In far too many cases, however, these achievements have been attained with very little professional support or guidance. In recent years experimental and research studies have greatly increased our understanding of the 'enigma' that is autism. If, in the future, such knowledge can be used to influence practice more widely, then the outlook for all those affected by this condition may be more positive. Thus, growing awareness of the communication and social deficits of young children with autism should result in the development of more appropriate and relevant teaching strategies. In particular, recognition of the need to encourage *functional communication* skills, at whatever level of competence is appropriate, may help to reduce the myriad problems that result from impairments in understanding and communication. Early training in social skills, and in the ability to understand how others think, feel or believe, may also have a long-term impact on individuals' acceptance into society. Also, support and advice for families *from the earliest years* on how to minimise the impact of obsessional and ritualistic behaviours may avoid the development of seriously disruptive behaviour patterns later.

However, in order to implement such strategies there needs to be much greater acknowledgement of the need to make professional and educational support available *before* problems become apparent. Once disruptive or inappropriate patterns of functioning are established they can become extremely difficult to change. Thus, intervention in early childhood to prevent or minimise the emergence of difficulties resulting from social, communication and ritualistic problems may have a major impact on the quality of life in later years. Financial support for early intervention and education is, in the long term, likely to prove far more cost-effective than crisis management in later life; and certainly, as far as autism is concerned, a focus on the prevention of problems will undoubtedly be more productive than fruitless searches for cures.

Bibliography

Abramson R., Wright H. H., Cuccara M. L., Lawrence L. G., Babb S., Pencarinha D., Marstella F. and Harris E. C. (1992). Biological liability in families with autism. *Journal of the American Academy of Child and Adolescent Psychiatry*, 31, 370–371.

ACE (Advisory Centre for Education), 1B Aberdeen Studios, London N5. www.ace-ed.org.uk

Akuffo E., MacSweeney D. A. and Gajwani A. K. (1986). Multiple pathology in a mentally handicapped individual. *British Journal of Psychiatry*, 149, 377–378.

American Academy of Pediatrics (1998). Auditory Integration Training and Facilitated Communication for Autism. *Pediatrics*, 102, 431–433.

American Psychiatric Association (1980). *Diagnostic and Statistical Manual of Mental Disorders (DSM-III)*, 3rd edn. Washington DC. APA.

American Psychiatric Association (1994). *Diagnostic and Statistical Manual of Mental Disorders (DSM-IV)* 4th edition. Washington DC. APA.

American Psychiatric Association (2000). *Diagnostic and Statistical Manual of Mental Disorders – Text Revision* 4th edn. (DSM-IV-TR). Washington DC. APA.

Anderson S. R., Avery D. L., DiPietro E. K., Edwards G. L. and Christian W. P. (1987). Intensive home-based early intervention with autistic children. *Education and Treatment of Children*, 10, 352–366.

Anderson S. R. and Romanczyk R. G. (1999). Continuum-based behavioral models, *Journal of the Association for Persons with Severe Handicaps*, 24, 162–173.

Andreasen N. C. (1979). The scale for the assessment of negative symptoms (SANS): conceptual and historical foundations. *British Journal of Psychiatry*, 155 (Suppl. 7), 59–62.

Asperger H. (1944). Autistic psychopathy in childhood. Translated and annotated by U. Frith (ed.) in *Autism and Asperger Syndrome* (1991). Cambridge. Cambridge University Press.

Aston M. (2003). *Aspergers in Love*. London. Jessica Kingsley Publishers.

Atkinson D., Gingell A. and Martin J. (1997). *I Have the Right to Know*, A course on sexuality and personal relationships for people with learning disabilities.

Attwood T. (2000). Strategies for improving the social integration of children with Asperger syndrome. *Autism: International Journal of Research and Practice*, 4, 85–100.

Attwood T., Frith U. and Hermelin B. (1988). The understanding and use of interpersonal gestures by autistic and Down's syndrome children. *Journal of Autism and Developmental Disorders*, 18, 241–257.

Ayres J. A. (1979). *Sensory Integration and the Child*. Los Angeles. Western Psychology Service.

Baladerian N. (1991). Sexual abuse of people with developmental disabilities. *Sexuality and Disability*, 9, 323–329.

Ballaban-Gil K., Rapin I., Tuchman R. and Shinnar S. (1996). Longitudinal examination of the behavioral, language, and social changes in a population of adolescents and young adults with autistic disorder. *Pediatric Neurology*, 15, 217–223.

Bandura A. (1969). *Principles of Behavior Modification*. New York. Holt, Rinehart & Winston.

Barnard J., Broach S., Potter D. and Prior A. (2002). *Autism in schools: crisis or challenge?* National Autistic Society.

Barnard J., Prior A. and Potter D. (2000). *Inclusion and Autism: Is it Working?* London. National Autistic Society.

Baron-Cohen S. (1988). Assessment of violence in a young man with Asperger's Syndrome. *Journal of Child Psychology and Psychiatry*, 29, 351–360.

Baron-Cohen S. (1995). *Mindblindness: An Essay on Autism and Theory of Mind*. Cambridge. MIT Press.

Baron-Cohen S. (2001). Theory of mind and autism: a fifteen-year review in *Understanding Other Minds, Perspectives from Developmental Cognitive Neuroscience*, 2nd edn. Baron-Cohen S., Tager-Flusberg H. and Cohen D. H. (eds), pp. 3–20. Oxford. Oxford University Press.

Baron-Cohen S. (2002). *Mind Reading – The Interactive Guide to Emotions, User Guide and Resource Pack*. Cambridge. University of Cambridge.

Baron-Cohen S. and Howlin P. (1993). The theory of mind deficit in autism: Some questions for teaching and diagnosis. In S. Baron-Cohen., H. TagerFlusberg and D. J. Cohen (eds.), *Understanding Other Minds: Perspectives from Autism*, (pp. 466–481). Oxford. Oxford University Press.

Baron-Cohen S., Joliffe T., Mortimore C. and Robertson M. (1997). Another advanced test of theory of mind: evidence from very high-functioning adults with autism or Asperger Syndrome. *Journal of Child Psychology and Psychiatry*, 38, 813–822.

Baron-Cohen S., Mortimore C., Moriarty J., Izaguirre J. and Robertson M. (1999a). The prevalence of Gilles de la Tourette's syndrome in children and adolescents with autism. *Journal of Child Psychology and Psychiatry*, 40, 213–218.

Baron-Cohen S., Scahill V. L., Izaguirre J., Robertson M. M. (1999b). The prevalence of Gilles de la Tourette syndrome in children and adolescents with autism: a large-scale study. *Psychological Medicine*, 29, 1151–9.

Baron-Cohen S., Tager-Flusberg H. and Cohen D. H. (eds.) (2001a). *Understanding Other Minds. Perspectives from developmental cognitive neuroscience.* Second edn. Oxford. Oxford University Press.

Baron-Cohen S., Wheelwright S., Skinner R., Martin J. and Clubley E. (2001b). The Autism-Spectrum Quotient (AQ): Evidence from Asperger Syndrome/ high-functioning autism, males and females, scientists and mathematicians. *Journal of Autism and Developmental Disorders,* 31, 5–17.

Bartak L. and Rutter M. (1973). Special educational treatment of autistic children: A comparative study. I. Design of study and characteristics of units. *Journal of Child Psychology and Psychiatry,* 14, 161–179.

Bauminger N. (2002). The facilitation of social-emotional understanding and social interaction in high-functioning children with autism: intervention outcomes. *Journal of Autism and Developmental Disorders,* 32, 283–298.

Bauminger N. and Kasari C. (2000). Loneliness and friendship in high-functioning children with autism. *Child Development,* 71, 447–456.

Beadle-Brown J., Murphy G., Wing L., Shah A. and Holmes N. (2000). Changes in skills for people with intellectual disability: a follow-up of the Camberwell Cohort. *Journal of Intellectual Disability Research,* 44, 12–24.

Bender L. and Faetra G. (1972). The relationship between childhood and adult schizophrenia. In A. R. Kaplin (ed.), *Genetic Factors in Schizophrenia,* Springfield, IL. C. C. Thomas.

Bernal J. (1994). *Psychiatric illness in learning disability* (unpublished article, St George's Hospital Medical School), London University.

Bettelheim B. (1967). *The Empty Fortress: Infantile Autism, and the Birth of the Self.* New York. Free Press.

Biersdorff K. (1994). Incidence of significantly altered pain experience among individuals with developmental disabilities. *American Journal on Mental Retardation,* 98, 619–631.

Biklen D. (1990). Communication unbound: autism and praxis. *Harvard Educational Review,* 60, 291–315.

Billstedt A., Gillberg C. and Gillberg C. (2003). Autism after adolescence, population-based 13–22 year follow-up study of 118 individuals with autism diagnosed in childhood (in press).

Birnbrauer J. S. and Leach D. J. (1993). The Murdoch early intervention program after 2 years. *Behavior Change,* 10, 63–74.

Boatman M. and Szurek S. (1960). A clinical study of childhood schizophrenia. In D. Jackson (ed.), *The Etiology of Schizophrenia.* New York. Basic Books.

Bolton P., Pickles A., Murphy M. and Rutter M. (1998). Autism, affective and other psychiatric disorders: patterns of familial aggregation. *Psychological Medicine,* 28, 385–395.

Bondy A. S. and Frost L. A. (1994). PECS: *The Picture Exchange Communication System Training Manual.* Cherry Hill, NJ. Pyramid Educational Consultants Inc.

Bondy A. and Frost L. (1996). Educational approaches in pre-school: behavior techniques in a public school setting. In E. Schopler and G. B. Mesibov (eds.), *Learning and Cognition in Autism*, (pp. 311–334). New York. Plenum Press.

Bowler D. M., Stromm E. and Urquhart L. (1993). Elicitation of first-order 'theory of mind' in children with autism. Unpublished MS, Department of Psychology, City University, London.

Bregman J. D. (1991). Current developments in the understanding of mental retardation. Part II: Psychopathology. *Journal of the American Academy of Child and Adolescent Psychiatry*, 30, 861–872.

Brown W. H. and Odom S. L. (1991). Strategies and tactics for promoting generalization and maintenance of young children's social behaviour. *Research in Developmental Disabilities*, 12, 99–118.

Burack J. A., Root R. and Zigler E. (1997). Inclusive education for children with autism: reviewing ideological, empirical and community considerations. In D. Cohen and F. Volkmar (eds.), *Handbook of Autism and Pervasive Developmental Disorders*, 2nd edn, (pp. 796–807). New York. Wiley.

Butera G. and Haywood H. C. (1995). Cognitive education of young children with autism: an application of Bright Start. In E. Schopler, and G. Mesibov (eds.), *Learning and Cognition in Autism*. New York. Plenum Press.

Campbell M. (1978). Pharmacotherapy. In M. Rutter and E. Schopler (eds.), *Autism: A Reappraisal of Concepts and Treatment*, (pp. 337–355). New York. Plenum Press.

Campbell M. and Cueva J. E. (1995). Psychopharmacology in child and adolescent psychiatry. A review of the past seven years. Part 1. *Journal of the American Academy of Child and Adolescent Psychiatry*, 34, 1124–1132.

Campbell M., Schopler E., Cueva J. E. and Hallin A. (1996). Treatment of autistic disorder. *Journal of the American Academy of Child and Adolescent Psychiatry*, 35, 134–143.

Capps L., Sigman M. and Yirmiya N. (1995). Self-competence and emotional understanding in high-functioning children with autism. *Development and Psychopathology*, 7, 137–149.

Carey T., Ratliff-Schhaub K., Funk J., Weinle C., Myers M. and Jenks J. (2002). Double-blind placebo-controlled trial of secretin: effects on aberrant behavior in children with autism. *Journal of Autism and Developmental Disorders*, 32, 161–167.

Carr E. G., Langdon N. A. and Yarbrough S. (1999). Hypothesis-based intervention for severe problem behavior. In A. C. Repp and R. H. Horner (eds), *Functional Analysis of Problem Behavior: From Effective Assessment to Effective Support*. Belmont CA. Wadsworth Publishing.

Charlop-Christy M. H., Carpenter M., LeBlanc L. A. and Kellett K. (2002). Using the Picture Exchange Communication System (PECS) with children with autism: Assessment of PECS acquisition, speech, social-communicative behavior, and problem behavior. *Journal of Applied Behavior Analysis*, 35, 213–231.

Chen S. and Bernard-Opitz V. (1993). Comparison of personal and computer-assisted instruction for children with autism. *Mental Retardation*, 31, 368–376.

Chesterman P. and Rutter S. C. (1994). A case report: Asperger's syndrome and sexual offending. *Journal of Forensic Psychiatry*, 4, 555–562.

Chez M. G., Buchanan C. P., Bagan B. T., Hammer M. S., McCarthy K. S., Ovrutskaya I., Nowinski C. V. and Cohen Z. S. (2000). Secretin and autism: a two-part clinical investigation. *Journal of Autism and Developmental Disorders*, 30, 87–94.

Chock P. N. and Glahn T. J. (1983). Learning and self-stimulation in mute and echolalic children. *Journal of Autism and Developmental Disorders*, 14, 365–381.

Chung S. Y., Luk F. L. and Lee E. W. H. (1990). A follow-up study of infantile autism in Hong Kong. *Journal of Autism and Developmental Disorders*, 20, 221–232.

Clare I. C. G. and Gudjonsson G. H. (1993). Interrogative suggestibility, confabulation, and acquiesence in people with mild learning disabilities (mental handicap): implications for reliability during police interrogations. *British Journal of Clinical Psychology*, 32, 295–301.

Clarke D. J. (1996). Psychiatric and behavioural problems and pharmacological treatments. In H. Morgan (ed.), *Adults with Autism*. Cambridge. Cambridge University Press.

Clarke D. J., Littlejohns C. S., Corbett J. A. and Joseph S. (1989). Pervasive developmental disorders and psychoses in adult life. *British Journal of Psychiatry*, 155, 692–699.

Clements J. and Zarkowska E. (2000). *Behavioural Concerns and Autistic Spectrum Disorders*. London. Jessica Kingsley Publishers.

COPE (2000). Compendium of Post-16 Education and Training in Residential Establishments for Young People with Special Needs. Trowbridge. Lifetime Carers.

Creak M. (1963). Childhood psychosis: A review of 100 cases. *British Journal of Psychiatry*, 109, 84–89.

Cumine V., Leach, J. and Stevenson, G. (1998). *Asperger Syndrome: A Practical Guide for Teachers*. London. David Fulton Publishers.

Cumine V., Leach J. and Stevenson G. (2000). *Autism in the Early Years: A Practical Guide*. London. David Fulton Publishers.

Cummins R. A. (1988). *The Neurologically Impaired Child: Doman-Delacato Techniques Reappraisal*. London. Croom Helm.

Dahl B. (1976). A follow-up study of a child psychiatric clientele with special regard to the diagnosis of psychosis. *Acta Psychiatrica Scandinavica*, 54, 106–112.

Dalrymple N. J. (1995). Environmental support to develop flexibility and independence. In K. A. Quill (ed.), *Teaching Children with Autism: Strategies to Enhance Communication and Socialization*, (pp. 219–242). New York. Delmar.

Darr G. C. and Worden F. G. (1951). Case report twenty-eight years after an infantile autistic disorder. *American Journal of Orthopsychiatry*, 21, 559–569.

Dawson G. and Osterling J. (1997). Early intervention in autism. In Guralnick, M. (ed.), *The Effectiveness of Early Intervention*, (pp. 307–326). Baltimore, MD. Brookes Publishing Co.

Dawson G., Osterling J., Meltzoff A. N. and Kuhl P. (2000). Case study of the development of an infant with autism from birth to two years of age. *Journal of Applied Developmental Psychology*, 21, 299–313.

Dawson G. and Watling R. (2000). Interventions to facilitate auditory, visual and motor integration in autism: a review of the evidence. *Journal of Autism and Developmental Disorders*, 30, 415–422.

Delacato C. H. (1974). *The Ultimate Stranger: The Autistic Child.* New York. Doubleday.

DeMyer M. K., Barton S., DeMyer W. E., Norton J. A., Allan J. and Steele R. (1973). Prognosis in autism: A follow-up study. *Journal of Autism and Childhood Schizophrenia*, 3, 199–246.

Department of Health (2001). *Valuing People: A New Strategy for Learning Disability for the 21st Century.* London. Department of Health White Paper.

Dewey M. (1991). Living with Asperger's syndrome. In U. Frith (ed.), *Autism and Asperger Syndrome*, (pp. 184–206). Cambridge. Cambridge University Press.

Directory of Social Change (2003). www.dsc.org.uk.

Dixon D. (1994). *From claim to appeal: a guide to disability appeal tribunals for disabled people and their advisers.* London. Disability Alliance ERA.

Dixon H. (1990). *Sexuality and Mental Handicap: An Educator's Resource Book.* Cambridge. Learning Development Aids.

Donaghy V., Bernal J., Tuffrey-Wijne I. and Hollins S. (2002). *Getting on with Cancer.* London. Gaskell Press/St George's Hospital Medical School.

Drury J., Hutchinson L. and Wright J. (2000). *Holding on, Letting Go: Sex, Sexuality and People with Learning Disabilities.* London. Souvenir Press.

Dugan E., Kamps D., Leonard B., Watkins M., Rheinberger A. and Stackhaus J. (1995). Effects of cooperative learning groups during social studies for students with autism and fourth grade peers. *Journal of Applied Behaviour Analysis*, 28, 175–188.

Dunlap G. and Fox L. (1999). A demonstration of behavioral support for young children with autism. *Journal of Positive Behavior Intervention*, 1, 77–87.

Durand B. M. and Crimmins D. B. (1988). Identifying the variables maintaining self-injurious behavior. *Journal of Autism and Developmental Disorders*, 18, 99–117.

Durand V. M. and Merges E. (2001). Functional Communication Training: A Contemporary Behavior Analytic Intervention for Problem Behavior. *Focus on Autism and Other Developmental Disorders*, 16, 110–119.

Dykens E., Volkmar F. and Glick M. (1991). Thought disorder in high-functioning autistic adults. *Journal of Autism and Developmental Disorders*, 21, 303–314.

Ehlers S., Nyden A., Gillberg C., Sandberg A. D., Dahlgren S. O., Hjelmquist E. and Oden A. (1997). Asperger syndrome, autism and attention disorders: A comparative study of the cognitive profiles of 120 children. *Journal of Child Psychology and Psychiatry*, 38, 207–217.

Einfield S. L. and Tonge B. J. (2002). *The Developmental Behaviour Checklist for Adults* (DBC-A). University of New South Wales and Monash University.

Eisenberg L. (1956). The autistic child in adolescence. *American Journal of Psychiatry*, 1112, 607–612.

Eisenberg L. (1972). The classification of childhood psychosis reconsidered. *Journal of Autism and Childhood Schizophrenia*, 2, 338–342.

Eisenmajer R., Prior M., Leekham S., Wing L., Gould J., Welham M. and Ong B. (1996). Comparison of clinical symptoms in autism and Asperger's disorder. *Journal of the American Academy of Child and Adolescent Psychiatry*, 35, 1523–1531.

Elliott R. O., Dobbin A. R., Rose G. D. and Soper H. V. (1994). Vigorous aerobic exercise versus general motor training: Effects on maladative and stereotypic behavior of adults with autism and mental retardation. *Journal of Autism and Developmental Disorders*, 25, 565–576.

Evans G. (1995). Leisure activities for people with autism. In P. Howlin, R. Jordan and G. Evans, *Life Skills for People with Autism*. Distance-learning course, University of Birmingham School of Education.

Evans J., Castle F. and Barraclough S. (2001). Making a difference: early interventions for children with autistic spectrum disorders. Local Government Association. NFER.

Everall I. P. and Le Couteur A. (1990). Fire-setting in an adolescent boy with Asperger's syndrome. *British Journal of Psychiatry*, 157, 284–287.

Fenske E. C., Zalenki S., Krantz P. J. and McClannahan L. E. (1985). Age at intervention and treatment outcome for autistic children in a comprehensive intervention program. *Analysis and Intervention in Developmental Disabilities*, 5, 49–58.

Findling R. L., Maxwell K., Scotese-Wojtila L., Husang J., Yamashita T. and Wiznitzer M. (1997). High-dose pyridoxine and magnesium administration in children with autistic disorder: An absence of salutary effects in a double-blind, placebo-controlled study. *Journal of Autism and Developmental Disabilities*, 27, 467–478.

Fine J., Bartolucci G., Szatmari P. and Ginsberg G. (1995). Cohesive discourse in pervasive developmental disorders. *Journal of Autism and Developmental Disorders*, 14, 315–329.

Fombonne E. (1999). The epidemiology of autism: a review. *Psychological Medicine*, 29, 769–786.

Fombonne E. (2001). What is the prevalence of Asperger disorder? *Journal of Autism and Developmental Disorder*, 31, 363–364.

Fombonne E. (2003). Epidemiological surveys of autism and other pervasive developmental disorders: an update. *Journal of Autism and Developmental Disorders*, 33, 365–382.

Frith U. (1991). *Autism and Asperger Syndrome*. Cambridge. Cambridge University Press.

Further and Higher Education Act (1992). London. Her Majesty's Stationery Office.

Gaboney P. (1993). *Coping with Challenging Behaviour*. Unpublished MS. Portfield School. Hampshire, UK.

Gabriels R. L. and Hill D. E. (2001). *Autism – From Research to Individualized Practice*. London and Philadelphia. Jessica Kingsley Publishers.

Gerland G. (1997). *A Real Person – Life on the Outside*. London. Souvenir Press.

Ghaziuddin M. and Butler E. (1998). Clumsiness in autism and Asperger Syndrome: a further report. *Journal of Intellectual Disabilities Research*, 42, 43–48.

Ghaziuddin M., Butler E., Tsai L. and Ghaziuddin N. (1994). Is clumsiness a marker for Asperger's Syndrome? *Journal of Intellectual Disabilities Research*, 38, 519–527.

Ghaziuddin M., Ghaziuddin N. and Greden J. (2002). Depression in Persons with Autism: Implications for Research and Clinical Care. *Journal of Autism and Developmental Disorders*, 32, 299–306.

Ghaziuddin M. and Gerstein L. (1996). Pedantic speaking style differentiates Asperger syndrome from high-functioning autism. *Journal of Autism and Developmental Disorders*, 26, 585–595.

Ghaziuddin M., Leininger L. and Tsai L. (1995a). Brief report: thought disorder in Asperger syndrome: comparison with high-functioning autism. *Journal of Autism and Developmental Disorders*, 25, 311–317.

Ghaziuddin M., Shakal J. and Tsai L. (1995b). Obstetric factors in Asperger Syndrome: comparison with high-functioning autism. *Journal of Intellectual Disabilities Research*, 39, 538–543.

Ghaziuddin M., Tsai L. Y. and Ghaziuddin N. (1991). Brief report. Violence in Asperger Syndrome: A critique. *Journal of Autism and Developmental Disorders*, 21, 349–354.

Ghaziuddin M., Tsai L. Y. and Ghaziuddin N. (1992a). Brief report: A comparison of the diagnostic criteria for Asperger's Syndrome. *Journal of Autism and Developmental Disorders*, 22, 643–651.

Ghaziuddin M., Tsai L. Y. and Ghaziuddin N. (1992b). Co-morbidity of autistic disorder in children and adolescents. *European Journal of Child and Adolescent Psychiatry*, 1, 209–213.

Ghaziuddin M., Weidmer-Mikhail E. and Ghaziuddin N. (1998). Comorbidity in Asperger Syndrome: a preliminary report. *Journal of Intellectual Disability Research*, 42, 279–283.

Ghaziuddin M., Ghaziuddin N. and Greden J. (2002). Depression in Persons with Autism: Implications for Research and Clinical Care. *Journal of Autism and Developmental Disorders*, 32, 299–306.

Gilchrist A., Green J., Cox A., Rutter M. and Le Couteur A. (2001). Development and current functioning in adolescents with Asperger Syndrome: A comparative study. *Journal of Child Psychology and Psychiatry*, 42, 227–240.

Gillberg C. (1984). Infantile autism and other childhood psychoses in a Swedish urban region: Epidemiological aspects. *Journal of Child Psychology and Psychiatry*, 25, 35–43.

Gillberg C. (1992). Epilepsy. In C. Gillberg and M. Coleman (eds.), *The Biology of the Autistic Syndromes*, 2nd edn (pp. 60–73). Oxford. MacKeith Press.

Gillberg C. (1985). Asperger's syndrome and recurrent psychosis – a case study. *Journal of Autism and Developmental Disorders*, 15, 389–397.

Gillberg C. and Coleman M. (2000). *The Biology of the Autistic Syndromes*, 3rd edition, Oxford. MacKeith Press.

Gillberg C. and Gillberg I. C. (1989). Asperger's syndrome: Some epidemiological considerations: A research note. *Journal of Child Psychology and Psychiatry*, 30, 631–638.

Gillberg C., Gillberg C., Råstam M. and Wentz E. (2001). The Asperger Syndrome (and high functioning autism) Diagnostic Interview (ASDI): a preliminary study of a new structured clinical interview. *Autism: International Journal of Research and Practice*, 5, 57–66.

Gillberg C. and Steffenberg S. (1987). Outcome and prognostic factors in infantile autism and similar conditions: a population-based study of 46 cases followed through puberty. *Journal of Autism and Developmental Disorders*, 17, 272–288.

Goldfarb W. (1961). *Growth and Change of Schizophrenic Children*. New York. Wiley.

Goldstein H. (2002). Communication intervention for children with autism: a review of treatment efficacy. *Journal of Autism and Developmental Disorders*, 32, 373–396.

Graham J. (1999). *The INTERACT Centre*. Hanwell Community Centre: London.

Grandin T. (1991). An inside view of autism. In E. Schopler and E. B. Mesibov (eds.), *High-Functioning Individuals with Autism*, (pp. 10–124). New York. Plenum Press.

Grandin T. (1995). The learning style of people with autism. An autobiography. In K. A. Quill (ed.), *Teaching Children with Autism: Strategies to Enhance Communication and Socialization*, (pp. 33–52). New York. Delmar.

Gray C. A. (1995). Teaching children with autism to 'read' social situations. In K. A. Quill (ed.), *Teaching Children with Autism: Strategies to Enhance Communication and Socialization*, (pp. 219–242). New York. Delmar.

Gray C. (1998). Social stories and comic strip conversations with students with Asperger Syndrome and High Functioning Autism in E. Schopler., G. Mesibov and Kunce L. J. (eds.), *Asperger's Syndrome or High Functioning Autism?* New York. Plenum.

Gray C. and White A. L. (2002). *My Social Stories Book*. London. Jessica Kingsley Publishers.

Green G. (1994). The quality of the evidence. In H. C. Shane (ed.), *Facilitated Communication: the Clinical and Social Phenomenon*, (pp. 157–226). San Diego, CA. Singular Press.

Greenberg M. S. and Beck A. T (1990). *Cognitive apporaches to psychotherapy: Theory therapy*. In R. Plutchik and H. Kellerman (eds.), Emotion and Psychopathology, 5 (pp. 177–194). San Diego, CA. Academic Press.

Greenspan S. J. and Wieder S. (1999). A functional developmental approach to autism spectrum disorders. *Journal of the Association for Persons with Severe Handicap*, 3, 147–161.

Gresham F. M. and Macmillan D. L. (1998). Early Intervention Project: can its claims be substantiated and replicated? *Journal of Autism and Developmental Disorders*, 28, 5–13.

Gringras P. (2000). Practical paediatric psychopharmacological prescribing in autism: the potential and the pitfalls. *Autism: International Journal of Research and Practice*, 4, 229–243.

Gunsett R. P., Mulick J. A., Fernald W. B. and Martin J. L. (1989). Brief report: Indications for medical screening prior to behavioral programming for severely and profoundly mentally retarded clients. *Journal of Autism and Developmental Disorders*, 19, 167–172.

Haddock G. and Slade P. D. (eds.) (1995). *Cognitive-Behavioural Interventions with Psychiatric Disorders*. London. Routledge.

Hadwin J., Baron-Cohen S., Howlin P. and Hill K. (1996). Can we teach children with autism to understand emotions, belief and pretence? *Development and Psychopathology*, 8, 345–365.

Happé F. G. E. (1994). Current psychological theories of autism: the 'Theory of Mind' account and rival theories. *Journal of Child Psychology and Psychiatry*, 35, 215–230.

Haracopos D. and Pendersen L. (1992). Sexuality and autism: A nationwide survey in Demark. Copenhagen. Preliminary report, unpublished manuscript.

Hardy C., Ogden J., Newman J. and Cooper S. (2002). Autism and ICT: A Guide for Teachers and Parents. London. David Fulton Publishers.

Hare D., Jones J. P. R. and Paine C. (1999). Approaching reality: the use of personal construct assessment in working with people with Asperger syndrome. *Autism: International Journal of Research and Practice*, 3, 165–176.

Harris S. L. and Handleman J. S. (2000). Age and IQ at intake as predictors of placement for young children with autism: A four- to six-year follow-up. *Journal of Autism and Developmental Disorders*, 30, 137–141.

Harris S. L., Handleman J. S. and Alessandri M. (1990). Teaching youths with autism to offer assistance. *Journal of Applied Behavior Analysis*, 23, 297–305.

Harris S. L., Handleman J. S., Belchic J. and Glasberg B. (1995). The Vineland Adaptice Behavior Scales for young children with autism. *Special Services in the Schools*, 10, 45–52.

Harris S., Handleman J. S., Gordon R., Kristoff B. and Fuentes F. (1991). Changes in cognitive and language functioning of preschool children with autism. *Journal of Autism and Developmental Disorders*, 21, 281–290.

Harrison J. (1996). Accessing further education: views and experiences of FE students with learning difficulties and/or disabilities. *British Journal of Special Education*, 23, 187–196.

Heavey L., Phillips W., Baron-Cohen S. and Rutter M. (2000). The Awkward Moments Test: A Naturalistic Measure of Social Understanding in Autism. *Journal of Autism and Developmental Disorders*, 30, 225–236.

Hermelin B. (2001). *Bright Splinters of the Mind. A Personal Story of Research with Autistic Savants.* London. Jessica Kingsley Publishers.

Hesmondhalgh M. and Breakey C. (2001). *Access and Inclusion for Children with Autistic Spectrum Disorders.* London. Jessica Kingsley Publishers.

Hingsburger D. and Ludwig S. (1992). *Being sexual: An illustrated series of sexuality and relationships.* Toronto: SEICCAN.

Hirtz D., Berg A., Bettis D., Camfield C., Camfield P., Crumrine P., Gralliard W. D., Schneider S. and Shinnar S. (2003). Practice parameter: Treatment of the child with a first unprovoked seizure. *American Academy of Neurology*, 60, 166–175.

Hobson P. (2002). *The Cradle of Thought.* London. Macmillan.

Hodgdon L. (1996). *Visual Strategies for Improving Communication. Volume 1: Practical Supports for School and Home.* Troy, MI. QuirkRoberts.

Holliday Willey L. (1999). *Pretending to be Normal.* London. Jessica Kingsley Publishers.

Holliday Willey L. (2001). *Asperger Syndrome in the Family.* London. Jessica Kingsley Publishers.

Hollins S., Clare I. and Murphy G. (1996). *You're Under Arrest.* Books Beyond Words. London. Gaskell Press/St George's Hospital Medical School.

Hollins S. and Curran J. (1996). *Depression in People with Learning Disabilities.* Leaflet for the 'Defeat Depression' Campaign. London. Royal College of Psychiatrists and Down Syndrome Association.

Hollins S., Horrocks C. and Sinason V. (2002). *Mugged.* London. Books Beyond Words. Gaskell Press/St George's Hospital Medical School.

Hollins S. and Howlin P. (1996). Learning Disability and Autism. *Medicine International*, 24, 47–49.

Hollins S. and Hutchinson D. (1993). *A New Home in the Community.* London. Sovereign Series.

Hollins S., Murphy G. and Clare I. (1996). *You're on Trial.* London. Books Beyond Words. Gaskell Press/St George's Hospital Medical School.

Hollins S. and Roth T. (1994). *Hug Me – Touch Me.* London. Sovereign Series.

Hollins S. and Sinason V. (1992). *Jenny Speaks Out.* London. Books Beyond Words. St George's Hospital Medical School.

Hollins S., Sinason V. and Boniface J. (1994). *Going to Court.* London. Gaskell Press/St George's Hospital Medical School.

Hollins S. and Sireling L. (1994). *When Mum Died/When Dad Died.* London. Sovereign Series.

Horvath K., Stefanotos G., Sokolski K. N., Wachtel R., Nabors L. and Tildon T. (1998). Improved social and language skills after Secretin administration in patients with autistic spectrum disorders, *Journal of the Association of the Academy of Minority Physicians*, 9, 9–15.

Howlin P. (1996a). *Auditory Integration Training. Report on the Light and Sound Centre.* London. National Autistic Society Publications.

Howlin P. (1996b). Asperger Syndrome: Differential diagnosis and current treatment strategies. *Directions in Psychiatry*, 16, no. 20, 1–12.

Howlin P. (1996c). Some approaches to modifying problem behaviours in autism. Occasional Papers, no 13: *Advances in the Assessment and Management of Autism*. London. Association of Child Psychology and Psychiatry.

Howlin P. (1997a). Recent advances in psychological understanding and treatment for people with autism. *Advances in Psychiatric Treatment*, 3, 94–102.

Howlin P. (1997b). *Autism: Preparing for Adulthood*. London. Routledge.

Howlin P. (1997c). Prognosis in autism: do specialist treatments affect outcome? *European Child and Adolescent Psychiatry*, 6, 55–72.

Howlin P. (1998a). Practitioner Review: Psychological and educational treatments of autism. *Journal of Child Psychology and Psychiatry*, 39, 307–336.

Howlin P. (1998b). *Children with Autism and Asperger Syndrome: A Guide for Practitioners and Carers*. London. Wiley.

Howlin P. (2002a). Special educational treatment. In M. Rutter and E. Taylor (eds.), *Child and Adolescent Psychiatry: Modern Approaches*, 4th edn. Oxford. Blackwell.

Howlin P. (2002b). Interventions and Outcome in Autism. In Singh N. N., Ollendick T. H. and Singh A. N. (eds), *International Perspectives on Child Adolescent Mental Health Volume 2. Selected proceedings of the Second International Conference on Child and Adolescent Mental Health, Kuala Lumpur, Malaysia*. London. Elsevier Science.

Howlin P. (2002c). Autism-Related Disorders. In O'Brien G., *Behavioural Phenotypes in Clinical Practice*. London. Mac Keith Press.

Howlin P. (2003). Outcome in high-functioning adults with autism with and without early language delays: Implications for the differentiation between autism and Asperger syndrome. *Journal of Autism and Developmental Disorders*, 33, 3–13.

Howlin P. and Asgharian A. (1999). The diagnosis of autism and Asperger syndrome: findings from a survey of 770 families. *Developmental Medicine and Child Neurology*, 41, 834–839.

Howlin P., Baron-Cohen S., Hadwin J. and Swettenham J. (1998). *Teaching Children with Autism to Mindread. A Practical Manual for Parents and Teachers*. Chichester. Wiley.

Howlin P. and Clements J. (1995). Is it possible to assess the impact of abuse on children with pervasive developmental disorders? *Journal of Autism and Developmental Disorders*, 25, 1–17.

Howlin P., Goode S., Hutton J. and Rutter M. (2004). Adult outcome for children with autism. *The Journal of Child Psychology and Psychiatry*, 45, 212–229.

Howlin P., Mawhood L. M. and Rutter M. (2000). Autism and Developmental Receptive Language Disorder – A follow-up comparison in early adult life. II, social, behavioural and psychiatric outcomes. *Journal of Child Psychology and Psychiatry*, 41, 561–578.

Howlin P. and Peacock G. (1994). Supported employment. *Communication*, 28, 2, 3–4.

Howlin P. and Rutter M. (1987). *Treatment of autistic children*. Chichester. Wiley.

Howlin P. and Yates P. (1999). The potential effectiveness of social skills groups for adults with autism. *Autism: International Journal of Research and Practice*, 3, 299–307.

Hoyson M., Jamieson B. and Strain P. S. (1984). Individualised group instruction of normally developing and autistic-like children: A description and evaluation of the LEAP curriculum model. *Journal of the Division of Early Childhood*, 8, 157–171.

Hoyson M., Jamieson B. and Strain P. S. (1984). Individualised group instruction of normally developing and autistic-like children: A description and evaluation of the LEAP curriculum model. *Journal of the Division of Early Childhood*, 8, 157–171.

Hughes-Brown C. and Rusch F. R. (1996). People with challenging behaviour in integrated work environments. In *People with Disabilities Who Challenge the System*, D. H. Lehr and F. Bow (eds) (pp. 307–330). Baltimore, MD. Paul H. Brookes.

Hutton J. (1998). *Cognitive Decline and New Problems Arising in Association with Autism*. Doctor of Clinical Psychology Thesis: Institute of Psychiatry, University of London.

Irlen H. (1995). Viewing the world through rose-tinted glasses. *Communication*, 29, 8–9.

Isager T., Mouridsen S. E. and Rich B. (1999). Mortality and causes of death in pervasive developmental disorders. *Autism: International Journal of Research and Practice*, 3, 7–16.

Iwanaga R., Kawasaki C. and Tsuchida R. (2000). Comparison of sensory-motor and cognitive function between autism and Asperger syndrome in pre-school children. *Journal of Autism and Developmental Disorders*, 30, 169–174.

Jacobson J. W., Mulick J. A. and Schwartz A. A. (1995). A history of facilitated communication: Science, pseudoscience, and anti-science. *American Psychologist*, 50, 750–765.

Jolliffe T., Lansdown R. and Robinson T. (1992). *Autism: A Personal Account*. London. National Autistic Society.

Jones R. S. P. and McCaughey R. E. (1992). Gentle teaching and applied behavior analysis. A critical review. *Journal of Applied Behavior Analysis*, 25, 853–867.

Jordan R. and Jones G. (1999). *Meeting the Needs of Children with Autistic Spectrum Disorders*. London. David Fulton Publishers.

Jordan R. and Powell S. (1995). *Understanding and Teaching Children with Autism*. Chichester. Wiley.

Kamps D. M. Barbetta P. M., Leonard B. R. and Delquardri J. (1994). Classwide peer tutoring: An integration strategy to improve reading skills and promote peer interactions among students and promote peer interactions among students with autism and general education peers. *Journal of Applied Behavior Analysis*, 27, 49–61.

Kanner L. (1943). Autistic disturbances of affective contact. *Nervous Child*, 2, 217–250.

Kanner L. (1946). Irrelevant and metaphorical language in early infantile autism. *American Journal of Psychiatry*, 103, 242–245.

Kanner L. (1949). Problems of nosology and psychodynamics of early infantile autism. *American Journal of Orthopsychiatry*, 19, 416–426.

Kanner J. (1951). The conception of wholes and parts in early infantile autism. *American Journal of Psychiatry*, 108, 23–26.

Kanner L. (1971). Follow-up study of eleven autistic children originally reported in 1943. *Journal of Autism and Childhood Schizophrenia*, 1, 119–145.

Kanner L. (1973). *Childhood Psychosis: Initial Studies and New Insights*. New York. Winston/Wiley.

Kanner L. and Eisenberg L. (1956). Early infantile autism 1943–1955. *American Journal of Orthopsychiatry*, 26, 55–65.

Kaufman B. N. (1977). *To Love is To Be Happy With*. New York. Fawcett Crest.

Kaufman B. N. (1981). *A Miracle to Believe in*. New York. Doubleday.

Keel J. H., Mesibov G. and Woods A. V. (1997). TEACCH-supported employment programme. *Journal of Autism and Developmental Disorders*, 27, 3–10.

Kerbeshian J. and Burd L. (1987). Are schizophreniform symptoms present in attenuated form in children with Tourette's disorder and other developmental disorders? *Canadian Journal of Psychiatry*, 32, 123–135.

Kerbeshian J. and Burd L. (1996). Case Study: Comorbidity among Tourette's Syndrome, Autistic Disorder, and Bipolar Disorder. *Journal of the American Academy of Child and Adolescent Psychiatry*, 35, 681–685.

Kerbeshian J., Burd L., Randall T., Martsolf J. and Jalal S. (1990). Autism, profound mental retardation and atypical bipolar disorder in a 33-year-old female with a deletion of 15q12. *Journal of Mental Deficiency Research*, 34, 205–210.

Kern J. K., Miller V. S., Evans P. A. and Trivedi M. H. (2002). Efficacy of Porcine Secretin in Children with Autism and Pervasive Developmental Disorder. *Journal of Autism and Developmental Disorder*, 32, 153–160.

Kilsby M. and Beyer S. (1996). Engagement and interactions: A comparison between supported employment and day service provision. *Journal of Intellectual Disability Research*, 40, 348–358.

Kim J. A., Szatmari P., Bryson S., Streiner D. L. and Wilson F. (2000). The prevalence of anxiety and mood problems among children with autism and Asperger syndrome. *Autism: International Journal of Research and Practice*, 4, 117–132.

Kitahara K. (1983). *Daily Life Therapy* (Vol. 1). Tokyo. Musashino Higashi Gakuen School.

Kitahara K. (1984a). *Daily Life Therapy* (Vol. 2). Tokyo. Musashino Higashi Gakuen School.

Kitahara K. (1984b). *Daily Life Therapy* (Vol. 3). Tokyo. Musashino Higashi Gakuen School.

Klin A., Jones W., Schultz R., Volkmar F. and Cohen D. (2002). Visual fixation patterns during viewing of naturalistic social situations as predictors of social competence in individuals with autism. *Archives of General Psychiatry*, 59, 809–16.

Klin A., Volkmar F. R. and Sparrow S. S. (eds.) (2000). *Asperger Syndrome.* New York. Guildford Press.

Klin A., Volkmar F. R., Sparrow S. S., Cicchetti D. V. and Rourke B. P. (1995). Validity and neuropsychological characterization of Asperger syndrome: convergence with nonverbal learning disabilities syndrome. *Journal of Child Psychology and Psychiatry*, 36, 1127–1140.

Kobayashi R., Murata T. and Yashinaga K. (1992). A follow-up study of 201 children with autism in Kyushu and Yamaguchi, Japan. *Journal of Autism and Developmental Disorders*, 22, 395–411.

Koegel L. K. (2000). Interventions to facilitate communication in autism. *Journal of Autism and Developmental Disorders*, 30, 383–392.

Koegel R. L. and Koegel L. K. (1995). *Teaching Children with Autism: Strategies for Initiating Positive Interactions and Improving Learning Opportunities.* Baltimore, MD. Brookes.

Koegel L. K., Koegel R. L., Harrower J. K. and Carter C. M. (1999). Pivotal response intervention I: Overview of approach. *Journal of the Association for Persons with Severe Handicaps*, 24, 174–185.

Kohn Y., Fahum T., Ratzoni G. and Apter A. (1998). Aggression and sexual offences in Asperger's Syndrome. Israel. *Journal of Psychiatric and Related Science*, 35, 293–9.

Komoto J., Usui S. and Hirata J. (1984). Infantile autism and affective disorder. *Journal of Autism and Developmental Disorders*, 14, 81–84.

Konstantareas M. M. and Hewitt T. (2001). Autistic disorder and schizophrenia: diagnostic overlaps. *Journal of Autism and Developmental Disorders*, 31, 19–28.

Konstantareas M. M. and Lunsky Y. J. (1997). Sociosexual knowledge. Experience, attitudes, and interests of individuals with autistic disorder and developmental delay. *Journal of Autism and Developmental Disorders*, 27, 397–413.

Krantz P. J. and McClannahan L. E. (1998). Social interaction skills for children with autism: a script-fading procedure for beginning readers. *Journal of Applied Behavior Analysis*, 31, 191–202.

Kravitz T. E., Kamps D. M., Kemmerer K. and Potucek J. (2002). Brief report: increasing communication skills for an elementary-aged student with autism using the picture exchange communication system. *Journal of Autism and Developmental Disorders*, 32, 225–230.

Kunce L. J. and Mesibov G. B. (1998). Educational approaches to high functioning autism and Asperger syndrome. In E. Schopler, G. B. Mesibov and L. J. Kunce (eds.), *Asperger Syndrome or High Functioning Autism* (pp. 227–262), New York. Plenum.

Kuperman S., Black D. W. and Burns T. L. (1988). Excess mortality among formerly hospitalized child psychiatric patients, *Archives of General Psychiatry*, 45, 277–282.

Kurita H. (1997). A comparative study of Asperger syndrome with high-functioning atypical autism. *Psychiatry and Clinical Neuroscience*, 51, 67–70.

Lainhart J. E. (1999). Psychiatric problems in individuals with autism, their parents and siblings. *International Review of Psychiatry*, 11, 278–298.

Lainhart J. E. and Folstein S. E. (1994). Affective disorders in people with autism: A review of published cases. *Journal of Autism and Developmental Disorders*, 24, 587–601.

Larsen F. W., Dahl V. and Hallum E. (1990). A thirty-year follow-up study of a child psychiatric clientele. I: demographic description, *Acta Psychiatrica Scandinavica*, 81, 39–45.

Larsen F. W. and Mouridsen S. E. (1997). The outcome in children with childhood autism and Asperger syndrome originally diagnosed as psychotic: A thirty-year follow-up study of subjects hospitalized as children. *European Child and Adolescent Psychiatry*, 6, 181–190.

Lawson W. (1998). *Life Behind Glass: A Personal Account of Autistic Spectrum Disorder*. Lismore, Australia. Southern Cross University Press.

Lawson W. (2002). *Understanding and Working with the Spectrum of Autism – An Insider's View*. London. Jessica Kingsley Publishers.

Layton T. L. and Watson L. R. (1995). Enhancing communication in nonverbal children with autism. In K. A. Quill (ed.), *Teaching Children with Autism: Strategies to Enhance Communication and Socialization* (pp. 73–104). New York. Delmar.

Leekham S., Libby S., Wing L., Gould J. and Gillberg C. (2000). Comparison of ICD–10 and Gillberg's criteria for Asperger syndrome. *Autism: International Journal of Research and Practice*, 4, 11–28.

Leicestershire County Council and Fosse Health Trust (1998). *Asperger Syndrome: Practical Strategies for the Classroom*: National Autistic Society.

Linter C. M. (1987). Short-cycle manic-depressive psychosis in a mentally handicapped child without family history: A case report. *British Journal of Psychiatry*, 151, 554–555.

Lockyer L. and Rutter M. (1969). A five- to fifteen-year follow-up study of infantile psychosis: III Psychological aspects. *British Journal of Psychiatry*, 115, 865–882.

Lockyer L. and Rutter M. (1970). A five- to fifteen-year follow-up study of infantile psychosis: IV Patterns of cognitive ability. *British Journal of Social and Clinical Psychology*, 9, 152–163.

Lord C. (1984). The development of peer relations in children with autism. In F. J. Morrison, C. Lord and D. P. Keating (eds.) *Applied Developmental Psychology* (pp. 166–230). New York. Academic Press.

Lord C. (1995). Facilitating social inclusion: Examples from peer intervention programs. E. Schopler and G. Mesibov (eds.) *Learning and Cognition in Autism* (pp. 221–239). New York. Plenum Press.

Lord C. (1995). Follow-up of two-year-olds referred for possible autism. *Journal of Child Psychology and Psychiatry*, 36, 1365–1382.

Lord C. (2000). Commentary: Achievements and future directions for intervention research in communication and autism spectrum disorders. *Journal of Autism and Developmental Disorders*, 306, 393–398.

Lord C. and Bailey A. (2002). Autism Spectrum Disorders. In M. Rutter and E. Taylor (eds.), *Child and Adolescent Psychiatry*, 4th edition. Oxford. Blackwell.

Lord C., Risi S., Lambrecht L., Cook E. H., Leventhal B. L., DiLavore P. C., Pickles A. and Rutter M. (2000). The Autism Diagnostic Observation Schedule-Generic: A standard measure of social and communication deficits associated with the spectrum of autism. *Journal of Autism and Developmental Disorders*, 30, 205–223.

Lord C., Rutter M. and Le Couteur A. (1994). Autism Diagnostic Interview – Revised: A revised version of a diagnostic interview for care-givers of individuals with possible pervasive developmental disorders. *Journal of Autism and Development Disorders*, 24, 659–686.

Lord C. and Schopler E. (1985). Differences in sex ratios in autism as a function of measured intelligence. *Journal of Autism and Development Disorders*, 15, 185–193.

Lord C. and Venter A. (1992). Outcome and follow-up studies of high functioning autistic individuals. In E. Schopler and G. B. Mesibov (eds.), *High Functioning Individuals with Autism* (pp. 187–200). New York. Plenum Press.

Lotter V. (1966). Epidemiology of autistic conditions in young children: 1 Prevalence. *Social Psychiatry*, 1, 124–137.

Lotter V. (1974a). Factors related to outcome in autistic children. *Journal of Autism and Childhood Schizophrenia*, 4, 263–277.

Lotter V. (1974b). Social adjustment and placement of autistic children in Middlesex: A follow-up study. *Journal of Autism and Childhood Schizophrenia*, 4, 11–32.

Lotter V. (1978). Follow-up studies. In M. Rutter and E. Schopler (eds.), *Autism: A Reappraisal of Concepts and Treatment*. New York. Plenum Press.

Lovaas O. I. (1993). The development of a treatment – research project for developmentally disabled and autistic children. *Journal of Applied Behavior Analysis*, 26, 617–630.

Lovaas O. I. (1996). The UCLA young autism model of service delivery. In C. Maurice (ed.), *Behavioral Intervention for Young Children with Autism* (pp. 241–250). Austin, Texas. Pro-Ed.

Loveland K., Tunali-Kotoski B., Chen R., Bresford K. and Ortegon J. (1997). Emotion recognition in autism: Verbal and non-verbal information. *Development and Psychopathology*, 9, 579–593.

Lowndes B. (1994). Supported living for people with Asperger's syndrome. *Communication*, 28, 13.

McCabe P., McCabe E. and McCabe J. (2003). *Living and Loving with Asperger Syndrome: Family Viewpoints*. London. Jessica Kingsley Publishers.

Macintosh K. E. and Dissanayake C. (2004). The similarities and differences between autistic disorder and Asperger Disorder: A review of the empirical evidence. *Journal of Child Psychology and Psychiatry*, 45, 421–434.

McCaughrin W. B., Ellis W. K., Rusch F. R. and Heal L. W. (1993). Cost-effectiveness of supported employment. *Mental Retardation*, 31, 41–48.

Macdonald H., Rutter M., Howlin P., Rios P., Le Couteur A., Evered C. and Folstein S. (1989). Recognition and expression of emotional cues by autistic and normal adults. *Journal of Child Psychology and Psychiatry*, 30, 865–878.

McDougle C. J. (1997). Psychopharmacology. In D. J. Cohen and F. R. Volkmar (eds), *Handbook of Autism and Pervasive Developmental Disorders*, 2nd edn (pp. 707–729). New York. John Wiley.

McDougle C. J., Kresch L. E. and Posey D. J. (2002). Repetitive thoughts and behavior in pervasive developmental disorders: treatment with Serotonin Reuptake Inhibitors. *Journal of Autism and Developmental Disorders*, 30, 427–435.

McGee J. J. (1985). Gentle teaching. *Mental Handicap in New Zealand*, 9, 13–24.

McGee J. J., Menolascino P. E., Hobbs D. C. and Menousek P. E. (1987). *Gentle Teaching: A Non-Aversive Approach to Helping Persons with Mental Retardation*, New York: Human Science Press.

McGee R., Prior M., William S., Smart D. and Sanson A. (2002). The long-term significance of teacher-rated hyperactivity and reading ability in childhood: findings from two longitudinal studies, *Journal of Child Psychology and Psychiatry*, 43, 1004–1017.

Magiati I. and Howlin P. (2001). Monitoring the progress of preschool children with autism enrolled in early intervention programmes. *Autism: International Journal of Research and Practice*, 5, 399–406.

Manjiviona J. and Prior M. (1995). Comparison of Asperger Syndrome and high-functioning autistic children on a test of motor impairment. *Journal of Autism and Developmental Disorders*, 25, 23–40.

Manjiviona J. and Prior M. (1999). Neuropsychological profiles of children with Asperger syndrome and autism. *Autism: International Journal of Research and Practice*, 3, 327–354.

Marcus L. M., Kunce L. J. and Schopler E. (1997). Working with families. In D. Cohen and F. Volkmar (eds.), *Handbook of Autism and Pervasive Developmental Disorders*, 2nd edn (pp. 631–649). New York. Wiley.

Marriage K., Miles T., Stokes D. and Davey M. (1993). Clinical and research implications of the co-occurrence of Asperger's and Tourette Syndrome. *Australian and New Zealand Journal of Psychiatry*, 30, 666–672.

Martin M., Scahill L., Lawrence M. S. N., Klin A. M. and Volkmar F. R. (1999). Higher functioning pervasive developmental disorders: rates and patterns of psychotropic drug use. *Journal of the American Academy of Child and Adolescent Psychiatry*, 38, 923–931.

Matthews A. (1996). Developing a support model within employment for adults with autism and Asperger's syndrome. In H. Morgan (ed.), *Adults with Autism*. Cambridge. Cambridge University Press.

Mawhood L. M. and Howlin P. (1999). The outcome of a supported employment scheme for high-functioning adults with autism or Asperger syndrome. *Autism: International Journal of Research and Practice*, 3, 229–253.

Mawhood L., Howlin P. and Rutter M. (2000). Autism and developmental receptive language disorder – a follow-up comparison in early adult life. I: Cognitive and language outcomes. *Journal of Child Psychology and Psychiatry*, 41, 547–559.

Mawson D., Grounds A. and Tantam D. (1985). Violence in Asperger's syndrome: A case study. *British Journal of Psychiatry*, 147, 566–569.

Mayes S. D., Calhoun S. L. and Crites D. L. (2001). Does *DSM-IV* Asperger's Disorder exist? *Journal of Abnormal Child Psychology*, 29, 263–271.

Melone M. B. and Lettick A. L. (1983). Sex education at Benhaven. In E. Schopler and G. B. Mesibov (eds.), *Autism in Adolescents and Adults* (pp. 169–186). New York. Plenum Press.

MENCAP (1989). *A London-wide Directory of Opportunities in Employment for People with a Learning Disability*. MENCAP, London Division, London. (Directories for other areas also available.)

MENCAP (1990a). *A London-wide Directory of Opportunities in Adult Education for People with a Learning Disability*. MENCAP, London Division, London. (Directories for other areas also available.)

MENCAP (1990b). *A London-wide Directory of Specially Designed Courses in Further Education for People with a Learning Disability*. MENCAP Education, Training and Employment Services, London. (Directories for other areas also available.)

Mesibov G. B. (1984). Social skills training with verbal autistic adolescents and adults: a program model. *Journal of Autism and Developmental Disorders*, 14, 395–404.

Mesibov G. B. (1990). Normalization and its relevance today. *Journal of Autism and Developmental Disorders*, 20, 379–390.

Mesibov G. B. (1992). Treatment issues with high-functioning adolescents and adults with autism. In E. Schopler and E. B. Mesibov (eds.), *High-Functioning Individuals with Autism* (pp. 143–156). New York. Plenum Press.

Mesibov G. B., Schopler E., Schaffer B. and Michal N. (1989). Use of the Childhood Autism Rating Scale with autistic adolescents and adults. *Journal of the American Academy of Child and Adolescent Psychiatry*, 28, 538–541.

Meyer R. N. (2000). *Asperger Syndrome Employment Workbook: An Employment Workbook for Adults with Asperger Syndrome*. London. Jessica Kingsley Publishers.

Miller J. N. and Ozonoff S. (1997). Did Asperger's cases have Asperger Disorder? A research note. *Journal of Child Psychology and Psychiatry*, 38, 247–251.

Miller J. N. and Ozonoff S. (2000). The external validity of Asperger disorder: lack of evidence from the domain of neuropsychology. *Journal of Abnormal Psychology*, 109, 227–238.

Milton J., Duggan C., Latham A., Egan V. and Tantam D. (2002). Case history of co-morbid Asperger's Syndrome and paraphilic behaviour. *Medical Science Law*, 42, 237–244.

Minshew N. J., Sweeney J. A. and Bauman M. L. (1997). Neurological aspects of autism. In D. J. Cohen and F. R. Volkmar (eds.), *Handbook of Autism and Pervasive Developmental Disorders*, 2nd edn (pp. 344–369). New York. John Wiley.

Mittler P., Gillies S. and Jukes E. (1966). Prognosis in psychotic children: Report of a follow-up study. *Journal of Mental Deficiency Research*, 10, 73–83.

Moon M. S., Inge K. J., Wehman P., Brooke P. and Barcus J. M. (1990). *Helping Persons with Severe Mental Retardation Get and Keep Employment: Supported Employment Strategies and Outcomes*. Baltimore, MD. Paul H. Brookes.

Morgan H. (1996) (ed.). *Adults with Autism*. Cambridge. Cambridge University Press.

Moss S. C., Prosser H., Costello H., Simpson N., Patel P., Rowe S., Turner S. and Hatton C. (1998). Reliability and validity of the PAS-ADD Checklist for detecting psychiatric disorders in adults with intellectual disability. *Journal of Intellectual Disability Research*, 42, 173–183.

Mostert M. P. (2001). Facilitated Communication since 1995: a review of published studies. *Journal of Autism and Developmental Disorders*, 31, 287–313.

Mudford O. C., Cross B. A., Breen S., Cullen C., Reeves D., Gould J. and Douglas J. (2000). Auditory integration training for children with autism: no behavioral benefits detected. *American Journal of Mental Retardation*, 105, 118–129.

Muller J. (1993). Swimming against the tide. *Communication*, 27, 6.

Murphy G. and Clare I. (1991). MIETS: A service option for people with mild mental handicaps and challenging behaviour or psychiatric problems. 2: Assessment, treatment, and outcome for service users and service effectiveness. *Mental Handicap Research*, 4, 80–206.

National Autistic Society (1997). *Approaches to Autism*. London. National Autistic Society.

National Autistic Society (2001). *Schools, Units and Classes for Children with Autism and Asperger Syndrome*. London. National Autistic Society.

National Autistic Society (2003). Publications Catalogue. London. National Autistic Society.

National Research Council (2001). *Educating Children with Autism*. Committee on Educational Interventions for Children with Autism. Division of Behavioral and Social Sciences and Education. National Research Council. Washington, DC. National Academy Press.

Newport J. and Newport M. (2002). *Autism/Asperger's and Sexuality: Puberty and Beyond*. Newport. Future Horizons.

Newson E., Dawson M. and Everard T. (1982). The natural history of able autistic people: their management and functioning in a social context. Unpublished report to the Department of Health and Social Security, London. Summary published in four parts in *Communication*, 19–21 (1984–1985).

Newton C., Taylor G. and Wilson D. (1996). Circles of friends: An inclusive approach to meeting emotional and behavioural needs. *Educational Psychology in Practice*, 11, 4.

New York State Department of Health Early Intervention Program (1999). *Clinical Practice Guideline. Autism/Pervasive developmental disorders, assessment and intervention for young children (Age 0–3 years)*. Albany, New York.

Nordin V. and Gillberg C. (1998). The long-term course of autistic disorders: update on follow-up studies. *Acta Psychiatrica Scandinavica*, 97, 99–108.

Nye C. and Brice A. (2003). Combined vitamin B6-magnesium treatment in autism spectrum disorder. *Cochrane Database of Systematic Reviews*, 4 CD003497.

O'Gorman G. (1970). *The Nature of Childhood Autism*, 2nd edn. London. Butterworth.

Oliver C. (1995). Self-injurious behaviour in children with learning disabilities: Recent advances in assessment intervention. Annotation: *Journal of Child Psychology and Psychiatry*, 36, 909–928.

Östman O. (1991). Child and adolescent psychiatric patients in adulthood. *Acta Psychiatrica Scandinavica*, 84, 40–5.

Ousley O. Y. and Mesibov G. (1991). Sexual attitudes and knowledge of high-functioning adolescents and adults with autism. *Journal of Autism and Developmental Disorders*, 21, 471–481.

Owens R. G. and MacKinnon S. (1993). The functional analysis of challenging behaviours: some conceptual and theoretical problems. In R. S. P. Jones and C. B. Eayrs (eds.), *Challenging Behaviour and Intellectual Disability: A Psychological Perspective*. Clevedon, Avon. BILD Publications.

Ozonoff S. and Cathcart K. (1998). Effectiveness of a home program intervention for young children with autism. *Journal of Autism and Developmental Disorders*, 28, 25–32.

Ozonoff S., Dawson G. and McPartland J. (2002). *A Parent's Guide to Asperger Syndrome and High-Functioning Autism*. New York. Guildford Press.

Ozonoff S. and McMahon Griffith E. (2000). Neuropsychological Function and the External Validity of Asperger Syndrome. In A. Klin, F. R. Volkmar and S. S. Sparrow (eds.), *Asperger Syndrome* (pp. 72–96). New York. Guildford Press.

Ozonoff S. and Miller J. N. (1995). Teaching theory of mind: A new approach to social skills training for individuals with autism. *Journal of Autism and Developmental Disorders*, 25, 415–433.

Ozonoff S., Rogers S. J. and Pennington B. F. (1991). Asperger's Syndrome: Evidence of an empirical distinction from high-functioning autism. *Journal of Child Psychology and Psychiatry*, 32, 1107–1122.

Ozonoff S., South M. and Miller J. N. (2002). DSM-IV defined Asperger Syndrome: cognitive, behavioural and early history differentiation from high-functioning autism. *Autism Journal of Research and Practice*, 4, 29–46.

Paradiž V. (2002). *Elijah's Cup, A Family's Journey into the Community and Culture of High-Functioning Autism and Asperger's Syndrome*. New York. Free Press.

Park C. (1992). Autism into art: A handicap transfigured. In E. Schopler and G. B. Mesibov (eds.), *High-Functioning Individuals with Autism* (pp. 250–258). New York. Plenum Press.

Perry D. W., Marston G. M., Hinder S. J., Munden A. C. and Roy A. (2001). The phenomenology of depressive illness in people with a learning disability and autism: seven case studies. *Autism: International Journal of Research and Practice*, 5, 265–275.

Peterson C. C. and Siegal M. (1995). Deafness, conversation and theory of mind. *Child Psychology and Psychiatry*, 36, 459–474.

Petty L. K., Omitz E. M., Michelman J. D. and Zimmerman E. G. (1984). Autistic children who become schizophrenic. *Archives of General Psychiatry*, 41, 129–135.

Piven J., Arndt S., Bailey J. and Andreasen N. (1996). Regional brain enlargement in autism: A magnetic resonance imaging study. *Journal of the American Academy of Child and Adolescent Psychiatry*, 35, 530–536.

Piven J., Harper J., Palmer P. and Arndt S. (1996). Course of behavioral change in autism: a retrospective study of high-IQ adolescents and adults. *Journal of the American Academy of Child Psychiatry*, 35, 523–529.

Piven J. and Palmer P. (1999). Psychiatric disorder and the broad autism phenotype: evidence from a family study of multiple-incidence autism families. *American Journal of Psychiatry*, 156, 557–563.

Pomeroy J. C. (1998). Subtyping of pervasive developmental disorders: issues of validity and implications for child psychiatric diagnosis. In E. Schopler, G. B. Mesibov and L. J. Kunce, *Asperger Syndrome or High Functioning Autism?* New York. Plenum.

Posey D. and McDougle C. (2000). The pharmacotherapy of target symptoms associated with autistic disorder and other pervasive developmental disorders. *Harvard Review of Psychiatry*, 8, 45–63.

Powell A. (2002). Taking Responsibility: Good Practice Guidelines for Services – Adults with Asperger syndrome. London. National Autistic Society.

Powell S. and Jordan R. (eds.) (1997). *Autism and Learning: A Guide to Good Practice*. London. David Fulton.

Pozner A. and Hammond J. (1993). *An Evaluation of Supported Employment Initiatives for Disabled People*. Sheffield. Employment Department.

Prekop J. L. (1984). Zur Festhalte Therapie bei Autistischen Kindern, *Der Kinderarzt*, 15, 798–802.

Prince-Hughes D. (2002). *Aquamarine Blue 5: personal stories of college students with autism*. Ohio. Ohio University Press.

Prizant B. M. and Rubin E. (1999). Contemporary issues in interventions for autism spectrum disorders: a commentary. *Journal of the Association for Persons with Severe Handicaps*, 24, 199–208.

Prizant B., Schuler A., Wetherby A. and Rydell P. (1997). Enhancing language and communication development: Language approaches. In D. Cohen and F. Volkmar (eds.) *Handbook of Autism and Pervasive Developmental Disorders*, 2nd edn (pp. 572–605). New York. Wiley.

Prosser H., Moss S. C., Costello H., Simpson N., Patel P. and Rowe S. (1998). Reliability and validity of the Mini PAS-ADD for assessing psychiatric disorders in adults with intellectual disability. Journal of Intellectual Disability Research, 42, 264–272.

Pyles L. (2002). *Hitchhiking through Asperger Syndrome*. London. Jessica Kingsley Publishers.

Queen Elizabeth Foundation for Disabled People Directory of Opportunities for School Leavers with Disability. www.qefd.org.uk.

Quill K. A. (1995a). *Teaching Children with Autism: Strategies to Enhance Communication and Socialization*. New York. Delmar.

Quirk-Hodgson L. (1995). Solving social-behavioral problems through the use of visually supported communication. In K. A. Quill (ed.), *Teaching Children with Autism: Strategies to Enhance Communication and Socialization* (pp. 265–286). New York. Delmar.

Realmuto G. M. and August G. J. (1991). Catatonia in autistic disorder: a sign of comorbidity or variable expression. *Journal of Autism and Developmental Disorders*, 21, 517–528.

Realmuto G. M. and Ruble L. A. (1999). Sexual behaviors in autism: problems of definition and management. *Journal of Autism and Developmental Disorders*, 29, 121–127.

Reaven J. and Hepburn S. (2003). Cognitive behavioural treatment of obsessive compulsive disorder in a child with Asperger syndrome: a case report. *Autism: International Journal of Research and Practice*, 7, 145–164.

Reid A. H. (1976). Psychiatric disturbances in the mentally handicapped. *Proceedings of the Royal Society of Medicine*, 69, 509–512.

Richer J. and Zappella M. (1989). Changing Social Behaviour. The Place of Holding. *Communication*, 23, 35–39.

Rimland B. (1988). Physical exercise and autism. *Autism Research Review International*, 2, 3.

Rimland B. (1994a). Comparative effects of treatment on child's behavior (drugs, therapies, schooling, and several non-treatment events). *Autism Research Review*, Publication 34b.

Rimland B. (1994b). Information pack on drug treatments for autism. *Autism Research Review International*, Information Pack P6.

Rimland B. (1994c). Information pack on vitamins, allergies and nutritional treatments for autism. *Autism Research Review International*, Information Pack P24.

Rimland B. (1995). *Studies of High-Dose Vitamin B6 in Autistic Children and Adults – 1965–1994*. San Diego, CA. Autism Research Institute.

Rimland B. (1998). The use of secretin in autism: some preliminary answers. *Autism Research Review International*, 12, 3.

Rimland B. (2000a). 'Garbage science', brick walls, crossword puzzles, and mercury. *Autism Research Review International*, 14, 3.

Rimland B. (2000b). *Autism Treatment Evaluation Checklist* (ATEC) CA. California Autism Research Institute.

Rimland B. and Edelson S. M. (1994). The effects of Auditory Integration Training on autism. *American Journal of Speech-Language Pathology*, 5, 16–24.

Rimland B. and Edelson S. M. (1995). Brief report: A pilot study of Auditory Integration Training in autism. *Journal of Autism and Developmental Disorders*, 25, 61–70.

Rinehart N. J., Bradshaw J. L., Moss S. A., Brereton A. V. and Tonge B. J. (2001). A deficit in shifting attention present in high-functioning autism but not Asperger's disorder. *Autism: International Journal of Research and Practice*, 5, 67–80.

Ringman J. M. and Jankovic J. (2000). Occurrence of tics in Asperger's Syndrome and autistic disorder. *Journal of Child Neurology*, 15, 394–400.

Rogers S. J. (1996). Brief Report: Early intervention in autism. *Journal of Autism and Developmental Disorders*, 26, 243–246.

Rogers S. J. (1998a). Empirically supported comprehensive treatments for young children with autism. *Journal of Clinical Child Psychology*, 27, 168–179.

Rogers S. J. (1998b). Neuropsychology of autism in young children and its implications for early intervention. *Mental Retardation and Developmental Disabilities Research Reviews*, 4, 104–112.

Rogers S. J. (2000). Interventions that facilitate socialization in children with autism. *Journal of Autism and Developmental Disorders*, 30, 399–410.

Rogers S. J., Ozonoff S. and Maslin-Cole C. (1987). An effective procedure for training early special education teams to implement a model program. *Journal of the Division of Early Childhood*, 11, 180–188.

Rosenthal-Malek A. and Mitchell S. (1997). The effects of excercise on the self-stimulatory behaviours and positive responding of adolescents with autism. *Journal of Autism and Developmental Disorders*, 27, 203–212.

Ruble L. and Dalrymple N. (1993). Social/sexual awareness of persons with autism: A parental perspective. *Archives of Sexual Behavior*, 22, 229–240.

Rumsey J. M., Rapoport J. L. and Sceery W. R. (1985). Autistic children as adults: Psychiatric social and behavioural outcomes. *Journal of the American Academy of Child Psychiatry*, 24, 465–473.

Rutherford M. D., Baron-Cohen S. and Wheelwright S. (2002). Reading the mind in the voice: a study with normal adults and adults with Asperger Syndrome and high-functioning autism. *Journal of Autism and Developmental Disorders*, 32, 189–194.

Rutter M. (1970). Autistic children: Infancy to adulthood. *Seminars in Psychiatry*, 2, 435–450.

Rutter M. (1972). Childhood schizophrenia reconsidered. *Journal of Autism and Childhood Schizophrenia*, 2, 315–337.

Rutter M. (1983). School effects on pupil progress: research findings and policy implications. *Child Development*, 54, 1–29.

Rutter M. and Bartak L. (1973). Special educational treatment of autistic children: A comparative study. II Follow-up findings and implications for services. *Journal of Child Psychology and Psychiatry*, 14, 241–270.

Rutter M., Greenfield D. and Lockyer L. (1967). A five- to fifteen-year follow-up study of infantile psychosis: II Social and behavioural outcome. *British Journal of Psychiatry*, 113, 1183–1199.

Rutter M. and Lockyer L. (1967). A five- to fifteen-year follow-up study of infantile psychosis: I Description of sample. *British Journal of Psychiatry*, 113, 1169–1182.

Rutter M., Tizard J. and Whitmore K. (1970). *Education, Health and Behaviour*. London. Longman.

Rydell P. J. and Mirenda P. (1994). The effects of high and low constraint utterances on the production of immediate and delayed echolalia in young children with autism. *Journal of Autism and Developmental Disorders*, 24, 719–730.

Rydell P. J. and Prizant B. (1995). Assessment and intervention strategies for children who use echnialia. In K. A. Quill (ed.), *Teaching Children with Autism: Strategies to Enhance Communication and Socialization* (pp. 105–132). New York. Delmar.

Sacks O. (1993). A neurologist's notebook: An anthropologist on Mars. *New Yorker*, 27 December, pp. 106–125.

Sainsbury C. (2000). *Martian in the Playground: Understanding the School Child with Asperger's Syndrome* Bristol. Lucky Duck Publishing.

Sandler A. D., Sutton K., De Weese J., Girardi M. A., Sheppard V. and Bodfish J. W. (1999). A double-blind placebo-controlled trial of synthetic human secretin in the treatment of autism and pervasive developmental disorder. *Journal of Developmental and Behavioral Paediatrics*, 20, 400.

Schopler E. (ed.) (1995). *Parent Survival Manual: A Guide to Crisis Resolution in Autism and Related Developmental Disorders*. New York. Plenum.

Schopler E. (1997). Implementation of TEACCH Philosophy. In D. J. Cohen and F. R. Volkmar (eds.), *Handbook of Autism and Pervasive Developmental Disorders*, 2nd edn (pp. 767–798). New York. John Wiley.

Schopler E. and Mesibov G. B. (1983). *Autism in Adolescents and Adults*. New York. Plenum Press.

Schopler E. and Mesibov G. B. (1986). Introduction to social behavior in autism. In E. Schopler and G. B. Mesibov (eds.), *Social Behavior in Autism* (pp. 1–11). New York. Plenum Press.

Schopler E. and Mesibov G. B. (1992). *High Functioning Individuals with Autism*. New York. Plenum Press.

Schopler E. and Mesibov G. B. (eds.) (1995). *Learning and Cognition in Autism*. New York. Plenum Press.

Schopler E., Mesibov G. B. and Kunce L. J. (1998). *Asperger Syndrome or High Functioning Autism?* New York. Plenum Press.

Schreibman L. (2000). Intensive behavioral/psychoeducational treatments for autism: research needs and future directions. *Journal of Autism and Developmental Disorders*, 30, 373–378.

Schuler A. L. and Fletcher E. C. F. (2002). Making Communication meaningful: Cracking the language interaction code. In Gabriels R. and D. Hill (eds.), *Autism: From Research to Practice*. London. Jessica Kingsley Publishers.

Schuler A. L., Peck C. A., Willard C. and Theimer K. (1989). Assessment of communicative means and functions through interview: Assessing the communicative capabilities of individuals with limited language. *Seminars in Speech and Language*, 10, 51–61.

Scott F., Baron-Cohen S., Bolton P. and Brayne C. (2002). The CAST (Childhood Asperger Syndrome Test); preliminary development of a UK screen for mainstream primary-school-age children. *Autism: International Journal of Research and Practice*, 6, 9–31.

Scott L. and Kerr-Edwards L. (1999). *Talking Together about Growing Up – A Workbook for Parents of Children with Learning Disabilities*. London. Family Planning Association.

Scragg P. and Shah A. (1994). Prevalence of Asperger's Syndrome in a secure hospital. *British Journal of Psychiatry*, 161, 679–682.

Seltzer M. M., Krauss M. W., Shattuck P. T., Orsmond G., Swe A. and Lord C. (2003). The symptoms of autism spectrum disorders in adolescence and adulthood. *Journal of Autism and Developmental Disorder* (in press).

Sequeira H., Hollins S. and Howlin P. (2003). Symptoms of psychological disturbance associated with sexual abuse in people with intellectual disabilities. *British Journal of Psychiatry*, 183, 451–456.

Shavelle R. M., Strauss D. J. and Pickett J. (2001). Causes of death in autism. *Journal of Autism and Developmental Disorder*, 31, 569–576.

Sheinkopf S. J. and Siegel B. (1998). Home-based behavioral treatment for young children with autism. *Journal of Autism and Developmental Disorders*, 28, 15–23.

Sheldon B. (1995). *Cognitive-behavioural therapy: Research practice and philosophy*. London. Routledge.

Sherratt D. (2002). Developing pretend play in children with autism. *Autism: International Journal of Research and Practice*, 6, 169–179.

Shields J. (2001). The NAS Early Bird Programme: partnership with parents in early intervention. *Autism: International Journal of Research and Practice*, 5, 49–56.

Short A. (1984). Short-term treatment outcome using parents as therapists for their own autistic children. *Journal of Child Psychology and Psychiatry*, 25, 443–485.

Sigafoos J., Kerr M. and Roberts D. (1994a). Inter-rater reliability of the Motivation Assessment Scale: Failure to replicate with aggressive behaviour. *Research in Developmental Disabilities*, 15, 333–342.

Sigafoos J., Roberts D., Kerr M., Couzens D. and Baglioni A. J. (1994b). Opportunities for communication in classrooms serving children with developmental disabilities. *Journal of Autism and Developmental Disorders*, 24, 259–280.

Sigman M. (1998). The Emanuel Miller Memorial Lecture 1997, Change and continuity in the development of children with autism. *Journal of Child Psychology and Psychiatry*, 39, 879–891.

Sigman M. and Ruskin E. (1999). Continuity and change in the social competence of children with autism, Downs' syndrome, and developmental delays. *Monographs of the Society for Research in Child Development*, 64 (1, serial no. 256).

Simpson R. L. and Myles B. S. (1993). Successful integration of children and youth with autism in mainstreamed settings. *Focus on Autistic Behavior*, 7, 1–13.

Sinclair J. (1992). Bridging the gap: An inside out view of autism (Or, do you know what I don't know?). In E. Schopler and G. B. Mesibov (eds.), *High-functioning individuals with Autism* (pp. 294–302). New York. Plenum Press.

Skill: the National Bureau for Students with Disabilities. London. www.skill.org.uk.

Slater-Walker G. and Slater-Walker C. (2002). *An Asperger Marriage*. London. Jessica Kingsley Publishers.

Smalley S., McCracken J. and Tanguay P. (1995). Autism, Affective Disorders, and Social Phobia. *American Journal of Medical Genetics (Neuropsychiatric Genetics)*, 60, 19–26.

Smith M., Belcher R. and Juhrs P. (1995). *A Guide to Successful Employment for Individuals with Autism*, Balitmore, MD. Paul H. Brookes.

Smyth J. and Wallace K. (1997). *A Guide to Grants for Individuals in Need*. London. Directory of Social Change.

Snow M. E., Hertzig M. E. and Shapiro T. (1987). Expression of emotion in young autistic children. *Journal of the American Academy of Child and Adolescent Psychiatry*, 26, 836–838.

Sovner, R. (1986). Limiting factors in the use of DSM-III criteria with mentally ill/mentally retarded persons. *Psychopharmacology Bulletin*, 22, 1055–1059.

Sovner R. (1988). Anticonvulsant drug therapy of neuropsychiatric disorders in mentally retarded persons. In S. McElroy and H. G. Pope, Jr (eds.), *Use of Anticonvulsants in Psychiatry* (pp. 169–181). Clinton, NJ. Oxford Health Care.

Sovner R. (1989). The use of valporate in the treatment of mentally retarded persons with typical and atypical bipolar disorders. *Journal of Clinical Psychiatry*, 50 (Suppl. 3), 40–43.

Spence S. H. (1991). Developments in the assessments of social skills and social competence in children. *Behaviour Change*, 8, 148–166.

Stanford A. (2003). Asperger Syndrome and long-term relationships. London. Jessica Kingsley Publishers.

Starr E. (1993). Teaching the appearance – reality distinction to children with autism. Paper presented at the British Psychological Society, Developmental Psychology Section Annual Conference. Birmingham.

Stehli A. (1992). The Sound of a Miracle: A Child's Triumph over Autism. Fourth Estate.

Stein D., Ring A., Shulman C., Meir D., Holan A., Weizman A. and Barak Y. (2001). *Journal of Autism and Developmental Disorders*, 31, 355–360.

Steingard R. and Biederman J. (1987). Lithium responsive manic-like symptoms in two individuals with autism and mental retardation. *Journal of American Academy of Child and Adolescent Psychiatry*, 26, 932–935.

Stevens P. and Martin N. (1999). Supporting individuals with intellectual disability and challenging behaviour in integrated work settings: an overview and a model for service provision. *Journal of Intellectual Disability Research*, 43, 19–29.

Stoddart K. (1999). Adolescents with Asperger syndrome: 3 case studies of individual and family therapy. *Autism: International Journal of Research and Practice*, 3, 255–272.

Stone W. L. and Yoder P. J. (2001). Predicting spoken-language level in children with autism spectrum disorders. *Autism: International Journal of Research and Practice*, 5, 341–361.

Strain P. S. and Hoyson M. (2000). On the need for longitudinal, intensive social-skill intervention: LEAP follow-up outcomes for children as a case in point. *Topics in Early Childhood Special Education*, 20, 116–122.

Strain P. S., Kohler F. W. and Goldstein H. (1996). Learning experiences – an alternative program: Peer-mediated interventions for young children with autism. In E. D. Hibbs and P. S. Jensen (eds.), *Psychosocial Treatment for Child and Adolescent Disorders: Empirically Based Strategies for Clinical Practice* (pp. 573–587). Washington, DC. American Psychological Association.

Sturmey P. (1998). Classification and diagnosis of psychiatric disorders in persons with developmental disabilities. *Journal of Developmental and Physical Disabilities*, 10, 4317–330.

Sugai G. and White W. J. (1986). Effects of using object self-stimulation as a reinforcer on the pre-vocational work rates of an autistic child. *Journal of Autism and Developmental Disorders*, 16, 459–474.

Sussman F. (1999). *More Than Words*. Toronto. The Hanen Program.

Sverd J., Montero G. and Gurevich N. (1993). Brief report: Case for an association between Tourette's syndrome, autistic disorder and schizophrenia-like disorder. *Journal of Autism and Developmental Disorders*, 23, 407–414.

Swettenham J. (1995). Can children with autism be taught to understand false beliefs using computers? *Journal of Child Psychology and Psychiatry*, 37, 157–166.

Swettenham J., Gomez J. C., Baron-Cohen S. and Walsh S. (1995). What's inside someone's head? Conceiving of the mind as a camera helps children with autism acquire an alternative 'theory of mind'. *Cognitive Neuropsychiatry*, 1, 73–88.

Szatmari P. (2000). Perspectives on the classification of Asperger syndrome. In A. Klin, F. R. Volkmar and S. S. Sparrow (eds.), *Asperger Syndrome* (pp. 403–417). New York. Guildford Press.

Szatmari P., Archer L., Fisman S. and Streiner D. L. (1994). Parent and teacher agreement in the assessment of pervasive developmental disorders. *Journal of Autism and Developmental Disorders*, 24, 703–717.

Szatmari P., Archer L., Fisman S., Streiner D. and Wilson F. (1995). Asperger's syndrome and autism: differences in behaviour, cognition and adaptive functioning. *Journal of the American Academy of Child and Adolescent Psychiatry*, 34, 1662–1670.

Szatmari P., Bartolucci G. and Bremner R. S. (1989a). Asperger's syndrome and autism: A comparison of early history and outcome. *Developmental Medicine and Child Neurology*, 31, 709–720.

Szatmari P., Bartolucci G., Bremner R. S., Bond S. and Rich S. (1989b). A follow-up study of high-functioning autistic children. *Journal of Autism and Developmental Disorders*, 19, 213–226.

Szatmari P., Bartolucci G., Finlayson A. and Krames L. (1986). A vote for Asperger's syndrome. *Journal of Autism and Developmental Disorders*, 16, 515–517.

Szatmari P., Tuff L., Finlayson M. A. J. and Bartolucci G. (1990). Asperger's syndrome and autism: Neurocognitive aspects. *Journal of the American Academy of Child and Adolescent Psychiatry*, 29, 130–136.

Szivos S. E. (1990). Attitudes to work and their relationship to self-esteem and aspirations among young adults with a mild mental handicap. *British Journal of Mental Subnormality*, 36, 108–117.

Szurek S. and Berlin I. (1956). Elements of psychotherapeutics with the schizophrenic child and his parents. *Psychiatry*, 19, 1–19.

Tanguay P. E., Robertson J. M. and Derrick A. M. (1998). A dimensional classification of autism-spectrum disorder by social communication. *Journal of Academy of Child and Adolescent Psychiatry*, 37, 271–277.

Tantam D. (1991). Asperger's Syndrome in adulthood. In U. Frith (ed.), *Autism and Asperger Syndrome* (pp. 147–183). Cambridge. Cambridge University Press.

The Times (July 13 2000) Law Report: The Family Division. *In re D (a child) Evidence: Facilitated Communication.*

Thorp D. M., Stahmer A. C. and Schreibman L. (1995). Effects of sociodramatic play training on children with autism. *Journal of Autism and Developmental Disorders*, 25, 265–283.

Tjus T., Heinmann M. and Nelson K. E. (1998). Gains in literacy through the use of a specially developed multimedia research strategy: positive findings from 13 children with autism. *Autism: International Journal of Research and Practice*, 1, 139–156.

Tjus T., Heimann M. and Nelson K. E. (2001). Interaction patterns between children and their teachers when using a specific multimedia and communication strategy: observations from children with autism and mixed handicaps. *Autism: International Journal of Research and Practice*, 5, 175–187.

Tolbert L., Brown R., Fowler P. and Parsons D. (2001). Brief report: lack of correlation between age of symptom onset and contemporaneous presentation. *Journal of Autism and Developmental Disorders*, 31, 241–245.

Tonge B., Brereton A. V., Gray K. M. and Einfeld S. (1999). Behavioural and emotional disturbance in high-functioning autism and Asperger syndrome *Autism: International Journal of Research and Practice*, 3, 117–130.

Toynbee P. (2003). *Hard work: Life in Low Pay Britain*. London. Bloomsbury.

Trevarthen C., Aitken K., Papoudi D. and Roberts J. M. (1998). 2nd edition *Children with Autism: Diagnosis and Interventions to Meet their Needs*. London. Jessica Kingsley.

Tryan G. S. (1979). A review and critique of thought-stopping research. *Journal of Behaviour Therapy and Experimental Psychiatry*, 10, 32–39.

Tuffreau R., Richard P., Chardeau P., Fortineau J., Morisseau L., Labastire P., Ross N. and Fombonne E. (1995). The outcome of severe developmental disorders in late adolescence. *Paper presented at the 10th International Congress of the European Society for Child and Adolescent Psychiatry*, Utrecht, Netherlands, 17–20 September.

Turk V. and Brown H. (1993). The Sexual Abuse of Adults with Learning Disabilities: Results of a Two-Year Incidence Survey. *Mental Handicap Research*, 6, 193–216.

Turner M. (1999). Repetitive behavior in autism: a review of psychological research. *Journal of Child Psychology and Psychiatry*, 40, 839–850.

Ullman L. P. and Krasner L. (1965) (eds.). *Case Studies in Behaviour Modification*. New York. Holt, Rinehart and Winston.

United States Bureau of Justice Statistics (1987). In *Adolescents* (Fall 1989) Princeton, NJ. Robert Wood Johnson Foundation.

Van Bourgondien M. E. and Mesibov G. B. (1987). Humor in high-functioning autistic adults. *Journal of Autism and Developmental Disorders*, 17, 417–424.

Van Bourgondien M. E., Reichle N. C. and Palmer A. (1997). Sexual behavior in adults with Autism. *Journal of Autism and Developmental Disorders*, 27, 113–125.

Venter A., Lord C. and Schopler E. (1992). A follow-up study of high-functioning autistic children. *Journal of Child Psychology and Psychiatry*, 33, 489–507.

Volkmar F. R., Carter A., Grossman J. and Klin A. (1997). Social development in autism. In D. J. Cohen and F. R. Volkmar (eds.), *Handbook of Autism and Developmental Disorders* (pp. 173–194). New York. Wiley.

Volkmar F. R. and Cohen D. J. (1991). Comorbid association of autism and schizophrenia. *American Journal of Psychiatry*, 148, 1705–1707.

Volkmar F. R., Klin A. and Cohen D. J. (1997). Diagnosis and classification of autism and related conditions. Consensus and issues. pp. 5–40 in *Handbook of Autism and Pervasive Developmental Disorders*, D. J. Cohen and F. R. Volkmar, eds. New York. John Wiley and Sons, Inc.

Volkmar F. R. and Dykens E. (2002). Mental Retardation in Rutter and Taylor, *Child and Adolescent Psychiatry* (pp. 697–710).

Volkmar F. R. and Klin A. (2000). Diagnostic issues in Asperger syndrome. In A. Klin, F. R. Volkmar and S. S. Sparrow (eds.), *Asperger Syndrome* (pp. 25–71). New York. Guildford Press.

von Knorring A-L. and Hägglöf B. (1993). Autism in northern Sweden: a population based follow-up study: psychopathology. *European Child and Adolescent Psychiatry*, 2, 91–97.

Walker M. (1980). Makaton Vocabulary (revised edition). Surrey, UK. The Makaton Vocabulary Development Project.

Watkins J. M., Asarnov R. F. and Tanguay P. (1988). Symptom development in childhood onset schizophrenia. *Journal of Child Psychology and Psychiatry*, 29, 865–878.

Wehman P., Moon M. S., Everson J. M., Wood W. and Barcus J. M. (1988). *Transition from School to Work. New Challenges for Youth with Severe Disabilities*. Baltimore, MD. Paul H. Brookes.

Welch M. (1988). *Holding Time*. London. Century Hutchinson.

Werry J. S. (1992). Child and adolescent (early onset) schizophrenia: a review in light of DSM-III-R. *Journal of Autism and Developmental Disorders*, 22, 601–624.

Werth A., Perkins M. and Boucher G. (2001). 'Here's the weavery looming up': verbal humour in a woman with high-functioning autism. *Autism: International Journal of Research and Practice*, 5, 111–125.

Wertheimer A. (1992). *Changing Lives: Supported Employment for People with Learning Disabilities*. Manchester. National Development Team.

Wetherby A. and Prizant B. (1999). Profiles of communicative and cognitive-social abilities in autistic children. *Journal of Speech and Hearing Research*, 27, 364–377.

Williams T. I. (1989). A social skills group for autistic children. *Journal of Autism and Developmental Disorders*, 19, 143–156.

Williams D. (1992). *Nobody Nowhere*. London. Corgi Books.

Williams D. (1994). *Somebody Somewhere*. London. Corgi Books.

Wiltshire S. (1987). Drawings, Selected and with an Introduction by Sir Hugh Cassaon. London. Dent.

Wimpory D. C., Hobson R., Williams J. and Nash S. (2000). Are infants with autism socially engaged? A study of recent retrospective parental reports. *Journal of Autism and Developmental Disorders*, 30, 525–536.

Wing L. (1981). Asperger's syndrome: A clinical account. *Psychological Medicine*, 11, 115–129.

Wing L. (1986). Clarification on Asperger's syndrome, Letter to the editor. *Journal of Autism and Developmental Disorders*, 16, 513–515.

Wing L. (2000). Past and future of research on Asperger syndrome. In A. Klin, F. R. Volkmar and S. S. Sparrow (eds.), *Asperger Syndrome* (pp. 418–432). New York. Guildford Press.

Wing L. and Gould J. (1978). Systematic recording of behaviors and skills of retarded and psychotic children. *Journal of Autism and Childhood Schizophrenia*, 8, 79–97.

Wing L. and Gould J. (1979). Severe impairments of social interaction and associated abnormalities in children: epidemiology and classification. *Journal of Autism and Developmental Disorders*, 9, 11–29.

Wing L. and Potter D. (2002). The epidemiology of autistic spectrum disorders; is the prevalence rising? *Mental Retardation and Developmental Disabilities Research, Reviews*, 8, 151–61.

Wing L. and Shah A. (2000). Catatonia in autistic spectrum disorders *British Journal of Psychiatry*, 176, 357–362.

Wolery M., Kirk K. and Gast D. L. (1985). Stereotypic behavior as a reinforcer: Effects and side-effects. *Journal of Autism and Developmental Disorders*, 15, 149–162.

Wolfberg P. (1995). Enhancing children's play. In K. A. Quill (ed.), *Teaching Children with Autism: Strategies to enhance communication and socialization* (pp. 193–218). New York. Delmar.

Wolfberg P. J. (1999). *Play and Imagination in Children with Autism.* New York. Teachers' College Press.

Wolff S. (1991). Schizoid personality in childhood and adult life. 1: The vagaries of diagnostic labelling. *British Journal of Psychiatry*, 159, 615–620.

Wolff S. (1995). Loners: *The life path of unusual children.* London. Routledge.

Wolff S. and Chick J. (1980). Schizoid personality in childhood: a controlled follow-up study. *Psychological Medicine*, 10, 85–100.

Wolff S. and McGuire R. J. (1995). Schizoid personality in girls: a follow-up study. What are the links with Asperger's syndrome? *Journal of Child Psychology and Psychiatry*, 36, 793–818.

World Health Organization (1992). ICD-10 *International Statistical Classification of Diseases and Related Health Problems*, 10th edn. Geneva. WHO.

Wozniak J., Biederman J., Faraone S. V., Frazier J., Kim J., Millstein R., Gershon J., Thornell A., Cha K. and Synder J. B. (1997). Mania in children with pervasive developmental disorder revisited. *Journal of the American Academy of Child & Adolescent Psychiatry*, 36, 1552–1559.

Zappella M. (1988). *Il legame genitore-bambino come base della terapia dei bambini autistici.* In P. De Giacomo and M. Scacella (eds.), '*Terapie dell'autismo*', Bari. Ed. Scientifi.

Zetlin A. and Murtaugh M. (1990). Whatever happened to those with borderline IQs? *American Journal on Mental Retardation*, 94, 463–469.

Zollweg W., Palm D. and Vance V. (1997). The efficacy of auditory integration training: a double blind study. *American Journal of Audiology*, 6, 39–47.

Index